THE CURE IS IN THE KITCHEN:

THE STRICT HEALING PHASE FOR THE MACROBIOTIC DIET

By Sherry A. Rogers, M.D.

For information address:

Prestige Publishers
3502 Brewerton Road
P.O. Box 3161
Syracuse, N.Y. 13220-3161

ISBN 0-9618821-3-1

Printed in the United States

THE CURE IS IN THE KITCHEN
The Strict Healing Phase For the Macrobiotic Diet

TABLE OF CONTENTS

DEDICATION

As this is my fourth book, most readers by now already know to whom it is dedicated. I can't help it. I'm incurably in love.

To LUSCIOUS
(who gets more luscious with the years)
and who is by far
God's greatest gift to me

Someone once said to me, "You don't get your reward here on earth, you know." But I'm afraid that was wrong. I got mine 22 years ago and I'm still basking in the 'lusciousness' of it all.

APPRECIATION

Thanks to Mrs. Shirley Gallinger, co-author of <u>MACRO MELLOW</u>, for her editorial comments. Far beyond that, however, is appreciation for her 15 years of selfless nurturing of our staff and patients, and the doctor. She has a wealth of wisdom regarding gardening, cooking, natural healing and the nurturing of the soul. She has grown with me as we travelled the globe, from multiple U. S. cities to Australia and the Caribbean, teaching environmental and nutritional medicine and macrobiotics.

All of this was a far greater gift than I ever imagined possible, and yet there is even a further unexpected bonus. She is a wonderfully loving friend.

ACKNOWLEDGMENT

Month after month after month, I would fly to Boston for the weekend to a renovated, unpretentious brick building in Brookline Village. Here from 8:00 in the morning until 10:00 at night, the Kushi Institute staff nurtured my mind as well as my body with my favorite foods, warm and generous hospitality, and most of all, the opportunity to learn macrobiotics from the master himself.

Mr. Michio Kushi may have been unaware of what he was getting into when he invited this doctor to his weekend seminars that provide a crash course for cancer patients who have been labelled by American medicine as terminal. Since he is a man of few words, I was intent upon not missing a single one. When he left the room after a consultation, I was right on his heels. Twice I followed him to the bathroom before I realized it. "Oh, I guess you can handle this by yourself," I flushed.

For me, being with Mr. Michio Kushi is a lot like being with Dr. William Rea. I'm flooded with strong emotions from every angle. First, there's the great admiration I have for both of them for their selfless sacrifices in becoming world-leaders in their respective fields, macrobiotics and environmental medicine. Second, there's the overwhelming gratitude I feel for both in that they have literally saved my life with their individual areas of expertise. Third, there's the unbridled enthusiasm and excitement of learning what new pearls they will share with me at each encounter.

How do I thank Michio for an open invitation to sit side-by-side with him as he sees his clients and for teaching me on a one-on-one level? If I started repeating every two seconds today, "Thank you, Michio," I couldn't begin to cover my feelings in a year. How do you thank a man who's greatest goal is to bring about world peace which must begin at the level of the individual's own personal health? I guess by what I am attempting to do in this book.

Thank you, Michio.

DISCLAIMER

Since, after reading this book, there has been no examination of your knowledge, plus there has been no examination of your body much less of your personal, medical and environmental history, nor has there been an assessment of your biochemical status, it would be potentially dangerous for you to use the enclosed information without COMPETENT MEDICAL SUPERVISION.

Also, I greatly appreciate the people who have shared their own stories with us in Chapter 9. But where they imply that I was instrumental in their getting well, I fear is an exaggeration. You see, I do not treat cancer, and in fact, do not even know how to treat cancer. Furthermore, I do not have any talents or medical abilities that any other doctors do not already have or cannot also acquire, if he or she chooses to learn this medical subspecialty. And I certainly do not have any medical secrets, as everything I believe in and do, is spelled out in my four books and dozens of scientific journals, publications and lay magazine articles.

Macrobiotics is not a diet to cure cancer. It is a diet, that along with other important lifestyle changes, enables some, but not all people to reach a state of wellness. In fact, the macrobiotic diet actually makes some people feel unwell or worse. Therefore, it definitely is not for everyone.

I feel compelled to warn the reader that although these kind people have accomplished what many doctors would consider the impossible, and have a few kind things to say about me, that these stories are not a testimony to me. Nor are they a testimony to macrobiotics. To believe this is to be mistaken. I cannot heal or cure anything, nor can macrobiotics. These stories, are in fact, solely a testimony to the uniqueness and perseverance of the human spirit and I thank these people again, with all my heart, for sharing their pain so that we might never lose hope regardless of the paths we choose to explore.

FOREWORD

The macrobiotic way of life is based on living in harmony with the natural environment. The environment has a profound influence on our health. The quality of air that we breathe and water we drink directly influence our condition, as does the human environment around us. A noisy, high-stress environment, for example, can interfere with our efforts to be healthy, while a quiet, natural environment supports well being. Daily food is a condensed form of the environment that we internalize each day, and thus has a decisive influence on health and well being.

Between this book, Tired Or Toxic?, You Are What You Ate, and The E.I. Syndrome, Dr. Sherry Rogers explores the relationship between diet, environment, and human health and sickness. She explains how an unnatural, overly artificial diet contributes to a variety of health problems, and how certain aspects of the modern lifestyle, including the use of artificial substances in our surroundings, can also weaken health.

It was through her study of environmental illness that Dr. Rogers discovered the macrobiotic approach. She has since deepened her understanding by participating in special seminars for physicians presented by the Kushi Institute, and by attending and assisting at the Macrobiotic Way of Life Seminars in Boston. She has also begun to offer macrobiotics to an increasing number of patients, and has witnessed numerous improvements in health as a result.

With her study and personal experience as a background, Dr. Rogers explains in her books how the macrobiotic diet, based on unrefined whole grains, beans and bean products, fresh local vegetables, sea vegetables and other whole natural foods, can prevent illness and restore health. She offers the case histories of her patients as proof of the efficacy of macrobiotics. Dr. Rogers also includes practical guidelines and suggestions designed to help readers embark on a new way of eating and living.

Dr. Rogers is a pioneer in the development of a new approach to healthcare, based on the synthesis of traditional and modern approaches. By emphasizing diet and way of life, she is pointing the direction toward an understanding of the most fundamental causes of sickness. And by presenting the macrobiotic diet within the context of prevention and recovery, she is furthering the development of a comprehensive system of healthcare that can solve society's most fundamental problems.

Like Dr. Rogers, hundreds of physicians throughout the world are pursuing the macrobiotic way of life, both in their own lives and as a solution to the modern health crisis. Macrobiotic study programs and seminars for doctors have been presented in the United States, France, in the Central African Republic of the Congo, and in Hungary and Yugoslavia.

Dr. Rogers is a leading member of the international network of macrobiotic physicians, and her efforts are supported by colleagues around the world. It is my hope that these ongoing efforts, including the publication of this new book, will serve for the development of a medicine of humanity that will contribute to health and peace throughout the world.

Michio Kushi
Brookline, MA
1990

CHAPTER 1
YOU CAN'T FIGHT SUCCESS

Every once in a while, I find myself sort of stepping out of my body to take a broader view of how I am relating with the world. It was one of these times when I found myself asking, "What in blazes are you doing, Sherry!?! Here you are a medical doctor for twenty years, and supposedly one of the leading specialists in the world in environmental medicine. You do not treat cancer patients, yet here you are in a renovated Boston warehouse/factory sitting with a Japanese man in his sixties, who forty years ago studied international law at Columbia.

"You've spent all evening furiously writing down every word he uttered as he saw a Harvard law professor, a New York City physician with AIDS, a Connecticut doctor with breast cancer, a Georgia accounting professor with cancer of the pancreas metastasized to the liver, a plumber with prostatic cancer metastasized to the kidney, a mid-western retired golf pro with cancer of the intestine metastasized to the bones and much more. If that isn't the most unlikely set of circumstances, not to mention that the day before, you saw people with him who had traveled from Hawaii, Michigan, Florida, California, Nova Scotia and Australia, Toronto and Ohio. How utterly unlikely that people would have traveled great distances to see this quiet, light-framed man of few words who isn't even a doctor!"

Why? Because there are many people who have kicked death in the teeth because of this man. Medicine may scorn and deride, but when they have labeled somebody medically terminal, that's when this man has taken over to accomplish the impossible: He has guided many terminal cancer patients back to total wellness. As I read Satillaro's and Nussbaum's books, I wanted the details of how they ate day to day. Since it wasn't there, I decided to go and work with the top expert in the world. I wanted the details of the secret. I wanted what medicine had not provided in 25 years of study: the secret to healing impossible conditions.

In my practice, we also see people who travel from all over the world and have reached the end of their diagnostic rope.

Medicine has nothing to offer them, either. The difference is, they are not terminal, just hopelessly incurable. But since 50% of the patients each day are from out-of-state and within one to three months, a majority are labelling themselves as 50%-90% better, we also have a system for the incurable (for information on how this system works, read The E.I. Syndrome, Box 3161, Syracuse, NY 13220).

But for the tough ones that even I could not help, or for those of us who were dramatically improved and now wanted to be even more well, I found that macrobiotics was the next answer. It brought hundreds of us to undreamed-of levels of wellness and we weren't even experts at doing it.

This drove me to want to hone my skills and knowledge of macrobiotics to a level comparable with my expertise in environmental medicine. What better place to start than at the top with Mr. Michio Kushi, and learn how people healed their cancers.

Many of you know from our first three books, that I was very ill for years with severe chemical sensitivities. I had been found wandering around the office one time not even knowing my name and address just because a water-proof paint had been used in the basement that you couldn't even smell upstairs. Another time I was found sitting in a corner at the Princeton Tailor in Hong Kong, crying and speaking irrationally because they were gluing down formica countertops. You can imagine my surprise when the third time I went to meet with Mr. Kushi, I walked into the Kushi Institute to find that they were actively painting and gluing down new carpet. I immediately thought it would be ridiculous for me to stay and that I might as well go right back to the airport and call it a major loss.

But before I knew it, I was whisked into the activities only to realize at the end of the day, and later on at the end of three days, that I had done the impossible. I had gotten so well with macrobiotics, that I had not one symptom during the time that all of this renovation was going on. Sure, I'll never be totally normal in that I'll be able to tolerate all of the xenobiotics, or foreign chemicals in the normal 20th century environment. But, I'm not so sure that it's good to be that clear. I think it's healthier for my body to alert me to get out of an area by giving a headache or brain fog rather than staying there and having that chemical later create genetic damage that can lead to cancer or other diseases.

But what impressed me more than my own improvement, which I had considered impossible, are the hundreds of other patients who have successfully implemented this program and have also become much less sensitive to Candida, molds, foods, electromagnetic fields and chemicals. To top this off, having witnessed scores of people who have cleared their own terminal cancers, has made me a real believer. I have reviewed their medical records and watched with wonder as they healed. I don't claim that this is a diet to cure all serious diseases. But I can verify that I have seen impossible terminal cases become totally healthy. And I have watched a few stop the diet and develop their problem all over again. Because we are all biochemically unique, I doubt it is appropriate for everyone, but I have no idea on the percentage. However, there is definitely something that we, as physicians, need to learn about this program.

THE PHASES OF THE MACROBIOTIC DIET

A macrobiotic program has two phases, each with varying levels of limitations. For as one becomes progressively healthier, he has fewer dietary limitations. In fact a truly healthy person can probably eat whatever he wants.

The transition phase enables one to gradually switch over from a standard American junk food and processed food diet, to macrobiotics. Or he can be in a strict, healing phase which is temporary, but necessary for a variety of months or years, depending on the individual's condition, to heal or clear a particular problem. After that, he can broaden and go back into a more transitional diet, which does not have the severe restrictions and limitations that the healing phase possesses.

The healing phase of a macrobiotic diet is meant to clear a particular condition. It is, necessarily, very strict and individualized and for this reason, you should see a doctor trained in macrobiotics or a qualified macrobiotic consultant. Since some who call themselves certified are really not, I would suggest you call or write the Institute and find out for yourself. In the meantime, you could begin a month on a strict healing phase while you are awaiting a consultation. You can't get into much trouble (imbalance) in a month, but do not go beyond that. And, of course, if you are worse, discontinue it until you have your consultation. For macrobiotics is not for everyone. In fact, nothing is.

Be aware that medications for diabetes or high blood pressure may not be needed after a while, so watch carefully for too low a pressure or low sugar as you heal naturally and no longer need as much medication. For example, medicine to lower your sugar is great if you have diabetes. But give it to a normal person and he can pass out or worse. Give it to someone who has normalized his sugar with the macrobiotic diet and you'll get the same effect. Tapering medications should be done with your regular physician or your macrobiotic physician. Also, do not eat anything that you know you react adversely to or that makes you worse. See Chapter 6 regarding the food allergic patient. It is not advised to stay on the diet in this book, unsupervised, beyond one month, especially if you do not feel progressively better. This book is meant to save you time and money in allowing you to get the fundamentals down before your personal consultation, so that you will have some of the basics down and get more from your consultation.

First you must understand the goals of the healing phase. Since most pesticides and other chemicals are stored in the lipids, or fat, you want to diet off as much fat as possible, and get below your desired weight. Then, when you put weight back on, it can be done with good, clean fat that is organic and not processed to promote arteriosclerosis (see Tired Or Toxic?, Prestige Publishing, Box 3161, Syracuse, NY 13220 for verification, scientific references and explanations of any statements in this book. We did not want to duplicate them in here). Naturally during this phase when you are progressively losing weight, everyone is going to ask you if you have cancer or if you're seeing a doctor. When they find out you're doing it intentionally with a diet that they have never heard of, they are usually aghast that you do not follow their advice and get off it.

For example, one young woman was an adorable, very attractive 36 year old with seven years of crippling rheumatoid arthritis. She shuffled in like the Tin Man from "The Wizard of Oz" with barely a moveable joint. Within eight months, she had dropped her weight from 135 to 86 pounds. She said it was really ironic because for seven years, she had been a prisoner in her body, trapped in the armor of daily pain and limitation of motion. Now that she had been macrobiotic, she had lost all of that pain and felt wonderful and could move freely. But, instead of being happy for her, all of her friends kept nagging her about when she was going to put her weight back on. Of course, the time eventually came (Chapter 9) when it was prudent for her to put the weight back on. But they didn't care enough to learn about her condition and the constant badgering became a negative for someone who was working against all odds and something she didn't need. Fortunately, she was able to see beyond their focus.

But don't worry, that's a more extreme case. Most of us did not lose proportionately that much, nor for that long. I'm 5' 2" and dropped 25 pounds the first month. As with most of us, it's effortless, happening in spite of eating a larger volume of food than ever before. When the medical condition is cleared and the diet broadens, the weight automatically returns to wherever you allow it.

Another goal of the diet, besides getting rid of stored chemicals, is to make the body chemistry as strong and healthy as possible. This includes the biochemical pathways for healing, regeneration, chemical detoxication and energy production. You make every single mouthful as utterly healthful as possible, and as high in nutrient density as possible, as well as being balanced with your needs. In other words, you eat as though your life depended upon it.

HOW MUCH CONVINCING DO WE NEED?

Frequently, I will encounter negativity from the medical profession about macrobiotics which really floors me when they have no alternative for the patient, and have not taken the time to learn that it is extremely healthful and logical. As I have said many times in the past, any therapy which has enabled some people to clear cancers and other "incurable" conditions that were labelled hopeless or medically terminal, should definitely not be ignored.

One of the most convincing cases that I read about was Elaine Nussbaum in her autobiography Recovery. She was a young woman in her thirties with cancer of the ovaries metastasized (spread) to the lungs and backbone. The bones eventually weakened and collapsed and she was bedridden. When she developed pneumonia, after two years of unsuccessful struggling with this, her medical doctors finally so much as said, "WHOA! We can't give you any more chemotherapy, any more surgery or any more radiation treatments. We don't even dare give you an antibiotic because you're so sick and so riddled with metastases. Anything we do is probably going to tip you over and cause your demise." It was with this generous two-month maximum life span, that she entered macrobiotics. She is totally clear to this day of all cancers, and is an active counselor in New Jersey. I recently had the pleasure of meeting her and was delighted to see that she is even more vivacious, younger and prettier than her book photographs, since she has had even additional time on the diet.

I have seen other people clear cancer of the breast, and I have even met people who cleared their brain tumors and resulting neurologic symptoms. While I was at a week-long seminar in the Berkshires, one young man from Europe had come there weeks prior, bedridden with a brain tumor. The week I was there was his first week out of bed. At the beginning of the week, he could barely walk, barely swallow and had an obvious facial paralysis on one side. When he closed his eyes to say prayer before dinner, he could not close the lid of one eye. Instead the eye rolled up into the head so the large, white globe was all that one could see. By the end of the week, he was walking, smiling, talking, had no facial paralysis and his eyes and lids were conjugate and normal.

While there, I met another young lady from South America who had been sent home by the most prestigious medical center in the U. S. to die of her brain tumor. Bedridden, she was taken to the Berkshires and today is beautifully healthy and has the nuclear magnetic resonance imaging scans to prove it.

There's one thing, however, that keeps cropping up among people who have cleared their cancers. One music professor who had cancer of the pancreas is a good example of this. All throughout his book on how he healed himself of his pancreatic cancer, he was always looking for ways to cheat or go off the diet, and indeed he did die within a few years. At the autopsy he was totally clear of cancer of the pancreas, but nonetheless, he had died of a pneumonia (which a normally strong body should be able to fight off). It appears that in the case of cancer, it's quite clear that many people have discontinued prematurely. Another example is Dr. Anthony Satillaro (whose well-publicized clearing of his cancer was published in Recalled By Life). He was advised to stay strictly on macrobiotics for seven years before he loosened up, or became more broad with his eating. However, after a few years, one could quickly see with the publication of his second book, which was more of a very liberal transition diet, that he had begun to fall off the wagon. He died a few years later with recurrence of his cancer after he had totally cleared it and all the bone metastases.

The same theme popped up as I watched people on return visits at the Kushi Institute. For example, one gal complained of an ovarian problem. As they looked over her chart, they noticed she had been there two years earlier for the same problem, and asked her what had happened. "Oh, I followed everything that you told me to," she said "and totally got rid of my problem. In fact, my gynecologist was amazed. But over the last year, I've resumed my old eating habits." And of course, back came her problem and here she was again ready to start over. It's amazing how much denial we all have and how strong our ties are to processed foods.

I myself was reluctant to evaluate macrobiotics, also, because I didn't want to change my eating habits. Besides that, I rationalized that I had already arrived. The special non-phenol titrated injections to the newer molds and pollens and dust had cleared my severe migraine headaches, burning eyes, asthma, chronic sinusitis and snorting, and hay fever. The food injections miraculously cleared my years of facial eczema which previously looked like I had a fire on my face that somebody had tried to beat out with an old golf shoe. Then the environmental controls (like getting rid of natural gas and carpets) and discovering and correcting my numerous biochemical defects (deficiencies of vitamins A, B1, B6, C, and minerals zinc, molybdenum, manganese, chromium , copper, magnesium and more) cleared the brain fog with the poor memory, poor concentration and mood swings plus the severe back pain (all of these details and instructions are in The E.I. Syndrome and Tired Or Toxic?). So I thought I had arrived.

Then I broke a corner of a tooth by accidentally biting on a nutshell. In retrospect I could relate major deteriorations in my health over the years to times following further amalgams. In my generation, they made huge amalgam fillings and over 50% of my teeth were filled. Replacements meant glues or adhesives of some type, all of which I have severe brain allergies to. So a mouthful of a chemical that one whiff of left me suicidally depressed was out of the question. Furthermore I reasoned that one more amalgam was a mere drop in the bucket. Within one month of the filling (mercury amalgam), I had spontaneous menopause and had only just turned forty-four and I had developed a severe shoulder pain which I'd never had before in my life. This shoulder was in the same acupuncture meridian as the tooth. I also had bloody colitis that had started. (Never before had I had a true appreciation of the pain of a dozen bloody bowel movements a day.)

After six months of intolerable and non-stop shoulder pain, I went on macrobiotics cold-turkey. Within one week the colitis was totally clear. Also I had more energy than I had had in years and felt terrific. I had what I call "macro mellowness." In fact, the office staff, accustomed to my flying off the handle at the slightest provocation, remarked to my husband, "Whatever she's on, keep her at it. We've never seen her so calm!" In less than three months, the shoulder was completely clear and I was windsurfing in the ocean. And within six months, I tried to go off the diet and developed severe diarrhea. Since I was in another country at the time, we immediately went out and bought a hot plate and some brown rice, and I got back on the diet and simmered down.

After a year, I tried again to go off the diet cold-turkey to see what would happen. It's not that I'm completely stupid, it's just that I was born with a little scientist inside me. Even as a child in junior high school, I would always pick the squeamish girls as my partners in biology so that I could have the whole earthworm or frog to myself. And so it was with macrobiotics. I wanted to see what would happen to someone if they discontinued the diet that they had thought was so healing.

My husband had won a business trip to Nassau and since no one there knew me, I thought I would go "incognito" as 'Mrs. Normal,' and not even let anyone know that I was a physician much less on any special diet. I was having a marvelous time, scuba diving, petting sting rays at a depth of 85 feet. Within four days I was totally bedridden with recurrence of my old back pain and had to be carried to the bathroom, and I had done nothing physical that would warrant the recurrence of this pain. But don't lose heart. After nearly two years, when I was lecturing in Australia, I had found the happy medium. I could eat a macrobiotic breakfast in the room while my husband had room service, pack enough for the trip on the road for a macrobiotic lunch, and at dinnertime have a full seven-course French meal complete with wine, French bread and pastries with no ill effects. And I did this for the several weeks that we were touring Australia after my four days of lectures. Even then, you see minor changes in yourself, though, and you realize that it's not something that you want to keep doing and that you do eventually, as soon as you get home, want to get right back into the stricter phase. It only makes sense that if we see such miraculous changes in ourselves occur within a few months or years of macrobiotics, then it behooves us to continue even longer to see how much healthier we can get.

After 2 1/2 years on macro, while lecturing in England, I was able to go off for 2 1/2 weeks with no problems. So don't worry that it is a life sentence. A diet that has the track record that this one does for actually clearing the impossible, should not be lightly passed by.

After 3 years, I found if I had wine, I would be drenched in sweat all night. My body was so healthy it could purge what it needed. However, I wouldn't advise this as a steady habit, since sweating is nutrient depleting for magnesium as an example.

Bear in mind also, that we are the first generation of man ever exposed to such an unprecedented level of chemicals. The body uses up precious nutrients in metabolizing and getting rid of these chemicals that we all breathe in every day (Tired Or Toxic? explains it). So being in this generation is nutrient depleting. If that were not enough of a burden on our bodies (being exposed to many new chemicals and getting nutrient depleted), we are also the first generation to eat so many processed foods. Both of these factors have a strong, causative effect in bringing about an inferior nutritional status in the body and fostering "mysterious" diseases. One common factor we see in nearly all of our patients, macrobiotic or not, has been many hidden nutrient deficiencies. It has made a great deal of sense to identify and correct these early on so healing can proceed that much faster. But more on that later.

CAUSES OF YOUR CONDITION:
Milk, Meat, Sugar, Salt, Alcohol, Flour Products and Fat

I know we're in deep trouble, when in 1990 in taking a dietary history on a thirty-four-year-old, college-educated engineer, I discovered he thinks a whole grain is shredded wheat! A whole grain is alive. It's actually the seed of the plant, housing the potential for a new life. Whole brown rice, oats, millet, barley, and wheat berries, are capable of growing. Put them in a saucer of water on the windowsill and they will sprout roots and green leaves in several days. If you put shredded wheat in a dish or 5-minute converted rice, pasta or white bread, they will only rot. They are not whole. They are not alive. They have been bleached and stripped of vitamins by chemicals so you can cook and eat them in five minutes versus forty-five.

What a tremendous benefit! To save forty minutes, they've removed vitamin E, B6, magnesium, and many other vitamins and minerals that prevent heart attacks, arteriosclerosis, and other degenerative diseases (for full explanation read Tired Or Toxic?). Because the resulting food is so devoid of nutrients, the government has made manufacturers add a few pennies' worth of the cheapest vitamins (the B's) that you see prominently displayed on the box, and which constitute the meaning of the word 'enriched.'

Not only does this devitalized product save forty minutes, but it lasts for ages in the pantry. Of course, fresh bread that you make at home won't last, because it's neither loaded with preservatives nor devoid of the nutrients that a growing bug needs. In the last ten years, we've measured vitamin and mineral levels in thousands of patients and rarely see anyone who's totally normal anymore. Certainly rampant, unrecognized nutritional deficiencies contribute to the many degenerative diseases which are on the rise, and can actually account for all the pathology of many diseases.

The question of what causes an illness is always addressed in the macrobiotic consultation, whereas in medicine, we're not so concerned by the cause, but only in covering up the symptoms with prescription drugs or surgery. For many people, for example, dairy causes the excessive formation of mucus. I have seen this in general allergy practice for twenty years. Many people who go on the diagnostic diets, as outlined in The E.I. Syndrome, will report that they no longer have as much nasal congestion after they discontinue milk products. Dairy is also responsible for many people having abdominal gas, bloating, indigestion, alternating diarrhea and constipation, and for many people having headaches as well. But medicine tends to ignore this time-honored cause of excessive mucus for many people. They prefer to treat chronic sinus problems as an antihistamine deficiency.

Another item that adds to physical decline and the development of symptoms in people is a diet high in sugars. Over the years, we have seen thousands of patients with Candida problems. Their lives have been dramatically changed. Most of them have been to at least a dozen physicians in search of an answer to their perplexing symptoms. Once they were on the Candida program, their symptoms of years disappeared within days. If we took them off the program, the symptoms recurred. In seeing thousands of these people, I would often ask "What part of the Candida program made the biggest difference to you? Was it going off sugars and ferments? Milk and wheat products? The addition of the acidophilus, or the further addition of Nystatin? Or was it the ketoconazole or other parts of the total load?" Invariably, 50% of the people had marked improvement as soon as they eliminated the sugars from their diets. We have since discovered why, since sugars, through non-enzymatic glycosylation can mimic any and all of the worst effects of any twenty-first century chemical on the body. This includes binding with DNA, the genetic material, to damage it to create cancer.

It's just common sense. Imagine if you took all of your savings out of the bank and you had to bet on which of two people hospitalized after an operation would heal the quickest. Would you bet on the one who ate ice cream and candy all day long, or the one who ate good, clean, wholesome macrobiotic food every day, with a diet of 50% whole grains and 50% vegetables?

We know, for example, that one of the common signs of

diabetes is poor healing, or inability to heal wounds as quickly as one should. Sugar is an extreme negative to the body because it actually uses up more precious vitamins and minerals in metabolizing it than it gives the body. Therefore, it leaves one in a deficit condition each time it's used. It's sort of like taking money out of the bank each time without ever putting any in. Sooner or later you have to pay up. The medical literature is full of papers on sugar showing that through the process of non-enzymatic glycosylation, it is one of the major causes of arteriosclerotic and vascular disease; not cholesterol. Cholesterol is merely a secondary cause (references and explanation for all this in Tired or Toxic?).

Another cause of many people's conditions is a high fruit diet. Many people proudly boast that they eat a lot of fruit, thinking that it means that they're having a healthful diet. In essence, they're only one step above the people who have a high sugar diet. I used to be upset with macrobiotic pronouncements that sugar, for example, was expansive and promoted disease, and that fruits were damaging and expansive as well. You can imagine my surprise when I stumbled across papers in the scientific literature that actually proved this. In Tired Or Toxic? we enumerated over thirty biochemical mechanisms of how macrobiotics is so healing. So that doctors could no longer denigrate it or put it down, we provided the scientific evidence with references.

For example, there are papers that show that if you give rats intravenous fructose (fruit sugar) and then dissect and analyze their livers under the microscope, indeed, the precious liver cells have become massively swollen or expanded with water. The endoplasmic reticulum (the delicate membranes where detoxification of chemicals takes place) have become so distorted with water uptake that they no longer function optimally. Indeed, this could be the precursor to chemical sensitivity. And we have seen this in practice over the years. People who eat a lot of fruit often have multiple dust, mold, pollen, Candida and chemical hypersensitivities.

Hypoglycemia, or low blood sugar can manifest as sugar cravings, weakness, headache, irritability, unexplained mood swings, sweats, fatigue, numbness and much more. It stems from poor pancreatic function. One way for the pancreas to become malfunctioning is through getting too tight or congested and contracted from too much meat, fats and salty cheeses. Having dry baked goods like rice cakes, and foods with a high content of natural oils like crackers, nuts, and other baked goods can retard the healing of an abused pancreas and make the condition worse. Hence, often when these are ingested, the symptoms actually do get worse. So avoidance of them in the beginning of the strict healing phase is necessary.

Also for proper pancreatic function, you need adequate levels of chromium, zinc, copper and magnesium for starters. These are measured by an RBC (red blood cell) chromium, RBC zinc, RBC copper and magnesium loading test (see <u>Tired Or Toxic?</u> for details). By not correcting these sooner, the hypoglycemia can drag on and drive one to eat the very things that make it worse.

As well, eating large amounts of meat not only provides a great deal of fat, which impairs the function of the endoplasmic reticulum, but has other deleterious effects on the system. Studies show that many spend their day, for example, in an average office where many modern-day chemicals outgas, such as formaldehyde, toluene, benzene, xylene and trichlorethylene. These come from the carpets themselves, the carpet glues, furniture and molding glues, the furniture stuffings, the papers, the plastics and the artificial rubber products in the business machines as well as the solvents and inks. These chemicals are in our bloodstream from breathing the room air. People in good health will metabolize, or detoxify and get rid of these chemicals. Much of the time, the chemical is hooked onto (conjugated with) a tripeptide in the liver called glutathione. This peptide hooks or conjugates onto the chemical, drags it out into the bile and then into the gut so that it can be lost with the stool and the body can effectively get rid of it. A substitute conjugate for some foreign chemicals is glucuronic acid.

When people eat a high-meat diet, there is excessive enzyme activity in the gut from beta-glucuronidase. This enzyme breaks the glucuronide conjugate bond, tearing off the chemical so that now the chemical is free to be reabsorbed into the person's bloodstream. In essence, they have used up energy and nutrients to get rid of the chemical, only to have it reabsorbed back into the body to give them a 'double-whammy' toxicant level. People, however, who have a low-meat diet have much less beta-glucuronidase and so they excrete their chemicals in a more normal fashion and are thus not wasting as much of the body's chemical energy. Furthermore, they are getting rid of the chemical more efficiently. We often observed this in clinical practice even before we recognized anything about macrobiotics. People who went on diets low in meat began suddenly becoming less chemically sensitive (because their detoxification mechanisms, in the endoplasmic reticulum were operating more effectively).

Of course, you are aware that a high-salt diet causes high blood pressure, and salt, indeed, is very contracting. It's just amazing to me that all of these properties of foods professed by macrobiotics were recognized years before these biochemical studies in the scientific literature came out for scientific validation. And these studies were done by people who had no concept of or idea that macrobiotics even existed. They were just studying these small isolated facets of a diet independently. I was fortunate enough, in perusing thousands of nutritional biochemistry articles to find them and make the connection.

Although dairy causes much mucus formation, chicken, beef, pork and other meats, plus oils and nuts account for much more of the fat. With the accumulation of fats, there is stagnation in the lymphatics and other tissues, resulting in poor circulation and decreased nutrients to the organs. Likewise, wastes that are not freely removed, accumulate and further hasten disease of the organ. Furthermore, eating high-sugar diets gets one further behind in many nutrients so that with combined poor circulation and nutrient deficiency, the stage is set for degenerative change and disease. For example, if it is the heart that is the predominant organ to be damaged, the person now has a label of heart disease.

Remember in 3rd grade we learned the 4 food groups?

> 1) dairy/eggs
> 2) meat/fowl/fish
> 3) fruits/vegetables
> 4) grains

Well, in this century those have eroded into:

> 1) fractured fats & oils (grocery store oils &
>   margarines stripped of B6, E, magnesium

and more)
2) high meat diets from animals bred to
have abnormal essential fatty acids and
high chemical overload (antibiotics,
hormones, pesticides)
3) purified sugar or fermented sugars
(alcohol)
4) broken or refined grains (again, stripped
of many nutrients to improve shelf life)

And this group of 4 processed food culprits constitutes as much as 50% of the American diet. Not only are these deficient in nutrients, but they require nutrients to metabolize them. Some even block many important biochemical pathways from functioning normally (Tired Or Toxic?).

Way back on August 6 1990, the cover article for U.S. News and World Report was "How to Reverse Heart Disease." This was a landmark for macrobiotics, for medicine is now ever so slowly beginning to catch up. Dr. Dean Ornish published in the Lancet how with diet (which is nearly a transitional macrobiotic diet), exercise, yoga and/or meditation, arteriosclerotic plaques were reversed or healed.

Prior to this, it was considered quackery to think it could be reversed. This justified $40,000 by-pass surgery and hundreds of dollars of cholesterol-lowering drugs a year.

Of course, cancer is still considered irreversible, but it will only be a matter of time before that paradigm, too, is rectified.

THE MACROBIOTIC VISUAL DIAGNOSIS

A macrobiotic visual diagnosis gives much clue to the foods that you have eaten in excess, although usually one's condition is a combination of these "wrong foods" that have brought about the total picture. It's interesting, though, how factual the visual diagnosis is. In the early days, I would sit on an airplane and try to guess what people would eat before their meals were served. One man sat down next to me and I was aghast at how utterly yin he appeared. I kept reprimanding myself saying, "This is ridiculous. You're just over-reacting." However when the mealtime came, he passed on dinner and ate only the brownie and ordered two large Cokes...a most extremely yin meal!

Another very pleasant man that I had sat next to on another flight struck me as being extremely yang. I timidly asked if he would mind if I told him what I thought he ate and if he would tell me if I was correct. He enthusiastically agreed and couldn't believe it when I told him that he loved meat and potatoes and hardly ever had any alcohol, coffee, sweets or fruits. He said, "You've hit the nail right on the head. That's exactly how I eat!"

As one studies visual diagnosis more and more, it becomes increasingly fascinating, especially to those of us who were trained in the strictly Western medicine mode, where such things are thought to be impossible. For example, one morning while observing at The Kushi Institute with Dr. Marc VanCauwenburghe, we sat across from our first consultation. I took one look at his face and enthusiastically asked, "Could I please try this one first?" I then told the gentleman that I thought his prostatic cancer had metastasized to his kidney, and he replied "Why, yes. You're right! I just got the results of the scan yesterday." "And it's your right kidney that's involved," I added. And he replied, "Why, yes! How did you know?"

Not all cases, however, are this easy or straightforward. But as you study more physical diagnosis, you will be better able to monitor your condition. As for other people, be very careful, because many are not interested. You have to remember that you're con-stantly bucking up against high-tech medicine, (which is analogous to an ambulance waiting at the foot of a cliff to rescue people who fall off). And very few people are interested in preventive medicine when they can have dramatic, high-tech medicine with fast, effortless results.

Just because it is not taught in American medical schools, we might have a tendency to think of Oriental physical diagnosis as less than scientific. So let me dispel that notion for you with two ex-amples so you can see for yourself.

It is said that the infraorbital (under the eyes) darkness is a sign of kidney trouble. You will notice one of the reasons a person who goes macro starts looking younger and healthier is the darkness under the eyes fades. But watch what happens after a day of reverting back to old habits with a beer and pizza or a bag of chips. It may take only one day or several weeks depending on his health level before he will begin to awaken with swelling and darkness under the eyes. This reflects the excess salt and water load that the kidneys are not able to handle.

Once you observe this you will begin to appreciate how a look at the face can often tell what the person eats as well as what organs are in trouble.

Let's take one more example. If a person who has improved (I use an improved example because it's easier for you to see as a beginner) starts getting into sweets and/or alcohol heavily again, the deep groove between the medial (inside) corner of the eye and the bridge of the nose darkens. You guessed it! This relates to the pancreas function.

Too much fats and oils can affect the pancreas, too, but not as fast and usually (in medicine there are never any absolutes or 'always') starts by producing heaviness or dull ache under the right ribs, where the gall bladder is.

And when the gall bladder becomes too overloaded with a high fat diet, you'll often find a problem along it's acupuncture meridian, which can range from shoulder pain to a lost 4th or 5th toenail. I've both witnessed this on others and experienced it with myself and the consistency of these findings far outweighs any haphazard explanation like sheer coincidence.

As I sat with Mr. Kushi in his consultations, I was constantly amazed at his perceptive powers. He would sit there and look at people across the desk and tell them which toenail, for example, had a fungal infection or was blackened or diseased. When I removed their shoes, sure enough, there it was! This is not black magic, but possible when one understands the acupuncture meridians of the body. Remember, Chinese medicine is based on these meridians, or this electrical circuitry of the body. This circuitry is what allows a New York City reporter to be able to have gall-bladder surgery while he's drinking a Coke and reading the "New York Times."

Acupuncture anesthesia and acupuncture treatment of disease is a very real entity. We only ignore it in the United States because (1) we are not trained in it, and (2) it requires time, and we like to do the quickest treatment possible so that we can fit many people into a day and (3) it doesn't sell drugs. But when you see warts and moles and blackened nails and bluish spots on various parts of the body, once you learn the meridians, you can better estimate what organ system is also beginning to get into trouble.

I have seen Mr. Kushi sit down with someone and say, "Why have you not told me about your pain right here?" as he touches their gall bladder, and they will say, "Oh! I forgot all about that. But yes, I have been having a lot of pain." These dysfunctions in the body are able to be read in the hands, face, skin and feet because the body is all interconnected. If one understands quantum physics, he will realize that the face or the hands or the feet or the iris is but a miniature representation of the entire body (read <u>Vibrational Medicine</u> in the Resources).

In essence, the food factor as one of the causes of disease is easy. When we eat excessive things the body doesn't like, it tries to get rid of them. When it is further overloaded, it gives us a symptom that is supposed to be a warning to us to analyze our lifestyle and make a change. When we ignore it or cover it up with medication, the excess gets stored. Excess fats plug the lymphatic circulation to the organ and it gets less oxygen and nutrients, then it starts failing. Excessive sweets, alcohols and chemical drugs are expansive (yin) and cause water retention or swelling and eventual weakness of the organ and symptoms. Excessive salts and baked goods are hardening to the fat, making it more dense and dangerous. And dairy causes mucous formation which also serves to congest organs and compromise their vitality and function.

The target organ predilection merely depends on a variety of things such as your heredity, your weakest point, diet, etc. It's too simple for high-tech medicine to buy, even though many have reversed arteriosclerosis, cancer, rheumatoid arthritis, multiple sclerosis, alopecia areata, food, Candida, electromagnetic and chemical sensitivities and more by using these principles. Why even now articles are popping up in the scientific literature showing that arteriosclerosis can be reversed and completely gotten rid of with diet. And they didn't even use macrobiotics, for they have slowly only adopted some of it's principles. But they are inching closer every year. It is only a short while before they will discover the same can apply to cancer.

So, it's obvious now, how sugar, dairy, fruit and meat have caused many of the conditions that we see. What's left? Those of you who read You Are What You Ate know the answer: grains, greens and beans. Now you can begin to moan and groan, or be thankful that you know what may have caused the diseases that you have. Now let's dig in and make it work for you.

CHAPTER 2

A HEALTHY PERSON CAN EAT ANYTHING

Now that you know the potential cause of many conditions, let's dig right into the very dogmatic, hard and fast rules of this strict healing phase diet. The reason we're doing this is that many people do not have the time or the money to attend courses to learn how to do this, nor the money for multiple consultations. But they need to get started getting well quickly. So we have spelled it out here. Once you have mastered the concepts in the book, then in one month of having started, you should have a consultation so that it can be personally adapted to your needs. Never lose sight of the fact that everything is constantly changing, including your body and it's environment. You might feel particularly well in the beginning of a diet like this, only to find that after a while you don't feel so well, in fact you feel worse. The diet must periodically change to adapt to your changing condition and needs. In fact, to stay on the healing phase for a prolonged period with minimal or no oil is very dangerous and will assuredly lead to disease. And never lose sight of checking those nutrient (vitamin, mineral, amino acid and essential fatty acid) levels, especially if you are not getting progressively better. Playing with a full deck can speed your progress (see Tired Or Toxic?).

I was surprised to hear a long-time macrobiotic editor say one time that macrobiotics was too dogmatic, when in essence, it is a very loose program once one is healed. But in this era with all of our instincts blunted by processed foods, we need strict guidance in the beginning to get those instincts back. Then you can eat as freely as you want, because your body never lies. A healthy body will tell you when you have wronged.

To look at it in another way, in the woods one does not see animals on crutches and sucking down Darvons or Tylenols, because animals eat by instinct. The sick raccoon or deer cannot go to the nearest doctor and say, "Take me, I'm yours. I don't want to have to change anything in my lifestyle or diet. Just make me well." Because he has to heal naturally, he has to rely on his own inner resources. When he is thirsty, he drinks. When he is sick, he doesn't eat. If he doesn't feel well, he changes his nest.

But us? We have no instincts. They've been blurred by our adulterated tastes. We drink to get high, we drink to wake up in the morning. We drink to satiate our sugar cravings and hypoglycemia, or because we have eaten too many salty foods. And then, we drink the wrong things. We drink fruit juices loaded with fructose sugar that further weaken our detox system and add too much sugar as well as pesticides and mold allergens from the stored fruits. These drinks have vitamin C artificially added because during pasteurization, all the natural vitamin C was destroyed. What else was destroyed that was not added, no one tells.

But on macrobiotics, you develop your instincts again after you become unmasked. So when you eat something wrong, just like an animal, you know right away; you don't have to second-guess. Many of you, after having been through The E.I. Syndrome, have felt what unmasking can be like. For example, you may have had years of arthritis pain, but you had French fries and steaks every week and never dreamed that beef and potato could be part of the causes of your pain. After you went off these for a few weeks and then back on them, your pain had ceased when you were off and came back very dramatically once you resumed eating them. You were indeed in the unmasked or natural instinctive state.

It is important for the body to be in the unmasked state, for it's nature's way of guiding us to the best foods for us. For example, after I had been on macrobiotics for half of a year, I went to the local organic bakery that I used to frequent in my pre-macro days every friday afternoon. I used to have a half dozen organic oatmeal cookies plus assorted muffins under the guise of my self-imposed belief that they were healthful for me. Now that I was unmasked and macro, I wanted to see what these had really been contributing to. The next morning when I awakened, having had a half dozen organic oatmeal cookies, I was totally congested as though I had the worst cold in the world, but I felt perfectly fine. By noon it had fully disappeared. Another time, I wanted to try ice cream after I had been macrobiotic for half a year. Within an hour of the ice cream, I had a three hour nap, and could not stay awake to save my soul. Yet a year later, when I was healthier, I could have one with no symptoms.

When you are really healthy and unmasked, your body is able to do what it is supposed to do, and that is to alert you to dangers to your health. That's why I think it's good that many of us who were highly chemically sensitive and are much better now, still are not totally insensitive to the 21st century chemicals. Indeed, I want my body to be able to give me a tiny headache or backache and tell me I have no business sucking down toluene fumes in a newly painted room ....especially since the scientific literature shows that most of these modern chemicals, encountered daily in our homes and offices, are potentially carcinogenic (can cause cancer).

Indeed, once someone is clear on a macrobiotic diet, he can eat anything he wants because his body will tell him immediately what is and what is not good for him. And your tolerance will vary with your state of health at the time. Just be sure you are indeed eating very well and are not fooling yourself by not having symptoms from excesses of known "bad" foods when you are not really un-masked. For now, since you have a tough condition that you need to heal, you need to eat as cleanly as possible right now, and in a fashion that many people have used that have successfully cleared their conditions.

An allergy is an overloaded, sick system. For example, before macrobiotics, if I ate the slightest amount of chocolate, my face would be a broken-out mess for three weeks. That's because I was in an overloaded, allergic state. Now, I can have a piece of chocolate and nothing appears to happen. However, if I keep doing it and get myself in a more unhealthy state, then my allergic symptoms manifest themselves. But to have a little bit of these things now and again does not cause an allergic response, since the total load is so vastly reduced and the healed detox system is functioning again. The amount of time during which you can tolerate previously intolerable foods is proportionate to how well you are to begin with. But beware of being downright foolish and getting masked again. Then it may take months or years, but eventually the dam will break and symptoms will resurface.

Since we have in macrobiotics, a system unmatched by anything else, in or out of medicine, that I have personally witnessed in its unique ability to clear incurable conditions, it behooves you and me to be very dogmatic while we follow this system. Oftentimes I will see people who say they are macrobiotic, when in essence they are no more macrobiotic than the ordinary vegetarian is. They have picked and chosen what they want to eat and have not cleared their condition first. **THIS IS NOT MACROBIOTIC.** This is one's illusion of how he would like macrobiotics to be. He would like to be able to have his cake and eat it too, and simultaneously feel he is doing the best for his body. So he fabricates all sorts of rationalizations, rules and excuses that allow him these indiscretions that only serve to further delay healing.

Right now, we're going to do a more logical approach. We're going to start you out on a strict phase; then within a month, you will need a consultation to have it personally tailored to your needs. Let's see how clear you can get of all your conditions. Only after you are totally well, does it make sense to then see how liberal you can be, or how much you can broaden your diet and for how long. In fact, the more variety, the better. And as you get healthier you will fill the need for more variety. But don't get caught in the trap of complacency. Suppose you broaden your diet for a few months and are having a ball eating foods you hadn't had in months. Slowly, months or years later, you start having symptoms, or not feeling as well, or are requiring more sleep. It is at this point that you should drop everything and go back to your former, stricter diet and get well again. But some find this too difficult to do. If it doesn't improve you within a few weeks, get your nutrient (vitamin and mineral) levels checked, for something is clearly missing.

Getting organized is the secret to any successful endeavor. An old Chinese saying says, "The bigger the back, the bigger the front." It might be translated here to mean the results are indeed proportionate to the efforts. Again, Alan Lakein's book, How To Get Control of Your Time and Your Life, is an excellent, very inexpensive paperback on time management.

TOOLS OF THE TRADE

It's ironic that women will think nothing of paying $100 for a dress that might be worn one or two seasons, but resent paying $60 for a pressure cooker that will be used daily for 30 years. Likewise, I struggled for ages with 5 pound bags of grains with twist-ties that invariably slipped off and messed up the pantry when I went to pick them up; finally I invested in storage jars. It also makes the pantry look much neater and more organized, and keeps the fresh grains bugproof.

Likewise, for two years, I avoided purchasing a macrobiotic knife. It had taken me twenty years to learn how to use a French chef's knife, so I thought that was the only knife necessary for cooking. However, when I bought the Mac knife (it looks like a miniature meat cleaver, and is the classic macrobiotic knife), it dramatically changed my cooking and the taste of things. Have you ever noticed how when you're out to dinner, some vegetables taste much better than yours just because of the mere change in the way they have been cut?

The Mac knife is sort of like a Cuisinart. Its razor-thin blade can produce very tiny slices so that there is more of the flavor and taste of the vegetables in the dishes as compared with the larger pieces which are only possible with a French chef knife. Also, the larger pieces take longer to cook and impart a different taste to dishes. Caution: I went through considerable 6-0 nylon suture material. So cut slowly while you are learning to use this knife. Also, we had several meals laced with fingernails since when you're chopping onions, it's very difficult to see the nails among them. This knife is much more dangerous than the other knives that you are accustomed to.

Also, many of us have experienced the frustration of trying to juggle the pots and pans because we simply needed one or two extra ones. Why put yourself through the frustration? It's easier at the beginning to have the tools of the trade rather than add to your frustrations in your new endeavor. I found that the all glass cooking pots were terrific. Also a glass cover to one of your fry pans is a great investment as you can see the instant your blanched greens reach their peak of perfection. You can see everything without having to remove the top and can monitor how the cooking is taking place and whether the water level is getting too low. Stainless steel is also excellent. Never buy aluminum or Teflon coated pans, however, since they get into the food and your body. Having destroyed four expensive pots, two chopping-block countertops and the kitchen floor, I'm glad I finally opted for the strategy of glass pots.

You might wonder how I destroyed the floor. Admittedly, that was a tough one. But if you burn a Cuisinart pan enough times, plus drop it a few times, you can dent the edge of the bottom which has a layer of aluminum sandwiched in between two layers of stainless steel. Then you must burn it royally one last time. When it is sufficiently hot and you go to rescue it from the stove, the molten aluminum runs out the dent hole and spatters all over the floor, igniting it simultaneously in about thirty spots where the molten globs land. It's quite an exciting effect seeing a sudden burst of thirty 8" flames appear on the floor, and guaranteed to make prospective dinner guests think twice about eating at your place again.

So a minimum of   2 frying pans,

2-3 saucepans,

1 pressure cooker,

1 large soup pan with insertable/removable steamer tray

would be ideal for starters. Glass jars for organization and storage of the grains, beans, seaweeds, mushrooms, kuzu, teas, seeds and nuts are also necessary. Also you will need knives:

1 paring knife,

1 Mac knife,

1 chef knife.

Also,   1 vegetable peeler,

1 grater,

1 suribachi,

2 timers with very loud bells,

1 tea strainer,

1 small colander,

1 large colander,

1 wire-mesh ladle, and

1 soup ladle.

A word about graters; I found an excellent German, hand-held grating board with extremely razor-sharp blades. It was one of those things advertised on T.V. at 6:30 a.m. with the 1-800 numbers. It's excellent and very fast for making shredded or julienned, grated or other cuttings of your vegetables, and extremely quick and durable. Or you can get the regular grater in the culinary section of the store, but it's not nearly as sharp.

Many of these things you can hold off on and get later. Then, like I and many others did, when you do, you will really appreciate them and you'll find yourself saying, "I wish I had done this earlier." For example, I held off on getting a pickle-press for a year and then I didn't use it for another year, while the plastic smell outgassed. Also, I held off getting a large wooden bowl for storage of the cooked grain and a pair of chicken shears for fine cutting of dry kombu to put into soups. Also you will need:

a cutting board

a wooden spoon

a wooden spatula

1 hand-held potato masher

3 sizes of stackable, covered glass refrigerator dishes

3 cute, little, covered condiment containers for the table

a stove-top heat dissipater

And for lunches at work, you'll need:

a wide-mouth thermos

a sectioned, covered container (it sort of looks like a T.V. dinner because of the sections), and

2 tiny, covered 1-2 oz. containers for dressing or condiments that you might want to take along

When you walk out of this office, you can begin your macro-biotics. Within three minutes of here is Nature Tyme (an extension of N.E.E.D.S.) where you can purchase your macrobiotic supplies. You can do this in person or by phone (1-800-634-1380 from anywhere in the U.S. including New York State). Like-wise, you can go to Nature's Pantry on Erie Blvd., the Natural Discount Store on East Genesee St., the Food Co-op on Kensington or Clear Eye in Savannah for your grains. If you want to send away for them, you can get them at N.E.E.D.S., Mountain Ark, Gold Mine Natural Foods, Natural Lifestyle, Walnut Acres, as examples.

When you are at the macrobiotic health store, you will want the following products. Things listed in brackets are some that you will not use right away either because you are yeast sensitive, or because you are generally not used in the first month of the strict healing phase, and so you can hold off on purchasing them. They will be used later on and they can be used now by people in the transition phase. Always get organic when possible, and eventually only shop where you can get organic.

GRAINS

Rice, short-grain brown	Amaranth
Millet	Tempeh
Barley	Mochi (plain)
Quinoa	{Oats}
Wheat berries	{Buckwheat}

{Flours}	BEANS
{Noodles}	Aduki (azuki, adzuki)
{Corn grits}	Chick-pea (also called garbanzo)
SEEDS	Lentil
Sesame	Black Soybean
Pumpkin	Natto
{Sunflower}	

SEA VEGETABLES OR SEAWEEDS

Nori	Hijiki (Hiziki)
Wakame	Kombu
Arame	Agar-Agar
Sea Palm	

CONDIMENTS/MISCELLANEOUS {Temporarily avoid ume plums, miso, shoyu (soy), pickles, tekka, vinegar and sauerkraut if you are yeast sensitive}

{Umeboshi plums}	{Pickles}

{2 year old barley miso}

{Sauerkraut (organic made with salt & cabbage only)}

{Johsen shoyu sauce}	Dried daikon
Dried lotus	{rice wine vinegar}

White sea salt	{Tekka}
Kuzu (also called kudzu)	
Dried chestnuts	{Umeboshi vinegar}
{Amasake}	{organic apple juice}
{Shiitake Mushroom (dried)}	

Now, go to the best green grocer in town and get the following vegetables (all will not be available at once):

ABOVE-GROUND	BELOW-GROUND
Hard squash	Turnips
Pumpkin	Onions
Brussel sprouts	Carrots
Cabbage	Parsnips
Cauliflower	Ginger
{Kohlrabi}	Radish
{Corn on the cob}	

GREENS	
Collards	Kale
Dandelion	Mustard
Parsley	Leeks
Watercress	Bok choy

Chinese Cabbage

At the Oriental grocery or some of the health food stores you can find daikon, burdock and lotus root depending on the season. Also, you may want to pick up some scrod, cod, haddock, halibut, trout, snapper, sole or flounder. Only one fish a week, and that is a small 3"x3" portion. But any of the above is fine. If you don't feel the need for fish or protein, however, don't eat any for now or only once a month. Once you have invested in your basic supplies, you will find that your weekly food bills are about a third less than usual and as you continue on macrobiotics, your doctor bills, likewise, will reduce.

BACK AT THE RANCH

Okay! You're home with bags of things you've never seen before, and you don't have the faintest idea of how to prepare them. First, clear a space in the refrigerator and pantry. Put boxed cereals, instant muffin mixes, Hamburger Helper, brownie mix, fake maple syrup, instant macaroni mix, and spices all in a box. You might as well give them away. Throw out items you haven't used in the last month, and find a new home (attic, garage, basement) for rarely used items for entertaining. Make the macro items that you will use daily readily accessible. Cooking can be a joy in an organized kitchen and sheer drudgery in a poorly planned one.

Arrange all the grains in one place, then all the beans, then all the seaweeds. You can put them in pretty jars or just use the twist-ties on the bags for now. It's best if you have an area where you can hang your pots rather than trying to rummage in the cupboard to find them. Also, buy a pot cover rack or organizer to slip inside the cabinet. This makes things handier. Now with the leftover space you will have more space to put your macrobiotic foods.

Okay, you have your kitchen supplies and foods. You now may need to read Macro Mellow to further learn how to organize the kitchen and cook the foods. Also we found in helping hundreds of people get started in macrobiotics, that there came a stage where the rest of the family had to be considered, hence, the birth of Macro

Mellow (affectionately known as "What the hell to feed the rest of the family who hates macro!"). It would be best if you read that book first because (1) you do have to feed the rest of the family and if you can use your macro ingredients it will be a lot easier for you , and (2) this book and You Are What You Ate introduce you to many techniques that I will assume here that you already know. The goal of The Cure Is In The Kitchen is to show you how to get the strict healing phase started. It is built on the foundation of knowledge gained from these two forerunners.

COOKING YOUR FIRST MEAL

Following is a quick summary page to copy and put on the refrigerator. Have magnets with comical or inspiring visions or sayings handy to put up your flow sheets and recipes. This will help you organize in the beginning. Any new endeavor requires much organization and repetition. Eventually you'll only need to spend 4 hours a week or less total cooking time to keep your macrobiotic meals going. In the beginning it will be longer because you are learning and don't have it memorized.

This will organize you for your first healing phase macrobiotic meal.

DISH	STEP #	TIME
Soak aduki beans & kombu	1	3 hours
Grate & press salad	2	2 hours
Clean veggies	3	10 minutes
Roast & cook rice	4	60 minutes
Make squash drink	5	45 minutes
Cut and start nishimi root veggies	6	30 minutes
Cook squash/aduki/kombu	7	45 minutes

Boil wakame, then vegetables for miso soup	8	25 minutes
Clean up kitchen, set table	9	15 minutes
Roast salt & sesame seeds	10	5 minutes
Steam greens, bancha tea	11	5 minutes
Transfer rice, wash salad	12	5 minutes

Later on you can factor in your:

Seaweed dishes

Pickles

Special baked casseroles and desserts

Play relaxing mood music and sing to yourself. Try not to become immersed in screaming kids and T.V. soaps while cooking.

First you are going to make breakfast for tomorrow (as well as lunch to carry to work and tonight's dinner).

STEP #1

Put 1/2 cup of dark, red aduki beans (washed, sorted for stones and drained) and a 3" piece of kombu seaweed in 1 1/2 cups of clean water in a bowl to soak.

STEP #2

Grate or finely chop 1 cucumber, 1 cup radishes, 1 stalk celery, sprinkle 1 tsp. salt over it, work in with hands, put in pickle press or in bowl covered by a dish (smaller than the opening) with a heavy weight on it (cans, pan filled with 5 lb. bag of flour, etc.). Set aside for your salad to get pressed. In 1/2 hr. if you do not see water forming when you tip the bowl, remove weight or unscrew press, mix in 1/2 tsp. more salt and press again.

STEP #3

Now it's time to clean the veggies and use what you need before you put everything away. Leave the bags from the grocery on the floor if you lack counter space and pull out all of the things you're going to need so you don't do double-duty opening and closing the refrigerator. Once the fridge is nearly emptied, it's a good time to clean some space off. How much of that processed food can you give away or pitch? What items have not been used in a month? This implies they have so much preservative, they probably can't go bad and will last forever. You'll recall that if the bugs don't want them, why should you? Make it easy on yourself by having enough space to put your veggies back so you know where they are and don't have to pull everything out to find them.

Wash and discard any discolored leaves from the greens. Put them in a Ziploc bag or glass covered ceramic dish. In the same bag, put an assortment of different cleaned vegetables: a couple of carrots, a turnip, some bok choy, onions, scallions, parsley, some of the kale, a quarter of the cabbage, one large hunk of the squash that would be the equivalent to two cups. Whatever vegetables you were able to procure, use a sampling of each in the bag including your greens, above-ground and below-ground vegetables. If you need, make up 2 bags, but keep the assortment varied. The rest of the produce can get stored as it comes from the grocery or however you normally store your vegetables. The object is to have a bag with an assortment of all of your vegetables cleaned and ready at all times so that you can just pluck it from your refrigerator for quick use in any dish. You don't have to rummage through the refrigerator looking for the greens, then the root veggies, etc. and then drag out everything to make your next meal. You'll probably in reality, want to keep one bag for your greens and all the other vegetables in another bag, since the greens take up so much room and you'll be having a green dish at every meal: breakfast, lunch and dinner.

Some of us who have organic gardens, have another refri-gerator in the basement which we traded in for the freezer we had for years. Mine contains huge bags of muddy carrots, for example. I pick them right in the garden, mud and all, and put them in the bags. They last well into spring and are nearly as fresh as the day I picked them. The mud from the garden keeps them surrounded by the bugs that they have become accustomed to and I just go down and grab a week's supply and wash them off for the week or as I use them.

STEP #4

Now you'll want to cut up equal amounts, half a cup each of an onion, carrot, cabbage and a hard winter squash. Add four cups of water, a pinch of salt and begin cooking it for half an hour. After it has come to a boil, turn it down to medium heat. This will be your sweet vegetable drink which helps with hypoglycemic symptoms and helps restore mineral content of the body to help you break down and metabolize or dislodge years of accumulated fats.

STEP #5

Now measure 2 cups of brown rice, rinse it in the colander several times. Preferred is to swirl it in a bowl first and pour it back into the colander to make sure that any stones and excess dirt are removed. Then roast it in a dry, hot skillet over medium heat until it has dried and has a rather nutty aroma. Keep stirring it so that it will not burn. Meanwhile, start 3 1/2 cups of water in the pressure cooker and add a stamp-size piece of kombu seaweed. When the rice is roasted dry and has a nutty flavor, add it to the pressure cooker that already has 4 cups of water and secure the cover. When it hisses, put the flame deflector between the stove burner top and the pressure cooker, turn the heat down to the lowest setting, and set your timer for 45 minutes.

STEP #6

Now cut up 2-3 root vegetables. You might take daikon, carrot, burdock, turnip, onion, parsnip or lotus root. Choose two or three from this category (except try to avoid carrots alone with daikon or turnip. Avoid using either of those two combinations if you can help it). Cut them into 1/2 inch chunks or wedges. Add a three inch piece of kombu, also some chunks of winter squash or cabbage if you like. Or you could use pre-soaked (15 minutes) dried daikon or dried tofu. Bring to a boil and simmer for fifteen to twenty minutes. Add a few drops of shoyu, simmer for three minutes and set aside. These will be ready as your nishimi dish. Always avoid stirring things up, but let them cook naturally without a massive mixing motion. You can take a peek easily under the glass pot bottom to see how things are coming along and make sure they're not sticking to the bottom.

STEP #7

Back to the soaking beans and kombu combination. Now cut up one butternut squash into 1 1/2" large chunks. This is that long, hard, pear-shaped, pale, yellow squash. Remove stem and seeds, but do not peel if it is organic. Add it to the pot. Next add the beans and kombu that were soaking plus the water they were soaking in. Add a little more water if you need, so that it comes just to the top of the beans. Bring the pot to a boil and then reduce to moderate heat to cook for forty minutes. Do not stir or mash. Add a little water to the top if you need to, but don't overdo because when these are done, you want most of the water to have been cooked out so that it's a combination of beans and very sweet squash, but it's not a soup.

STEP #8

For miso soup, soak a three inch piece of wakami seaweed for ten minutes. Bring the water to a boil and cook over a moderate heat for 15 minutes. Add a few shredded vegetables for just one or two minutes. These could be carrots, daikon, greens (even scallions, parsley or watercress), onions, turnips; anything you might have a little piece of that is leftover. Pour a little of the water into a cup. Add a half teaspoon of miso for every cup of soup (which will be for each person). Dissolve the miso in an aliquot of soup poured into a bowl. Add it back to the soup. Let it simmer lightly for just a minute or two. Chop a little fresh scallion or parsley for garnish, and voila! You have miso soup complete with parsley or scallion garnish. It should be a thin, delicate, light tasting soup, not overly hot, not crammed with vegetables and not too salty or heavy with miso. You may make this in the morning for breakfast (presoak your wakame overnight). It is a quick soup that can be made any time of day. Try to have two bowls or two cups a day, whichever your appetite seems to want (if you are not yeast sensitive and tolerate it. If in doubt, wait a couple of weeks before you try to add miso).

STEP #9

Now in a separate pan, roast 1 level tsp. of sea salt then grind it in the suribachi. Next wash 1 cup of sesame seeds (black is preferable to white), roast them in a hot pan until they are dry and have a nutty aroma. They will burn easier than the rice so give them more attention and a little lower heat. Add them to the roasted salt. Grind those in as well and you have pure gomashio or roasted sesame seed salt. You can usually turn the grinding over to any eager kitchen helper.

STEP #10

In between when you're cooking things, clean up the kitchen, wash and put away utensils and pans, set the table and make use of the normally less productive cooking times. If you wash and put away during preparation, there is barely anything left to do when you have finished.

STEP #11

Boil some water and steam your greens in a basket after having chopped them. Steam them lightly for only 2-3 minutes. Give coarser stems a head start and add the more tender leaves later. You can also just drop them into boiling water for one minute and blanch them and retrieve them with your mesh ladle. Whatever greens are cooked, always try to rescue them when they are at the peak of their bright green color, being brighter than when you started. Avoid overcooking them so that they have lost their bright green color. For this reason, remove the lid or they will keep cooking. You want to eat them when they are actually more green than when you started out.

You could also start some water now for your bancha tea. Don't ever worry about meals being lukewarm and not piping hot when you're cooking macrobiotically. With American cooking, we eat much meat and it's laden with much fat. Fat, of course, congeals when it cools. Therefore, we need to have our meals piping hot to keep the fat liquid and good tasting. With macrobiotics, there is so little fat that the goodness and taste come from the natural sweetness of the vegetables, beans and grains themselves. So lukewarm food is perfectly acceptable. In the beginning it will be difficult anyway for you to pull together a meal that is anything other than lukewarm.

STEP #12

When the rice is finished, put a chopstick or fork under the steam release valve and let the steam out after you have removed the pot from the burner. Remove the lid once the steam has gone and with your large wooden paddle, loosen the rice from the sides and bottom of the pressure cooker. Allow the steam to rise so it minimizes the sogginess of the rice, then transfer the rice to a wooden or ceramic storage bowl and cover it loosely with one of your bamboo nori mats.

For the pressed salad, remove the aliquot that you want to use for this evening's dinner. Put it in a small bowl. Add a cup or so of water and swish it around and then drain it in a colander. All you're trying to do is remove the salt used in pressing. Now you have your fresh, pressed salad.

The following is the menu that you have prepared for dinner.

Miso soup with garnish

Rice with gomashio

Steamed greens

Aduki squash kombu

Nishimi (root vegetable) dish

Pressed salad

Bancha tea

I can't believe how fantastic you are! You have pulled together an entire macrobiotic meal on your first day, something that took me a couple of years to accomplish. We'll go into how to eat your meal in the next chapter.

-37-

Gearing Up For the Next 24 Hours

Before turning in for the evening, briefly think about breakfast, lunch and dinner for the following day. For breakfast:

1) Do you have your bag of raw washed, uncut greens (greenie bag) ready? It should be leftover from the preparation of dinner greens.

2) Is the wakame soaking in a little pot?

3) Do you have a bag of scrubbed vegetables ready from which to choose one to be grated for your miso soup?

4) Do you have your grain and condiment ready for morning porridge (leftover from dinner)?

5) Take a sheet or two of nori out for each person so that it will be ready to toast and make into a "Herb Walley" for breakfast.

In case you're wondering what a "Herb Walley" is, when I first went to the Kushi Institute, they suggested I might want to stay with Virginia and Herbert Walley in Newton, Massachusetts. Since I hate hotels with windows that do not open, and these people lived macrobiotically and would provide the meals, I was already excited about the idea. However, I had no idea at that time how wonderful it would be. This couple is truly adorable. I felt like I was reliving "On Golden Pond." Also, they were extremely organized, loving and helpful. I would recommend anyone to stay there who is visiting the Kushi Institute or Boston itself.

In 1981, Herb had cancer of the prostate diagnosed by physical exam, blood test and positive biopsy. It was recommended he have an orchiectomy and a prostatectomy (surgical removal of testicles and prostate) and go on female hormones for two years. Since this did not appeal to him, he started looking for alternatives and read Dr. Satillaro's book (Recalled by Life). In the first month he had a discharge of depression so bad he was bedridden. It took real commitment to continue. Within nine months of the macrobiotic diet, his cancer was gone, the scans were negative, the prostatic acid phosphatase was normal and his physical exam was normal. After five years of macrobiotics, his recent physical examination, again by his internist, revealed absolutely no evidence of cancer of the prostate whatsoever. This man looks much healthier and much more handsome than his seventy-seven years would suggest he should. And yet, look at all of the men who have had years of female hormones with breast development as well as radiation and chemotherapy for secondary metastases and died anyway. But, does his internist recommend the macrobiotic diet for any of his other cancer patients?

Anyway, Herb has a little invention in the morning that he uses that all of us fell in love with. After he toasts the nori sheet, he will tear it into four squares. He then takes one square and rolls it into an ice cream cone shape and drops a little fingerfull of toasted pumpkin seeds into the funnel. He then folds over the top and wraps it up into a little, bite-size package and plops it in his mouth. This is wonderful since it satisfies our need for the crunchies, and the sweetness of the pumpkin seeds overrides the seaweed taste of the nori. It's a delightful combination. Many people who do not like seaweed, like what I call the "Herb Walleys".

If you haven't yet roasted any pumpkin seeds, it's very easy. Place a cupful in a colander, wash and drain and transfer to a moderately hot frying pan. Stir them frequently so that they don't burn, until they are light golden and fully dried and toasted. If they start popping, the heat is too high. Put them in a little covered jar, and you'll have them to last the whole week. They are also great on rice and other whole grains or soft grain ("breakfast porridge or cereal"), but limit yourself to 1-2 tsp. a day.

Now back to lunch tomorrow.

1) Do you have enough greens in your green bag to steam for breakfast and lunch?

2) Will you have enough grain to pack (as well as gomashio)?

3) You can add some of the aduki squash kombu dish to your lunchbox.

4)   You can wash the salt from a tablespoon of organic sauerkraut that you buy from a health food store. If the ingredients contain anything more than organic cabbage, sea salt and spring water, don't buy it. Use that for your pickles and wash off (in the morning) a cup of your pressed salad and add that to your lunchbox.

For dinner tomorrow evening, do you need to have any beans soaking or grains soaking so that they'll be ready and cook quicker when you get home?

Now you have accomplished what it took many of us years to do. You're learning that macrobiotics can be done, it's just that the focus changes. Instead of walking in the house in the evening and wondering, "Ugh! What am I going to fix for dinner? I'm starving and I need something right away," you're going to walk in the house and wonder, "What am I fixing for breakfast, lunch, and dinner the next day?" because usually you will already have something of your macrobiotics left from a previous meal to tide you over and also to help you cut down on the time for preparation of this meal. The beans and grains can last a day or two as well as the root vegetable dishes. However, the greens should be made fresh for every meal and prepared at the very last minute as much as possible. Now this doesn't mean you'll eat the same meal for breakfast, lunch and dinner. Although you can do this in the beginning, you'll learn how to implement variety and stagger your cooking so you don't run out of everything all at once. Every meal can be a unique treat.

BREAKFAST TIME

Normally, you will not want to spend any more than fifteen or twenty minutes on breakfast. Besides, it will take far more than the preparation time to eat it and you'll be packing your lunch for the office, also.

You already know how to prepare your miso soup (wakame soaked for ten minutes or overnight, cooked for ten or fifteen minutes, simmered with a few grated vegetables for a few minutes more, with the miso added the last few minutes and simmered again.

(All miso, shoyu, tamari and salt are always simmered in with food, never added without cooking). The garnish {finely chopped or grated daikon, carrot, parsley or scallion, etc.} is then added for the top). Your Herb Walleys should be ready except for just toasting the sheets of nori on the burner (which you could do earlier, but it's so quick, there is no need). Lightly hold your nori sheets over a hot burner (like the one boiling the wakame) until they turn a pale green. It's only necessary to heat them on one side, usually the dull side. You can tear them into fours and munch on them while you are preparing the rest of the breakfast, getting your 50 chews in.

Regarding the ferments, although they must always be cooked into a dish, never cook miso or shoyu or tamari sauce in a heat higher than low simmer since heat will destroy the active enzymes.

For the soft grain (porridge), take any leftover grain, 1/2 to 1 1/2 cups, depending on your appetite, and add it to an equal amount of water. This constitutes soft rice or soft grain. Cook it for about fifteen minutes. It improves the digestibility and is very much like a porridge. You can certainly add some of your leftover root vegetables or beans to it if you like. You can finish by sprinkling on top 1/2 tsp. gomashio or roasted pumpkin seeds or any garnish.

Take one to three minutes to water saute, steam or blanch some greens. It's a good time to use "strange greens" that you would not normally use like a handful of chopped parsley or scallion tops. Add your condiment to the soft rice. Have some bancha tea if you want, and you have just prepared a full course macrobiotic breakfast. If possible, try to have greens at every meal, including breakfast. If breakfast is rushed, you could make nori rolls the night before, or you could even have your porridge ready to just heat up and skip any of the other dishes. However, after a while, you will see how quick it is to make the miso soup along with the soft grain, Herb Walleys and steamed greens that it will be no problem.

The variations are endless. Continually strive for variation in cutting and cooking styles as well as variety of foods to tantalize your palate. Avoid getting into a rut or the monotony of the same foods. You can use any vegetables in the miso soup that you have. You can use a variety of different types of misos. For the soft grain, you can use any of your grains that you have, or mix them in various combinations. While breakfast is cooking, you can put your lunch together. Later on when you are more healed, breakfast becomes even more fun because then you can have bits of apple, nuts or raisin in your grain. But for now, you're going to forego those pleasures.

You might say, "What? Soup and green vegetables for breakfast?" But when you think about it, how utterly logical. Doesn't it make a lot more sense when you're trying to heal your body to put extremely nourishing, whole foods into it rather than a boxed, processed, enriched cereal made out of sugar and bleached flours (with vitamins and minerals removed), or worse yet, doughnuts and coffee? Or worse yet, nothing? If you have a delicate piece of machinery that has to last a lifetime (your body), do you forget to oil it, or do you use any old junk oil in it? Of course not. And your body is much more precious; it has to last a lifetime.

Breakfast Checklist

Miso soup (with grated daikon)
Herb Walley (seaweed dish)
Green, steamed
Porridge
Condiment (optional)
Bancha tea or medicinal prescribed drink like kombu tea and/or sweet vegetable drink (optional)

LUNCH TIME

If you have the opportunity to cook or go home for lunch, you can appreciate now that the varieties are endless. But if, as most people do, you need to carry your lunch, make it simple for yourself. Some of the leftover grain, a bean dish (optional), some blanched greens leftover from morning, some of the root vegetable dishes, some pressed salad, the condiment and maybe a pickle. A bancha tea bag can be tossed in for your "coffee-break," or better yet, a thermos of your sweet vegetable juice or a soup.

If there's a microwave available at work, try to avoid using it since the fields from it are destructive to the energies of foods. You have undoubtedly witnessed what it does to a reheated roll. It changes the molecular structure so that the texture is unrecognizable. You're better off eating your food lukewarm. Avoid putting it in the refrigerator at work so you won't have a cold lunch.

You don't necessarily need the bean dish at lunch. One grain and one vegetable dish will certainly suffice if that's all you can handle at this time. The pickles can be anything from a tablespoon of washed sauerkraut to your own pickles that you will later learn to make. There are quick pickles that can be made within an hour, others that can be made within half a day, and others within several days, depending upon your needs, tastes and talents. For now, there are also ready-made macro pickles like daikon pickled in rice bran which you can merely slice and serve. The condiments you should probably make up at least once or twice a week so that you always have them handy.

Just remember to try to keep your proportions balanced. You can eat as much or little as you want, just watch that it's 50:50 whole grains versus vegetables. You have already seen the circle that suggests that each day's total percentage of foods should be 50-60% whole cereal grains, 25-30% vegetables and 5-10% beans and sea vegetables and 5-10% soups. Occasional uses for fish, seasonal foods, nuts, seeds, natural snacks and daily use of condiments and beverages are also recognized. Just bear in mind that this circle is for the total day, not for each meal. Roughly try to balance each meal 50-50 grains and vegetables (this includes sea vegetables, soups, beans, condiments and everything else that is not whole grain). So if, for example, you have a busy morning and only have time for your porridge you made the night before, that breakfast was 100% grain. Make sure you have a lot more vegetables for lunch and dinner that day to balance it out.

Lunch Checklist

Soup (or have at dinner instead)
Grain
Condiment
Green
Root dish
Bean dish (or have at dinner instead)

Pickle
Seaweed dish
Special prescribed drink or tea

DINNER TIME

At dinner, again you want 50% whole grain. It need not always be rice. Try millet or quinoa or mixtures like hato barley and rice, 1:3.

You can make your miso soup or a heartier soup, especially if you did not have any for lunch, as you only need it one to three times a day.

Limit the beans to 1/2 to 1 cup per day total, and some days, if you have no beans, that is perfectly fine.

Try to have at least a steamed, blanched (boiled), water sauteed vegetable or pressed salad at every meal. In other words, you definitely want at least one portion of greens at every meal, even breakfast. For the other two meals you want to try to strive for at least two vegetable dishes. At the end of the day, if you have had a total of six vegetable dishes, three of which are greens, you have done a perfect job. It won't always work out that way with your busy life, but strive for it at least half the week. If you want to have a root vegetable for breakfast as well, then you could have two vegetables at every meal, or if preferred you could have three or four vegetables for dinner and two for lunch.

Again, the pickles, the condiments and the garnishes are needed.

Take time daily, or every other day, to prepare a quarter cup of a sea vegetable dish. This could be arame which cooks pretty quickly. It could be cooked with grated onions or carrots or any vegetable that you choose and seasoned with a few drops of shoyu sauce at the last moment, simmering for a couple of minutes. An additional 1/2 tsp. per serving sprinkling of sesame seeds is good. Later you will learn to make side dishes of hijiki and incorporate more kombu into your daily cooking. Try to have a sheet or two of nori each day (if you want more, that's fine), and at least the total of a one to five inch strip of kombu each day in your various cookings. A postage stamp size of kombu for the grains is sufficient and a two or three inch piece for various sea and bean and vegetable dishes is good (portions are per person served). Later you will learn how to factor in special remedies that will be prescribed for you individually as well, like kombu tea. The sea vegetables supply you with precious minerals.

As your health improves, then the combinations, permutations and possibilities expand enormously. In the beginning however, you will not be ready for any transition foods since you will be concentrating on healing. The dinner menu might look something like this:

Millet soup

Sweet rice with aduki beans

Brown rice with barley

Nishimi root vegetable

Arame with vegetable

Pressed Salad

Steamed greens

Scallion/Miso condiment

This is one menu that we learned in the cooking courses at the Kushi Institute in the two day seminars which provide an excellent crash course for people needing to get into macrobiotics quickly. Although you can read about these things here, there is no substitute for actually seeing the preparation first hand. Variety is very important, but basic technique is tantamount.

Dinner Checklist

Soup (if none at lunch)
Grain
Condiment
Green
Bean (if none at lunch)
Nishime Root vegetable
Another vegetable dish
Sea vegetable dish
Pickle
Beverage

HEALING MEALS SKELETON

opt.= optional and not necessary every day

Breakfast

1. Medicinal drink (opt.)

2. Miso soup with garnish

3. Soft grain with condiment

4. Green, steamed

5. Tea (opt.)

Lunch

1. Grain with condiment

2. Green (steamed, boiled, or water sauteed, etc.)

3. Pressed Salad (opt.)

4. Nishimi (root vegetable)

5. Bean dish (opt.)

6. Pickles, salt washed off (opt.)

7. Tea (opt.)

Dinner

1. Medicinal drink (opt.)

2. Soup with raw garnish

3. Pickles (opt.)

4. Grain

5. Green

6. Bean Dish (opt.)

7. Seaweed dish (opt.)

8. Vegetable (opt.)

9. Tea (opt.)

Eventually you will get to a point where you can handle having all of these things at most meals, but in the beginning remember, guilt is not a healthy emotion. So don't make yourself guilt-ridden by not attaining perfection. Some days you will just not feel like cooking or you will just not feel like eating. So just remember to balance yourself 50-50 with grains and greens and if you can throw in a few root vegetables, all the better. Eventually attempt to get six vegetable dishes a day, preferably two at each meal or three twice a day. Every day have some boiled, steamed, pressed or water sauteed greens; three dishes of them. Also try to have 2-3 servings of any one or more of the following each day; but for each item, have it only two or three times a week if you prefer.

Vegetable dishes aside from greens and pressed salad

1. Nishimi (root vegetables)

2. Squash-Aduki-Kombu

3. Dried daikon/kombu

4. Dried tofu stew

5. Roots with tops

6. Water Sauteed vegetables

And to avoid folic acid deficiency, have at least each of any two daily, 1-3 tbsp.: raw garnish (chives, scallions, parsley, watercress), 1/2 to 2 cups pressed salad, 1/2 to 2 cups stir-fry or blanched vegetables with minimum cooking time (cooking destroys folic acid).

To avoid B12 deficiency, one serving of fish a month will do.

Summary of the average guidelines for daily food servings:

Whole grain	50% of day, preferably 50% of each meal
Greens	3 times a day
Vegetable dishes	3 times a day (any of the 6 styles above)
Beans	0-2 servings, maximum 15% of total day
Sea vegetable	1 to 2 nori sheets, 1/4 to 1/2 cup sea vegetable side dish like arame or hijiki, a 3" to 6" strip of wakame (it can be cooked with sweet squash and onions and "lost", for example), and 1 to 6" kombu in grains, beans or soups. This is the average total for sea vegetables per day per person.
Condiments	Keep minimal, 1 to 2 tsp. miso a day total, and 1/2 tsp. shoyu, total.
Seeds	Maximum 1 tbsp. per day total for gomashio and pumpkin each. No sunflower yet.
Pickles	1-3 tsp., 1-2 times a day

| Beverages | 0-5 times a day, as needed |
| Medicinal | As prescribed. |

Try to never have a grain without condiment and never have a soup without garnish. It doesn't have to be much. Grate a teaspoon finely of any vegetable. Keep the condiments down to one to three teaspoons a day of gomashio, for example, and one to three teaspoons a day of the pumpkin seeds. Try to keep the meals to two or three times a day and pretty regular. You can eat as much as you want provided the proportions are correct and the chewing is thorough until the food is liquid. Avoid eating for approximately three hours before sleeping.

A FOUR DAY PLAN

Now we'll try to sort out the different variety of foods and how you might spread them out over four days.

GRAINS

	Breakfast	Lunch & Dinner
Day 1	Soft Grain	Organic Brown Rice
Day 2	"	Rice with 30% Millet
Day 3	"	Rice with 30% Barley
Day 4	"	Rice with 15% Chick Peas

Don't forget, 50% of each meal and at least 50% of the day should be a whole grain. You certainly can have all sorts of other varieties. One day for breakfast you may want 50-50 amaranth and teff, 1/2 cup of each with 2 cups water and in 15 minutes you have a deliciously new breakfast. Or use the same formula for buckwheat and quinoa (if buckwheat is allowed when you have your consultation), or quinoa and millet. There are many interesting and unusual combinations that you can create. For grain allergies, see the chapter on allergies.

BEANS (You may prefer to make 2-3 days' worth at a time to economize on cooking time)

Day 1-3 Black soy beans

Day 2-6 Aduki, squash, kombu dish

Day 3-9 Lentil Soup

Day 4-12 Chick peas (they could be in the rice if preferred, or in a salad or soup)

Remember 10-15% of the total daily food should be beans. That means that you can have anywhere from 0-1 cup of beans maximum a day. You don't necessarily have to have beans every day, and you could eat the same one for a couple of days, or dress it up with a dash of tamari, grated carrot and onion or mash it into a spread on the second day. Another day they could be added to a soup, blended or not.

GREENS

	Breakfast	Lunch	Dinner
Day 1	Pressed (because it can be pre-made)	Boiled	Blanched or steamed
Day 2	"	Carrot/ cabbage rolls	"
Day 3	Blanched or steamed	"	Pressed

Day 4   "   Boiled   "

This is just an example, as there are many other combinations that you can do with your greens, but just be sure you have them 3 times a day and don't cook all vegetables in the same style. For example, you can make carrot/cabbage rolls for the lunchbox and endless other combinations. The reason for cooking style variation is easy: different styles result in different nutrient and energy contents of the food as well as digestibility.

THE OTHER VEGETABLES

	Breakfast	Lunch	Dinner
Day 1	Nishimi	Roots w/leaves	Sauteed
Day 2	Roots w/leaves	Dried tofu	Kinpira
Day 3	Kinpira	Dried tofu	Sauteed
Day 4	Dried daikon	Dried daikon	Nishimi

Remember you want 3 other vegetable dishes a day and you only want a couple a week each of the nishimi, dried daikon, dried tofu, kinpira, roots with leaves or sauteed vegetables. Any combination of the vegetables that you are allowed is fine. All you are trying to do is vary the style of cutting, the length of cooking and the style of cooking, because different nutrients are preserved better with different styles. You're trying to get a good combination of many styles so that you can get the maximum nutrition. People have tried to clear cancers with vitamin pills and all sorts of diets, and macrobiotics has the best track record that I have seen, so it behooves us to not modify it. Rather it makes more sense for severe cases to stick to what we have observed works. Probably one reason it does is because it provides maximum nutrition from the foods themselves, while simultaneously optimizing the body's assimilation of them.

SEA VEGETABLES (Example of use)

	Breakfast	Lunch	Dinner
Day 1	Nori, 1 to 2 sheets. Wakame 2 to 3" piece in miso soup	1 to 2" piece kombu for every cup of rice or grain cooked	1/4 to 1/2 cup arame with sesame seeds as a side dish, wakame in miso soup
Day 2	"	"	1/4 to 1/2 cup hijiki as a side dish, wakame in soup, root dish or squash
Day 3	"	Green nori flakes condiment	1/2 cup arame/squash dish, wakame in miso soup
Day 4	"	"	Hiziki with onion and shoyu

You'll also be able to have kombu tea and various medicinal, prescribed remedies with kombu. You can make kombu/carrot rolls. Once or twice a week you could have sea palm, and every 1-2 weeks agar-agar (kanten, usually used as a thickener in desserts), kelp, Irish moss or mekabu. There are many ways to get the priceless minerals in you via the sea vegetables.

For example, one delicious way to use wakame is to soak a 6" strip snipped into 1/4" pieces. Cook with 1-2 cups chunked hard sweet winter squash and one chopped large, sweet onion for 40 minutes. Leave squash skins on if organic and not waxed. The sweetness of the squash masks the seaweed and satiates sweet cravings as well. If you really hate seaweed, cook it in broccoli or squash soup and run it through a blender.

Another way to "lose" it is cook a 4" piece of kombu with 1/2 cup marrow beans for 2 hours. Finely diced carrot and onion can be added for the last 20 minutes. The kombu disintegrates and mixes with the marrow bean exudate, making a great hearty soup.

PICKLES (wash off the salt from all of them for the first month, since part of the cause of most conditions is too much salt and hardening of accumulated fats)

One pickle dish (1-3 tsp.) a day is sufficient, two are OK.

Day 1- Sauerkraut (salt rinsed off)

Day 2- Quick Tamari Pickles

Day 3- Sauerkraut (salt rinsed off)

Day 4- Quick tamari pickles

CONDIMENTS These should be on the table at all times for flavoring. Try to keep the gomashio to 1 tsp. a day for each of 3 meals (total 3 tsp. or 1 tbsp. a day) or a total of 1 cup a week. The same goes for pumpkin seeds.

	Breakfast	Lunch	Dinner
Day 1	1-2 tsp. pumpkin seeds	1 tsp. gomashio	1/4 tsp. tekka
Day 2	"	shiso leaf powder	kombu or sea weed powder

-54-

Day 3	"	"	1/4 tsp. tekka
Day 4	"	umeboshi plum	kombu or seaweed powder

Other condiments include green nori flakes, scallions or parsley. Kombu or shiso leaf powder is made by roasting in a dry skillet until dark and crisp, then grinding it into a powder. They can be mixed 2:1 with sesame or umeboshi. Later on a few drops of brown rice vinegar, umeboshi vinegar, lime or lemon juice can add zest. For now, use ginger juice.

Remember, your food requirements will change (with your consultations) as your condition changes. They will also change with the seasons and with the environment. Rules are to be broken. But in general, try to be strict the first few months. Remember, one indiscretion can erase all of the good you have done. One day a week you can have foods that are on the occasional list, but avoid the foods on the forbidden list.

Vary the ingredients. Vary the cutting and cooking techniques. For example, one day you could dry roast your grain in a skillet before you pressure cook it. Or you can presoak your grain before you cook it. You can cook it in a pressure cooker or you can boil it. You can heat it slowly, or heat it fast. You can cook it with a stamp size piece of kombu for each cup of grain, or with a pinch of good quality sea salt. You can use other seaweeds, beans, chestnuts and mixtures of other grains. The quality of the water and the heat (gas vs. electric), salt and the grain (organic, fresh, freshly hulled) all make a difference. For example, the best rice I ever had in my life was at the Kushi Institute in the Berkshires. I found the secret was that they had a milling machine in the basement that is used to hull the rice weekly. As we have more people taking advantage of a macrobiotic way of life, there will be more demand and then more availability of such things as freshly hulled rice.

As you are beginning to appreciate, the healing phase is so different from how you now cook, that you'll need to read this book first to get set up, and then go over it once a month a few more times to be sure you are doing it correctly. It will make more sense after you have tried a few meals.

COOKING INSTRUCTIONS FROM SOUP TO SEEDS

GRAINS

For grains, usually 1 1/2 to 2 cups of water are needed for every cup of brown rice, depending on the amount of water pre-scribed for you. In the beginning, start with a 1:2 ratio until your consultation at the end of 1 month. Some grains, such as millet, require even more water and oftentimes a 1:2 1/2 or even 1:3 ratio. And of course, when mixed together, or when grains and beans are mixed, a little extra water will be necessary. Cooking of grains can also be done after pre-roasting them to enhance the flavor. Vary using an inch piece of kombu per cup of rice or a pinch of sea salt.

BASIC MISO SOUP

Basic miso soup: Basically, miso soup consists of a sea vegetable cooked for 15 minutes, usually wakame, and then vege-tables added that are finely grated that will only take a few minutes to cook. A small amount of miso, such as 1/2 tsp. to 1 tsp. per 1 cup of broth, a cup being one person's portion, is dissolved in a small bowl where some of the soup has been poured. Then all of this is added back to the soup and simmered (do not boil) 1-2 minutes. A small garnish (1 tbsp. or less) such as finely chopped parsley, grated carrot, or minced scallions, should be used in every dish. The types of beans, grains, and vegetables can vary every day. A small piece of carrot and daikon that were left over in your veggie bag, could be the soup one morning. Another day it could have a small amount of greens in it. Another day it could be some squash and turnip. The combinations are endless.

Don't forget to use the tops of carrots in your soups when you have them in the summer from your garden. Also, in the springtime, forage for dandelion greens and cook the greens as well as the roots. Try to get as much variety as possible. I like to forage for wild watercress along the stream banks.

VEGETABLES

Vegetables that you can have <u>daily</u> include carrots, collards, dandelion, kale, leeks, mustard greens, parsley, watercress, bok choy and Chinese cabbage, acorn squash, broccoli, Brussel sprouts, butternut squash, buttercup squash, cabbage, cauliflower, Hubbard squash, hokaido, pump-kin, onion, red cabbage, rutabaga, turnip, burdock, carrot, daikon, dandelion root, lotus root, parsnips, radish.

Vegetables that you should limit to <u>once or twice a week</u> include: celery, chives, cucumber, endive, escarole, green beans, green peas, iceberg lettuce, Jerusalem artichokes, kohlrabi, lambs quarters (this grows as a weed in my organic garden and it probably does in yours as well. Learn how to recognize it so that you can eat it), corn, shitake mushrooms, patty pan squash, Romaine lettuce, salsify, snap beans, snow peas, sprouts, summer squash, wax beans.

Avoid these vegetables for now: tomatos, potatoes, peppers, eggplant, spinach, asparagus, garlic, okra and vegetables not included in above lists.

NISHIMI DISHES (Waterless Cooking)

Basically, this is a root dish and should be had about three times a week at least. It takes about 20 minutes to cook and uses roots and round vegetables, any combination is fine. Normally, there is a 3" piece of kombu, cut into 1" squares, and slices or chunks of vegetables are used, usually 2 or 3 vegetables are included. A pinch of sea salt or tamari can be added during the last few minutes of cooking. If the water evaporates too quickly, more can be added. Remember to lower the flame for the last few minutes once you have added tamari. This dish can be eaten for several days. Common combinations would be:

1. Carrot, burdock and kombu

2. Burdock, lotus root and kombu

3. Carrot, parsnip and kombu

4. Squash, onion and kombu

5. Turnip, shitake mushroom and kombu

But nearly any combination is fine.

SQUASH/ADUKI/KOMBU

The squash, aduki bean and kombu dish should also be eaten 1-3 times a week, or even 5 times if someone has diabetes or high blood pressure. Basically, 1/2 cup of aduki beans is soaked with a 1" piece of kombu for 2-5 hours. 60% squash is used. Skins are left on and it is chopped fine, after removing stem and seeds. Onions could be used, carrots or parsnips if squash is not available. The squash and kombu are put in the pan first, the presoaked aduki beans and their water are poured in on top. If extra water is needed to bring it up to the level of the beans, this should be done. After 20 minutes, add a few pinches of sea salt, more water to bring the level to the top of the beans, cover and cook for another 10-15 minutes, or until all of the water has cooked down. This is a very crucial point since you want it to be soft and waterless, but not burned. Do not stir or it will become mushy.

DRIED DAIKON

Dried daikon with kombu is a dish that can be enjoyed as 1/2-1 cup servings 2-3 times a week. A 3" piece of kombu is soaked and then sliced. Dried daikon is likewise soaked and sliced. If it's dark, discard the soaking water. If it's yellow, keep it. Add just enough water to cover the daikon. Other vegetables can be added, especially onion and carrot if you don't care for the taste of dried daikon alone. This is cooked for 30-40 minutes until everything is tender. Other root or above ground veggies may be added for flavor.

ROOT WITH LEAVES

Another dish that is recommended 3 times a week is roots with leaves. This can be daikon with daikon leaves, carrots with carrot tops, or turnips and turnip greens, or dandelion roots with their leaves. Chop them and cook for about 10 minutes in water, depending on size and shape you prepared. A pinch of sea salt or shoyu afterwards is used and lightly simmered in. You can't always get these ingredients, but use them when available.

BOILED SALAD

Boiled salad should be used daily. When you boil multiple vegetables, only do one at a time, starting with the one with the most light and sweet flavor first so that you don't have the stronger flavors contaminating your milder tasting vegetables. Never add the vegetables to the cold water, but bring it to a boil first, to minimize cooking time. Once the water is boiling, add a pinch of sea salt and the vegetables, allowing them to boil for one minute. Then quickly remove them with your mesh ladle or strainer. Repeat the above for each vegetable. They should be crispy and fresh, not limp and dead colored. If your consultation permits, a few drops of umeboshi vinegar or brown rice vinegar can be added to this.

PRESSED SALAD

Pressed salad 1/2 cup once or twice a day minimum should be on everyone's list. Wash and finely slice the vegetables. Use your Mac knife or fine grater for this. Here is where you can use your radishes, cabbages, celery, cucumbers, carrots, daikon and vegetable leaves. Sprinkle 1/2 tsp. of sea salt per cup of chopped vegetables and use both hands to firmly mash and crunch as though you were kneading bread for just a few minutes. Try to break down the cellulose and mix the salt in with these. Then put on the pressure and let it sit for one or more hours. You can take out portions and wash them off or after 2-5 hours, add water and mix with your hands, drain off the water and salt, putting the rest of it in the refrigerator for use as you need (it lasts better if you wash off the salt the last minute before serving). Try to bring it to room temperature before you eat it. Depending on your condition, you might need more, but start with 2-3 times a week, one portion being about 1/2-1 cup.

Do not have any raw salads at this point in time; this means have only cooked or pressed (pickled) salads where some of the work of digestion has already been done before eating as these processes begin to break down the cellulose without sacrificing many nutrients.

SALAD DRESSINGS

Some conditions will permit salad dressing. If yours will, the following are some of the ideas that you can use.

1. One umeboshi plum mashed in a cup of water.

2. A few drops of rice wine vinegar.

3. A few drops of miso or shoyu with lemon juice or ginger juice.

4. Diluted miso in warm water, heated for a few minutes. A mashed umeboshi plum may be added to this. But limit your total plums to 1 or 2 a day, and 2 a day only a few times a week.

5. Blend sweet vegetable juice, tamari or miso or soy, ginger, sesame or pumpkin seeds.

6. Ginger, tamari and kuzu in kombu broth.

7. Blend 1/2 cup soft tofu with 1 minced, pitted umeboshi (apricot) and 3 tsp. fresh dill (optional) and/or a few drops of lemon or lime juice. Minimum 3 tsp. twice a week.

GREENS

For greens with tough center stems, cut out the stems and finely chop these and cook in a small amount of water for 2-3 minutes. Then coarse chop and add the remaining greens themselves for another minute or two. Or roll the leaves up like a cigar and finely slice into ribbons. Make sure that whenever you cook boiled salad (blanched vegetables) or the steamed green dish, that the vegetables are bright green and not dull green. If they are not fresh and bright, you have cooked them too long and some nutrients are destroyed, like folic acid.

SAUTEED VEGETABLES will be prepared with water in the healing phase and not with oil at this point. It's similar to the steamed greens. You should have one or the other or both every day.

SEA VEGETABLES

Sea vegetables should be used daily. One or two sheets of nori, a 3" strip of wakame in the miso soup daily, kombu daily in beans and other vegetable dishes as well as in your grain. Arame and hijiki, 1/2 cup can be had daily.

Once or twice a week you could have sea palm which is more easily tolerated by many or agar-agar (also called kanten and usually used in desserts as a thickener), kelp or Irish moss or mekabu. For sea palm, merely add 4-6 stalks (about 6" long) to any vegetable dish. You may need to presoak and precook it so the veggies do not get overcooked.

KINPIRA

Kinpira is a root dish, usually of burdock and carrot, shaved or cut into small matchsticks and sauteed in a skillet with the smallest amount of water and a pinch of sea salt or tamari. Sometimes a few drops of ginger juice can be used. When you can have oil at a later stage, then oil is used. The pan is lightly brushed with 1/2 tsp. of dark, unrefined sesame oil, then saute for a few minutes, then lightly cover the bottom of the skillet with water and cook for 20 minutes more. Onions, turnips or lotus root can be used or substituted. At the very end of cooking, a few drops of shoyu can be added and simmered in until all the water is cooked away. Then at the end, a few drops of grated ginger juice is added. Merely grate the ginger and put it either in a little tea strainer or squeeze it in your fingertips so that the juice drops on the vegetables.

In summary, for kinpira, substitute water for the oil. Use shaved burdock and carrot and sometimes lotus root. Cook gently for 40 minutes with minimum of water. Add a few drops of freshly grated and squeezed ginger juice at end with soy. Eat 3 times a week.

DRIED TOFU

Dried tofu with vegetable stew is another dish that can be eaten 2-3 times a week. Or dried lotus root can be substituted. Again a 3" piece of kombu is soaked and boiled for a few minutes in a couple cups of water. Sliced dried tofu or daikon, burdock, carrot or lotus root can be added. You can add other vegetables. This is cooked for 15 minutes. A few drops of shoyu may be added at the end. Cabbage, onions, Brussel sprouts or squash can be added in the last half of cooking. Do not use fresh tofu in the beginning for the healing phase.

WATER SAUTEED VEGETABLES

This is a different and quicker way to prepare vegetable mixtures. Merely use minimal water and keep adding more as needed. Just use the least you can get away with in order to cook the vegetables and have no liquid left.

BEANS

Aduki beans, chick peas, lentils (green, brown) and black soy beans are to be used regularly and one of them should be eaten every or every other day.

Black eyed peas, turtle beans, great Northern beans, marrow beans, kidney beans, lima beans, mung beans, navy beans, pinto beans, soy beans, split peas and whole dried peas are only for once a week. Any vegetables can be combined with these beans: carrot, onion and squash, chestnuts and kombu are the most common and all of them could be used at once.

CONDIMENTS

Scallion/miso condiment is good for the liver, 1 tsp. daily. Cook 1 cup chopped scallions with a few drops of sesame oil for 5 minutes, then add equal water and ume vinegar to make a paste. Simmer in 1 tsp. miso.

Kombu powder is made by roasting the sea-weed in a dry skillet until it is dark and crisp and then ground into a fine powder. It can also be mixed with toasted sesame seeds in a ratio of 2 parts seaweed to 1 part sesame. Other combinations can be 2 parts of a roasted ground sea-weed, 1 part sesame seeds and 1 part roasted umeboshi plum.

When making gomashio, roast the salt first and grind it in the suribachi. Next, wash the seeds to clean them; floating ones are usually dead and do not have any seed in them, so skim them off and discard. Then dry roast the rest in the skillet while you are grinding the salt. It's a good time to do your affirmations and meditations. If there's no aroma from the seeds, they're too old. After they are all browned (be sure to keep heat just below the point where they are popping), grind them in with the roasted, ground salt. A cup should last all week.

PICKLES

Regular use pickles can include organic sauerkraut. Be sure to wash off the salt. Or you can make quick tamari pickles. Slice any root or round vegetables. Cover with a mixture of 50/50 water and tamari. After 2 hours, remove the vegetables from the liquid and serve. If it's too salty, rinse these off.

Umeboshi pickles can be made by putting 1/2 dozen umeboshi plums in a large jar with 2 quarts of water. Shake and let sit for a few hours. Then place sliced vegetables in here and put the jar in a dark, cool place. They can be served in 4-5 days. See other cookbooks like Macro Mellow for other pickle recipes, but these will get you through the first few months.

When doing nishimi or root dishes, if you are using a small amount of sauerkraut for flavor, then you don't need soy, grated ginger or salt.

SEASONINGS

Basic seasonings for regular use would be barley miso (mugi

miso) and soy bean miso (hatcho), shoyu sauce and unrefined white sea salt. Ginger, horseradish and vinegars are more for occasional use (once a week). Some types of tamari contain mirin, an alcohol, and should be avoided for now or used occasionally and sparingly.

TEAS

Regular use teas would be bancha twig or stem teas or roasted barley tea or roasted brown rice tea, with spring water or well water.

SPECIAL DISHES

FISH AND CARROTS

Fish and carrots are good for vitality and people who are extremely ill. Chop the entire fish (that has already been scalded and gutted) including the head into 2-3" slices. The eyes may be removed if you wish. Chop an equal amount of carrot into thinly shaved slices. Put it in a pressure cooker with 1 cup of bancha twigs tied in cheesecloth. Add enough water to cover the fish and pressure cook for 1 1/2 hours. Add miso to taste as you would for regular miso soup and a small amount of grated ginger. Simmer for 5 minutes. Strain. Garnish with scallions.

SWEET RICE AND ADUKI BEANS

One variation that is popular is sweet rice and aduki beans. Wash 1/4 cup aduki beans and boil them in 1 cup water for 15 minutes. If they boil too long, the color will be lost. In the meantime, wash 1 1/2 cups organic rice, short grain brown, and 1/2 cup sweet rice and put with 3 1/2 cups of spring water plus the beans and the bean water. Add 3 pinches of sea salt and pressure cook. After the heat has come up, reduce it to low and add a flame deflector and pressure cook for 15 minutes. Bring the pressure down by releasing the gauge as usual and let sit 4-5 minutes and loosen from the pot as usual.

MILLET SOUP WITH VEGETABLES

Wash 1/2 cup of millet and dry roast it in a frying pan. Soak 1/2" piece of kombu in cold water and bring to a boil. Start adding 1/2 cup finely diced celery, 1/2 cup sliced onions, 1 cup finely cubed but not peeled butternut or buttercup squash, then the roasted millet and 4 cups spring water. If you have any soup stock or leftover vegetable juice from boiling, this will add an even better flavor. After the millet has become soft, put over medium heat. Cook millet and vegetables on low for 30-40 minutes. Mix in 1 tbsp. miso, pureeing it first in a separate dish with a little of the broth as usual. Simmer 3-5 minutes. Garnish the served soup with nori (cut into small strips) or parsley or scallions.

MILLET SOUP SUMMARIZED

Millet soup is higher in protein than brown rice, but not as balanced, so it's not a central grain but a side grain. Use a leek, celery, squash and kombu broth. Roast the millet before adding to the top. Simmer in salt or miso towards the end.

The principle is to layer the onions, celery, squash then roasted millet for the millet sweet vegetable soup. Then the sweetness of the veggies rises into the grain.

SOUP OF A THOUSAND CHEWS

Boil in 3 c. of water, 2 stalks of broccoli, a diced onion, a diced stalk of celery and a 3" piece of wakame for 30 minutes. Blend. Simmer in 1 c. cooked lentils and 1 tsp. shoyu. Float a thin slice of lemon on the top. The lentils in the soup remind the person to chew.

ARAME/ONIONS/CARROTS

One way to fix seaweed would be arame with onions and parsnips or carrots. Place one cup of dried arame in a pot and quickly rinse it twice and drain. Then let it soak for 5 min. and slice it. It does not have to be soaked as long as hiziki and should not be since it has been sliced or shredded and nutrients can be lost. Place 1/2 cup of spring water in a skillet. Layer in 1 cup sliced onion and 1 cup parsnips sliced into matchsticks. Set the arame on top of the vegetables with just enough water to cover the vegetables but not the arame. Add 1/2 tsp. shoyu. Bring to a boil. Reduce the flame to medium low and cook for 35 minutes. Add enough shoyu for taste. Cook the liquid until completely reduced and serve.

MISO CONDIMENT

Wash 1 cup scallions, thinly sliced including the roots. Layer roots then scallions in an oiled frying pan with 2 tsp. unrefined dark sesame oil. Add 1 tsp. miso that has been softened in 2 tbsp. water. Cover and simmer for 5 minutes. 2 tsp. roasted and mashed sesame seeds may be substituted for the oil for those who cannot yet have oil. Just a tsp. a day of this is all that is used (as with any condiment).

SWEET VEGETABLE DRINK

For sweet vegetable drink, chop finely 1/2 cup each of onions, carrots, cabbage, and sweet winter squash with skins. Add 4-6 cups boiling water and allow to boil 2-3 minutes. Reduce flame, cover and simmer for 20 minutes. Strain out the vegetables which can then be used in soups or stews if you like. Drink broth hot or warm or at room temperature. Have 1-3 cups a day. It may be refrigerated but remember to heat it before ingesting.

Some of the following may be prescribed and the directions for making them are included.

Ume-sho-bancha- Place 1/2 to 1 umeboshi plum in a tea cup with 1/2 to 1 tsp. of shoyu. Pour in hot bancha tea. Stir well, drink hot.

Ume-sho-kuzu- Dilute 1 heaping tsp. kuzu with 2 tsp. water. Add 1 cup water and 1/2 to 1 umeboshi plum. Bring to a boil, stirring constantly. Reduce flame and simmer until translucent. Add 1/2 tsp. shoyu. Simmer 1/2 minute longer. Drink while it's hot.

Ume-sho-kuzu with ginger is the above recipe with 1/8 tsp. fresh grated ginger juice added with the shoyu.

Mu tea comes in 2 forms, Mu-8 and Mu-16, and is available at macrobiotic stores.

Carrot daikon drink, grate 1 tbsp. each of carrot and daikon. Add 2 cups water. Boil 5 minutes with a pinch of sea salt or 5-10 drops tamari. One third of a sheet of nori may be added or 1/2 umeboshi plum cooked in with the vegetables.

Aduki bean tea- Put 1 cup of beans in a pot. Add 4 times more water and an 8" strip of kombu. Boil. Reduce flame. Simmer 45 minutes or 1 hour. Strain out the beans and drink the liquid, 1 cup per day.

Shiitake mushroom tea is 1 cup water and 1 shiitake mushroom in a saucepan. Boil. Reduce heat and simmer 15 minutes. Add a drop of shoyu and drink hot.

Kombu shiitake tea- Add a 3" strip of kombu and 1 shiitake mushroom to 4 cups water. Boil. Reduce flame. Simmer 20 minutes. Drink 1/2 to 1 cup per day as prescribed.

Ginger compress- Grate enough fresh ginger to equal the size of a baseball. Place inside of a cotton cloth or sack and tie. Bring 1 gallon water to a boil. Reduce flame to low and squeeze the ginger juice from the sack into the water by wrapping sack around a wooden spoon. Place the sack in the pot and let it simmer 5 minutes.

Hanging on to the ends, dip the middle section of a towel into the ginger water. Twist the ends so that it wrings the middle without having to touch it. It's too hot and you'll get burned. Place the towel, after it has cooled slightly, on the person's skin. Always test it carefully to be sure it will not burn him. Do not press it hard as it will still be too warm and can burn. As it cools you can press down. Be sure the other areas of the body are comfortably warm. Never use this for a cancerous condition. As it cools, put it back in the water. Wring it out again and carefully apply it. Never reuse the water, but discard it after each session.

FORGET IT! THIS DIET IS TOO COMPLICATED

Don't panic. So you don't have dried daikon, dried tofu, or

daikon roots and leaves. You will be doing great just by eating fresh vegetables, whole grains and your sea vegetables. With time those other items will appear as you grow more macrobiotic. In the meantime, just do what you can with what is available and keep reading and learning. That will be enough for most.

THE HEALING DIET IN A NUTSHELL

So many people have said, "Just tell me the whole diet in a nutshell." As you can see, it's complicated. But when you've practiced and learned it and start expanding your repertoire, it's a piece of cake (couscous cake, of course). And obviously there are a great many individual variations. But if we had to synopsize the healing diet that I have witnessed to benefit the most people, below is an example of what each day would be like. Keep the total daily and meal proportions 50:50 (grain:veggies).

ARISE	Skin brushing
	Singing
	Yoga, or meditation
BREAKFAST (5 items)	Nori/pumpkin seeds
	Soft grain/gomashio
	Miso soup
	Green, steamed
	Daikon tea
SNACK	Sweet vegetable drink
	Affirmations or
	visualizations
LUNCH (7 items)	Soup
	Grain
	Pickle
	Sea vegetable
	Green
	Other vegetable
	Root dish
	Kombu tea

SNACK	Sweet vegetable drink Singing, laughter
DINNER (9 items)	Soup w/garnish Bean Grain w/condiment Pickle Sea Vegetable Green Other vegetable (opt.) Root dish Ume/sho/kuzu
RETIRE	Body scrub Meditate and/or compresses Foot soak

Naturally, if one is very sick, he needs a full-time person to cook, do compresses, massages, stimulate laughing and singing, and perhaps reading to him.

If he is not that sick, he may need to stop work to devote all his energies to healing.

If he is like most of us, he must work and dovetail the above in an already overloaded schedule of someone who is so chronically exhausted and unwell that they can barely do what they have to. But probably that schedule had something to do with why we got so sick in the first place. So getting organized may mean cutting out something. Eventually you'll be so well you'll need less sleep and will have the time to pull it all off. Bear in mind if your top priority is not that of getting well this year, then you might reconsider doing this at all. If you're not that committed to getting more well this year than you have ever been in your life, and are going to moan and groan, and make everyone around you miserable, then why do it?

I know macro is tough the first two years. It's very antisocial for starters. (1) You can't go out and eat with people (until you get organized enough to take your own food in the beginning). (2) If you do eat with them you're so busy chewing 50-100 times you can't talk with them. (3) You can't do anything with them because you're too busy cooking and tending your garden. But when you get organized and get a group of friends who are macro, it actually becomes fun. And eventually when you feel what real vibrant health is all about, it becomes your chosen way of life. And when you are well, you can eat any way you choose.

Remember, you are eating as though your life depended upon it. Therefore, each mouthful is as nutritious as possible. It is planned maximal nourishment.

Now, back to the master plan. Remember variety of dishes, variety of cooking styles and variety of ingredients is tantamount to success. Variety is important to avoid boredom and to get maximal nutrition.

So for breakfast, you could have nori daily or use other seaweeds. The grain can be whatever is left, or you can cook it fresh. The miso is a basic wakame 3" strip cooked 10-15 minutes, grated vegetable cooked another minute and miso simmered in 2 minutes, served with a garnish. The green can be a strange one like scallion tops, parsley, watercress, or your old bok choy, collards, cabbage or kale. The daikon tea could be a cabbage tea, green juice, or kombu tea, or ume/sho/kuzu, or one of your prescribed medicinal teas.

The snack is any vegetable drink. Why drink water when you can get extra minerals and vitamins from greens or other vegetables?

For lunch, you need not have soup if you have it for breakfast and dinner. This soup could be a hearty stew-type with large chunks of vegetables and kuzu. Or it could be a puree of many vegetables, or broccoli and onion. Or you may want a very light miso soup with less than 1/4 cup of finely grated vegetable. Start learning to listen to your body. The possibilities are infinite. For those who do not like vegetables or seaweeds, soups can be pureed in a blender to hide many things. Then the right shoyu or miso, or garnish can make a world's difference. Finely chopped scallions, grated carrot, a twist of lemon or a squeeze of grated ginger can provide the dash and freshness you crave. The quality of the stock is a big factor in taste. And a little cooked blended or pureed oatmeal or other grain can give it a creamy texture as heavy cream used to.

Snack time is again a good time for any medicinal drink or remedy, compresses, affirmations or visualizations, singing and laughter.

Dinner does not need soup if you had 2 already that day. The beans are, you recall 15% of the total day. So you can have a fairly large amount to tide you through the night. Later on when you can have fish, it would replace the beans, since it is a more complete protein. The grain, greens, other vegetable dishes and root vegetable dishes are limitless. Just meticulously avoid a monotonous rut. Learn a new dish each week at least to build your repertoire.

The pickles are just a tablespoon, the garnish and condiments like gomashio or seaweed powders or tekka are kept under a teaspoon per meal and in some cases, under a tsp. per day.

And before retiring, do your scrubs and prescribed compresses. Meditation, singing, laughter, reading, catch-up cooking are all possible here, too.

So basically, if you have grains, greens, roots and sea vegetables, condiments and garnish at every meal, plus factor in root and other vegetable dishes for lunch and dinner, plus one soup and one bean dish for either or both of these, you'll be doing great. And for dinner, add a relaxing drink like green juice, sweet vegetable juices, kombu tea or ume/sho/kuzu or bancha.

So 5 items for breakfast, 7 for lunch and 9 for dinner is a rough guide. But if you prefer they can be more evenly averaged out to 7 items a meal. Realistically, every other day you may only be able to manage grain and green or you may not want so much food. If you can manage the elaborate meals even half of the week, you are doing great. The rest of the time, simple rice, steamed greens, water sauteed vegetables and a wakame/miso soup may be all you can handle. That's fine.

CHAPTER 3

CRUSHING CRAVINGS

Do you want to lose that urge to kill when someone gets between you and your favorite food? Do you want to stop being obsessed with where your next food fix will come from? Would you like to have days free of preoccupation with food so you could concentrate on more important things than when you'll get your next coke, coffee or goodie? Then first you need to understand why you have cravings.

We rarely see animals in the wild walking on crutches or sucking down Darvons. That's because they live by instinct. If they are thirsty, they drink. If they are sick they fast or change their nests. But we have lost many of our protective instincts. If we are thirsty it is usually because we need to balance too much salt, or we drink to satiate a sweet craving, or we drink to wake up or drink to relax. We rarely live by instinct, because it has been submerged by our addictions.

Now say an animal has been grazing in an area where the soil is lacking a particular mineral. The animal will forage to replace that mineral. But what happens to man when he lacks a specific nutrient? He also forages: in a refrigerator stocked with coke and ice cream! He is driven to find that something that makes him feel normal. But since we are surrounded by a myriad of processed foods, we often make an improper choice, and the craving never gets cured. And it can easily lead to overweight.

When you think about it, there are basically only five categories of causes for cravings commonly. One, the individual craves because he is eating out of balance. For example, the person who eats too many processed high salt foods will crave sugars to balance it. Too high a fat diet will also cause a craving of either sugars or salts or both. These people frequently disgust themselves because they eat to the point of pain even when they are not hungry. So to nip the cycle of too high a salt, fat, or sugar diet in the bud, one of the quickest things to do is start a diet of whole foods and greatly reduce the processed foods. What are whole foods? Things like brown rice and lots of vegetables and beans.

The second reason for cravings you could kill for is hypoglycemia, or low blood sugar. This can disguise itself as headaches, horrid fatigue, or vicious mood swings, for example. And hypoglycemia can have many causes, but the most common is a combination of too many sweets, coffee, alcohol and other processed foods.

A second cause is an overgrowth of a yeast called Candida in the intestines. This yeast often gets a head start in the gut after you have had a bout of antibiotics. But other medications such as ulcer and stomach prescriptions to decrease the acid in the stomach, birth control pills, and prednisone can do it. Since the yeasts thrive on sugars, but also need them to survive, they can cause you to crave sweets. But at the same time these very sweets cause the yeast to grow even faster, thus causing you to crave even more. You can padlock the refrigerator door, but it will be futile, for you are mercilessly driven to satisfy that craving. The treatment is to go on the yeast program that is outlined in The E. I. Syndrome, temporarily cut out all ferments and sweets (including fruits) and to replace processed foods with whole grains and vegetables.

The 4th most common reason for wicked uncontrollable cravings is by far the sneakiest: unidentified nutrient deficiencies. At first you might think that couldn't apply to you, because you live in the land of plenty and eat a wide variety of foods, and may even take supplements. But we have the dubious distinction of being the first generation of man ever to eat so many processed foods.

For example, to make bread nowadays, you first need white flour. To make this highly processed food, you take whole wheat and grind it into flour, then bleach it to make it white. Unfortunately, though, the minerals such as magnesium, chromium and copper are reduced 80%. And what can a chromium deficiency cause? The very hypoglycemia that caused your cravings, for starters. And a deficiency of all three minerals (which is very common, since most people eat bleached flour bread every day) can cause high cholesterol.

In fact the reason many people have high cholesterol is because they do not have all the minerals needed to metabolize the cholesterol properly. But instead of discovering the biochemical cause behind the high cholesterol, diets of more processed foods (margarines, egg beaters, etc.,) are prescribed along with expensive medications that can potentiate Alzheimer's (early senility) and early heart attacks through free radical degenerative disease.

So how do you correct this? Have your doctor draw your vitamin and mineral levels as described for him and you in Tired Or Toxic? Once they are diagnosed and corrected, make sure you are on a diet of whole real foods that are rich in these nutrients so you never get that way again.

There are other causes for cravings as well. But the fifth category is one of hidden or unsuspected food and chemical sensitivities. For example it is common for many people to be driven by cravings when they eat any food containing wheat or work around chemicals. And chemical overload can come from such common sources as from auto exhaust fumes, new carpet, paint, and other chemicals in the normal environment. They outgas formaldehyde, toluene, xylene and other hydrocarbons that abnormally stimulate the brain's appetite center in some of those affected.

All of the above have been detailed in Tired Or Toxic? As well, it contains the scientific references for statements made, for interested physicians.

So next time you have a craving, look at it as a gift or early warning. For it is the only way your body has of alerting you that you are eating wrong, have hypoglycemia, intestinal dysbiosis, or have an undiscovered nutrient deficiency or food or chemical sensitivity. And by discovering and correcting the cause early, you may just be staving off that first heart attack from an undiagnosed magnesium deficiency or whatever other symptom would have been next after having ignored the real cause and improperly fed your craving.

If you can't figure out your craving and correct it, write out a typical weekly menu and bring it in (to us or your doctor/counselor). We'll figure it out for you. The reason for writing it is to save you time and money. Once the foods can be seen at a glance, the proportions and how it is prepared can be gone over. Then if the problem is not apparent there, we should still have enough time to discern where the problem really stems from.

As an addendum, I personally would recommend that cancer patients only choose doctors or counselors who have not only successfully guided cancer patients but who also make available addresses and telephone numbers of these people. When your life depends on any treatment, you want to check it out thoroughly.

Once you can identify the type of craving you have, try these substitutes (brackets contain items that may not be recommended in the first few months).

Pungent
1. chopped scallion
2. grated daikon
3. ginger pickles
4. {wasabe (dry mustard)}
5. raw cabbage
6. {horseradish}

Salty
1. gomashio
2. miso
3. tamari pickles
4. sea salt
5. sea vegetables
6. kombu tea

Bitter
1. nori strips
2. parsley leaves
3. dandelion greens
4. mustard greens
5. {grain coffee}

Sweet
1. grated carrots {in sweet rice wine}
2. sweet vegetable drink
3. sweet squash puree
4. sweet potato
5. chestnut puree
6. yinnie syrup

Sour
1. sauerkraut
2. {umeboshi vinegar}
3. {lime, lemon}

Soon you'll be able to come up with others.

GIVE NEW MEANING TO A MAC-ATTACK

So you're having a craving and you don't want to blow it? Make ume/sho/kuzu/ginger/bancha. Often this will level you out. If it's sweets you crave, make brown rice with sweet vegetable juice and (presoaked) chestnuts. Or cook sweet rice and add a few raisins after, or cook it in diluted apple juice. Or cook an apple with water and a pinch of sea salt. To this you could also add a cup of boiling water and a cup of couscous, cover, turn off heat, and in 10 minutes you have a couscous "apple cake."

But most importantly, identify the cause, should a sugar craving emerge, rather than succumb to it. But when it does need satiating, you'll be able to do so in a less deleterious way.

As an example, if you crave sugar, have you had too much salt, seaweed, oil, or beans? Have you put too much shoyu in your dishes? And to feel more content, do you need a hot fudge sundae? Or could you be content with baked mochi pieces dipped in tahini/yinnie sauce? Or better yet, a piece of cooked fruit? Or best, your sweet vegetable drink and some sweet vegetable dishes like parsnips, pumpkin, sweet brown rice, or baked carrots?

If it is salt you need, make a wakame/cabbage/miso/ ginger soup, or substitute turnip or daikon for the cabbage. Make nori rolls or kombu tea. Ginger and lemon can help the pungent/sour craving. If you can get yourself back on the track by macro methods instead of a hot fudge sundae, you have progressed a great deal. And bear in mind that should you require frequent emergency dietary corrections, often you will need to isolate the cause. The more extreme the balancing, the more strain on the system and you are trying to unload it, not stress it further, in order to allow healing to take place.

YIN AND YANG

Balancing foods by the 5 phases and by yin and yang is more than the beginner in the strict healing phase can handle usually, and have been explored in other fine works. It will be necessary for continual improvement, however, to begin to appreciate these aspects.

At first yin and yang may seem very confusing and irrelevant, but they are not. In fact, they are the basis of macrobiotics and everyday life. You actually already use them to make everyday decisions, but may be unaware of it.

For example, if you were invited to go cross country skiing, would you eat beforehand hot porridge or stew, or salad or ice cream? You need body heat and energy, so you would choose a yang food.

Likewise, if you were trying to impress your boss with the facts of a tight new proposal, would you have alcohol before it? No, you would save yin, expansive, "air-head," giggly, playful foods for a time when you unwind with friends and let it all out. You would not have it during a time requiring tight precision. Macrobiotics merely takes these same yin and yang principles to a much deeper level.

You see? You really already understand much more about yin and yang than you thought. And in trying to identify with the concepts of yin and yang, don't get caught in the American frame of reference of good and bad. First of all, it doesn't exist. There is very little that is totally good or totally bad. For every bad or unfortunate event, there is nearly always something good that comes from it if you look hard enough and from enough perspectives. Likewise, nothing is ever totally yin or totally yang. Furthermore, yin and yang have nothing to do with good and bad, but with balance.

Since macrobiotics is really about living within the guidelines of nature and not violating the rules of nature, you can understand why balance is important. And since we are living beings, we are constantly changing in our attempt to adapt to the world: nothing is static. What is good for us this month or year may not be good for the state we will be in next month or year. We need to constantly adapt or balance with our internal state as well as external environment. If you are living in New England in February, you don't eat the same things you would on a Caribbean vacation. You adapt. You balance yourself with Nature. The degree of understanding of yin and yang makes this constant balancing act of life more sophisticated, so that higher levels of wellness are possible.

You probably also realize that because we all have a unique biochemistry, psyche, environment, climate, etc., there is no one perfect diet for everyone. And even when a diet is found that makes one feel great, he changes; thus, his needs change as well. With all this taken into consideration, how do I dare write a whole book with such precise diet recommendations?

Easy. I personally witnessed it turn around my life and the lives of hundreds of my patients and the lives of scores of people who had consulted Mr. Kushi for diet/lifestyle recommendations. And these were no ordinary people, but people who had exhausted all that medicine has to offer. We had come to a dead end. And many were not expected to live a year regardless of what was done.

I know of nothing else that has accomplished what I have observed (and that you will read about in this book in the personal stories). It goes without saying that an Eskimo could not survive on raw salads. He needs the blubber to keep him warm. And I have seen a Caribbean population increase their cancer rate as they became daily meat eaters.

Does this mean that a macrobiotic Eskimo should eat a persistently high fat diet to heal? I don't know. I never saw an Eskimo patient, and least of all one with cancer. And I never saw anyone clear a serious condition on a high fat diet. Nor have I seen a Caribbean native clear on fruits and vegetables.

So for now, there are many unanswered questions and even more unproven answers. For my money, I'll stick with what I have observed, and deal with the out-lyers as they present.

CATCH-UP COOKING

There are moments or days when you'll want to roast pumpkin seeds, clean out the refrigerator and make a new soup, make your veggie or greenie bag, make a new grain or new recipe you've never tried before. Or maybe you don't feel creative, so just soak beans, cook a stew or make your soup stock from your "compost soup" bag, or just make "green juice," or prepare the sweet vegetable drink. Or make a large amount of a dish to share or exchange with a macrobiotic friend. Do anything you can with moments that promise to be less productive to release the pressure on those extra busy days.

Catch-Up Cooking Checklist

Beans soaking or cooking
Root bag, veggie bag and green bags ready
Sea vegetable dish
Gomashio or pumpkin seeds
"Compost soup" bag or green juice cooking for future soup stock
A special new dish (casserole, stuffed squash, etc.)
Sweet vegetable drink

Clarification: Remember, all the 4 bags are designed for is to save time and help organize the refrigerator. It is far easier on a busy morn to pull out a bag of assorted cleaned veggies than to rummage through a refrigerator bulging with greens. There are two ways you could do it. (1) Have a separate bag for root vegetables, one for greens and one for others (squash, cauliflower, etc.), or (2) have separate bags (one for each day or 2) of a mixture of all 3 categories. Whichever appeals to your cooking style and logic is fine. You are just trying to "file" them after they have been cleaned so that you can grab them quickly for cooking and avoid rummaging through the frig for many uncleaned vegetables that were separately wrapped, and having to drag out numerous bags to fix a meal.

The compost soup bag is just your leftover vegetable parts that make great soup stock for boiling and discarding after their nutrients have been rendered. What's in the bag? Cauliflower and broccoli stalks, huge bunches of turnip, carrot and other leaves if you have more than you could ever eat in the garden, vegetable parts you do not like (I don't like the white stalks of bok choy), corn cobs, leftover pieces of veggies that were used in other dishes or grated. I call it the compost soup bag or the green juice bag. But it's really all the same: a good start for high nutrient soup/bean stock or cooking water.

-79-

WHAT YOU CANNOT HAVE

Some foods will be on temporary hold; others may be a life sentence. Most of the foods on the DO NOT HAVE list are only temporarily restricted. Usually after 3 months of the strict phase, many people are so well they can expand to other foods. In fact, to stay off oils, for example, more than 3 months would be dangerous and create new medical problems of serious nature. But once healthy enough, you can tolerate anything for a specified amount of time. And that's the goal; to get so healthy that you can eat a large variety of foods with no ill effects ever!

In the meantime, because you have years of damage to your body, you're going to want to be extremely strict in the beginning to attain maximum healing. There will be many exceptions to the following which will have to be individualized at consultations. For example, people with chemotherapy and irradiation are so utterly drained that they will need fruits and oils and much more fish proteins than the average very ill person.

For the majority of people in the first month of the healing phase, there will be no animal food, no dairy, no oils, no fruits and no baked flour products. In other words, nothing with broken grains. Also no spices, mustard, peppermint, herb teas, grain coffees, oils or nuts; no sweets, honey, maple syrup, vinegars or alcohols. Once a week, if you crave it, you could have some corn on the cob, a small amount of a seasonal, cooked fruit with a pinch of sea salt, a few slices of steamed sourdough bread or a serving of noodles with vegetables. You should not have any raw salad, oatmeal, or buckwheat, while the vitamins, minerals, hormones and medications will need to be individualized at your consultation.

Since there are many temporary rules that will need to be adhered to, try to avoid getting into the old, American idea of the fact that if something is good for you, then a lot of it must be even better, because this is just not true. Remember that there is a balance for everything. Everything has a bell-shaped curve. In other words, there's an ideal amount of food, water and air for you. But too little or too much of any of those is lethal. There is a large, bell-shaped curve at which point there is an optimum dose. And this holds true for everything in the universe. Some things just have a narrower peak of beneficial effect. For example, too much seaweed and miso can make you so tight that you will not discharge or heal. Too little will retard your buildup of minerals needed to detoxify, thereby also retarding healing.

If you lack strength when you do the diet, you should see the doctor or your certified macrobiotic counselor right away. Often the fish/carrot soup is helpful. Usually, the first thing you will want to check is whether you are having enough variety in your diet. Remember to vary the grains and vegetables tremendously. Also remember to check the quality of the salt. Is it the best grade white sea salt that you can find? Also check the quality of your foods. Are they organic and as free of pesticides as you can get? And if that doesn't provide an answer, look at whether the person preparing the food is happy and what type of energy is used for the cooking.

Always try to have a live garnish with your soup. It can be very simple such as a teaspoon of chopped scallion, parsley, or celery leaves. And always have condiment with your grain whether it's a little sprinkling of gomashio or pumpkin seeds. Pickles can be made, but in the beginning you'll probably want to buy some ready-made macrobiotic pickles or organic sauerkraut (N.E.E.D.S., Walnut Acres, Gold Mine Natural Foods, Mountain Ark, etc.) and just wash the salt off.

Your basic seasonings will be:

1. Salt (this needs to be cooked the longest)

2. Misos (there are a variety of flavors of these, and these must always be simmered for a couple of minutes at the end of the recipe)

3. Shoyu sauce (this requires the shortest cooking, but with just a minute or two simmering also)

4. Finely chopped raw scallions or parsley

5. Ginger juice (grate and squeeze)

But remember, too much of any of the seasonings #1-3 is very yang. You can become thin, very hungry, always eating and always losing weight and never satisfied with your diet.

Chewing is of utmost importance. I suggest you first purchase a three-minute egg timer and chew each mouthful of food until the egg timer is halfway through. This will give you well over one hundred chews. Often people are baffled as to how they can get so many chews from one mouthful of food. The trick is to keep pushing the food forward with your tongue and keep working it forward to the front of your mouth and not letting it slide down the hatch. You will quickly notice that most Americans chew their food less than 10 times a mouthful. In fact, many chew, chew, gulp. Chew, chew, gulp.

Chewing is extremely important for many reasons, and to chew for less than 50 times is to take the chance of not healing at all in spite of doing everything else well. (1) First of all, chewing breaks down the food to smaller size so that more nutrition can be obtained from it. (2) It also mixes the food well with saliva so that it takes the work away from the pancreas. (3) It also alkalinizes it so that there is less work for the blood buffering system and (4) reduces the molecular size so that it reduces the antigenicity, or allergic potential of the food. Many people swallow such large pieces of poorly chewed food that the whole food antigen is presented to the gut. Since this is abnormal for the gut, it recognizes it as foreign and hence, it is attacked as a foreign invader, antibodies are formed, and food allergies occur. If you chew it 50-100 times per mouthful, you reduce this allergenicity dramatically.

Even if you don't have good teeth, just masticate the food for two to three minutes for each mouthful. This way you will thoroughly mix it with saliva to begin the breaking down process. Don't forget, that as people age, 50% of the people over 50 have less of the gastric juices that they so importantly need in order to extract the nutrients from the food. So thorough chewing is an absolute must. Chewing over 100 times per mouthful will speed your healing even more so. It also turns out to be a good time to do your mental affirmations or meditation.

It's ironic that macrobiotics is so socially isolating because of the different foods that we eat, and next because of the extra time we spend cooking our foods. Now it seems that we're actually compounding the problem by not being able to talk with the people who are eating with us. However, in the beginning you are going to have to learn how to chew in preference to talking during the meals. To chew less than 50 times a mouthful is to waste all of your efforts.

So the healing phase is, for most, devoid, at least the first month (until your consultation) of:

Oils

Fruits (including raisins, lemon), fruit juices, vegetable juices

Meats

Shellfish

Flour products- noodles, crackers, rice cakes, pancakes, breads

Nightshades- tomatos, peppers, paprika, eggplant, tobacco, potatoes

Poultry, eggs

Dairy (milk, cheese, cream, ice cream)

Alcohol

Oatmeal or whole oats, buckwheat, corn

Commercial table salt

Nuts

Most seeds, such as sunflower seeds

Sugar, chocolate, honey, maple syrup, soda pop (It goes without saying that alcohol is omitted, I hope)

Spices, grain coffee, herb tea (It goes without saying that

mayonnaise, catsup, mustard and Worcestershire sauce
are omitted)

Raw salad

Bubbly or mineral waters, Perrier or carbonated waters
or club soda

For ferment sensitive patients, they will have to avoid miso, tamari,
shoyu and tekka until the consultation. Avoid eating for three hours
before bed. This gives the gut time to heal and rest. Avoid any oily
food as it can plug lymphatics and cause you to get worse. Avoid
nicotine and tar because it makes the fats harder and more difficult to
dislodge. Use the sweet vegetable drink to soften fats. Oatmeals are
too fatty, buckwheat is too yang. One tablespoon of pickles a day,
maximum. Have fresh soup twice daily and green vegetables thrice
daily. Beans should be restricted to half a cup a day, total. Increase
the variety in foods and decrease the salt and miso to decrease the
tightness.

WHAT IS TIGHTNESS?

For example, being tense, edgy, irritable, snappy, angry or
hostile can be a sign of tightness. It can be from too much yang, usually salty seasonings like miso, shoyu, tamari, tekka. The treatment is
to have more green vegetables and cut out the former for awhile until
mellowness occurs (usually days or weeks, otherwise see the doctor).

The contrast is when one is too laid back or mellow and can't
get anything done. Give more salt and/or protein.

There are three corrections of previous works that Mr. Kushi
made me aware of. One is, always be sure that miso, shoyu and tamari are simmered 2-3 minutes into any dish. They are not merely
added before serving. The second is that tamari sauce is not indicated for the healing phase. Johsen shoyu is probably the best quality
shoyu sauce and should be used in recipes that call for shoyu, tamari
or soy sauce. In the beginning, when macrobiotics was introduced to
the States, in order that people did not confuse Chef Boy Ar Dee or
Chun King commercialized soy sauces (with carmelized sugars and

corn syrups in them) for macrobiotic, organic, fermented bean products, the word tamari was used. However, then tamari started being imported into the United States in a variety of forms. It is no longer, however, the same product as the original shoyu sauce. Many tamaris nowadays even have mirin, which is an alcohol, added to them. This is emphatically contraindicated in the healing phase. Third, in the beginning, there was a slight mistranslation and the umeboshi plum is actually an apricot and not a plum.

Many times it was brought out in the consultations that if a person has one piece of cheese, one piece of chocolate a week or even one egg a month, he will not heal. Therefore, it is important to follow the rules, at least temporarily. For we should all bear in mind that as peculiar or contrary as some of the recommendations may seem, it is the only therapy that we have ever witnessed that could clear conditions that no one in the world could help. Therefore, it behooves us to try not to alter it in any way. (And actually as you will read, we do know why it works.) Furthermore, it goes without saying that if you are putting this much effort forth to get well, it's silly and counterproductive to sabotage your efforts. If cravings get out of hand, have your consultation earlier so the cause can be found and corrected.

In the first two months you should:

(1) be losing weight effortlessly
(2) be feeling more calm or a sense of well-being
(3) be feeling stronger or more rested

If you are not, here's a preliminary checklist of the more common reasons:

(1) Eating too much food
(2) Not balancing proportions
(3) Not enough seaweed
(4) Not chewing adequately
(5) Not addressing the psychological issues (job and marriage satisfaction, and self-image)
(6) Not skin brushing
(7) Not meditating
(8) Not singing and exercising
(9) Too much seasoning

(10) Still hooked on a particular food
(11) Eating before bed
(12) Not enough variety in foods and cooking styles
(13) Not having good quality organic food
(14) Not having good quality water
(15) Not having good quality salt
(16) Using microwave
(17) Using electric (you can cook rice on a backyard barbecue grill if gas sensitive)
(18) Having poor chemical, dust, mold environmental controls (the environment can put too much stress on the body to enable healing)
(19) Not having a loving, supportive environment and a loving cook with good energies
(20) Having undiagnosed nutrient deficiencies

As number 12 suggests, sooner or later you will need to learn more about cooking or you'll get too tight or bored or both.

As you get more sophisticated (and more well) in your cooking, you'll learn for example, to thicken soups with tofu, kuzu, "grain milk," "bean milk," roux (rice, whole wheat, etc. flours and arrowroot or corn starch), tahini and other seed and nut butters (for special occasions only, as these have too much fat) and cauliflower puree. Now you can begin to see how creativity can perk up the texture and tastes of meals.

With this little peek at what helps to make a gourmet macro cook, you can see that there is fun ahead once you master the basics. But should you stop at basics, you'll not only retard your chances of getting well, but deprive yourself of developing a new talent.

HOW STRICT DO I NEED TO BE?

Being in the strict healing phase of macrobiotics is a lot like being pregnant or having syphilis. You either are pregnant or you're not. You either have syphilis or you don't. You are in the strict healing phase, or you are not. So if you are going to make the effort, you might as well go all the way for a 6-12 month trial.

Perhaps understanding a little of some of the many reasons of why macro is so healing will help you appreciate this. In macro (strict healing phase we're talking of, not transition or already healed) you eat as though your life depended on it. In other words, every single mouthful is as nutritious as possible.

You never throw away the water that vegetables have been cooked in, but rather save it for a drink or soup stock. Having 2-3 soups a day expands the quantity of vegetables you consume but disguises them in a different form to please the palate. Also you can hide seaweeds in them.

The elimination of processed foods, especially flour products raises your mineral levels about five-fold and that doesn't even count the seaweeds. You are ingesting grains, greens, seaweeds and other vegetables at every meal, not to mention the daily beans.

The consistency of this high nutrient diet is one of the aspects that allows the body to not only heal but gear up for discharges and regeneration. Just imagine if you had a Rolls Royce car. You would not put the cheapest grade oil in it. You would use the most superior quality! Nor would you wait for the oil light (analogous to the warning symptoms we call disease) to go on. You would check it periodically.

Likewise, if you had an expensive bonsai (a miniature Oriental tree that is groomed and pruned for years to resemble a full grown tree with character---a real work of art) you would not haphazardly water it. Rather, you would check it daily, and water and feed it with consistency.

Or imagine a fine horse that you were raising or a precious child. You know that consistency is the key. If you let them misbehave one day and reprimand them on another day for the same act, you do not get the desired performance. But with consistency, you do.

If your body is receiving highly nutritious food at regular intervals, then all of a sudden has to "make do" with something of lesser value, you may set it back much more than you realize. Likewise, dieting off all the old fats that harbor the chemicals, drug residues and pesticides of a lifetime is crucial to recovery of the detox enzymes in the endoplasmic reticulum. A little bit of cheese or oil could reclog these important membranes.

One of the first things nearly all of us had to heal was the gut. By cutting out meat, you reduce the putrefaction metabolites peculiar to meats. This cuts down on inflammation of the gut and allows it to proceed with better absorption of nutrients. As well, (all of this is explained in detail with scientific references in Tired Or Toxic?) less meat makes the detox system healthier. Likewise, cutting out sugars slows the growth of undesirable organisms like Candida and also decreases gut inflammation so that improved nutrient absorption can occur. By eliminating processed foods, you avoid the chemicals, dyes and additives that overwork the gut detox pathways as well. Unburdened, the body can concern itself with detoxing some of your other stored chemicals.

A word about freshness is needed. Some of the worst vitamin and mineral levels I ever saw in a macrobiotic person were in a man who did not do his own cooking. He hired it done. But he was religious in trying to do his chewing and other aspects. This demonstrated that freshness, particularly where the greens are concerned is imperative.

Likewise, a famous macrobiotic case that cleared his cancer, eventually got his cancer back and died because he, too, had never gotten into the cooking. Even if you are well-to-do, I would suggest that you delegate or hire anything else out, but not your cooking. How can you justify letting someone else take responsibility for the most important aspect of your health—your food! You should oversee this yourself or share/trade a few dishes a week with someone else who is also motivated enough to do the strict healing phase. For example, you will probably, as we all have, occasionally find you have made enough grain or bean to last you for 2 weeks. This should be given away. It's best to eat fresh, and the favor will probably be returned. Or you make the root vegetable seaweed dish one week and share with a friend and he can make the bean dish. Then switch off the next week and you make the bean and he can make the grain, etc. (Don't say, "He?" We have doctors, dentists, attorneys and millionaire CEOs in our practice cooking their own macro because their wives won't.)

If you find yourself in a social situation where you did not plan and bring your food, it may be better to fast than set your progress back 2-4 weeks with an indiscretion that may only bring a few minutes of pleasure. And in the case of some cancers, the set back may irrevocably lead to your downfall. I have seen people clear a cancer, multiple sclerosis, chemical sensitivity and Candida hypersensitivity, then go off the diet and get the condition back. Then try as they may, they never could get rid of the condition again. It is almost as though there is no second chance. But lest this make you have second thoughts about beginning this program, these examples did not just loosen up, they completely went back to junk food.

Although it has been mentioned, it deserves repeating. Oil and fish are eliminated your first month until the consultation (unless you feel so awful without them that you cannot). But do not go more than a month on your own without oil. Oils or fatty acids are essential to life. They make up every cell membrane (sort of the computer keyboard of the cell where all the directions come from). They make up the mitochondrial wall (where energy is synthesized), they form the endoplasmic reticulum (where chemicals are detoxed) and they constitute the protection of every nerve, the brain, and all cells. You can get into serious symptoms without oil for a prolonged time.

Even though macro is so utterly rich in nutrients, we rarely see anyone who has normal vitamin and mineral levels, macro or not. I suspect this is because, as the first generation of man ever exposed to so many chemicals, our detox pathways are working overtime. And never forget that for every molecule of chemical you detox, you lose specific nutrients. So we as a generation are more nutrient deficient than previous generations because (1) we eat processed foods, and (2) our detox systems are losing nutrients trying to metabolize our chemical environment every moment of our lives, and (3) the whole foods we do buy may be grown on less nutritious soil than the same foods years prior.

So it is more difficult to heal in this era without addressing nutrient deficiencies. In fact, in people who only have a couple of months or less to live, it is even more imperative to check their nutrient levels. (1) You know they are low because of the severity of their medical problem. For example if the person has cancer, he most likely had some nutrient deficiencies that enabled him to get cancer. Then (2) the cancer itself through its growth has further depleted him of nutrients. I personally never saw a cancer patient with normal nutrient levels. Lastly, (3) since macrobiotics is a natural and slow process of healing and regeneration, doesn't it make more sense to correct the nutrient deficiencies so the person will be stronger, thereby increasing his chance of living long enough for the macro to help heal him? So even though macrobiotic practices have not included the recommendations of nutrient assessments, it makes a lot of sense to me and I have seen it work. One problem with them is they may force some of the dramatic discharges I have seen. Also some people absolutely have to have a course or two of radiation, chemo, and/or surgery to enable them to live long enough for macro to heal.

At one stage, some will become hostile and defiant regarding all of the forbidden foods. Sure man was definitely a hunter and meat eater. And the plains people did not eat seaweed. And yes, the West coast macrobiotic communities think the East coast is too rigid. You can find all sorts of excuses to not do the diet. And if you're looking for one, let me help you: Do not do the diet. There now, feel relieved?

For those who were like myself, and many of the others with the severest cancers, E.I., multiple sclerosis and other end of the road diseases, and for those for whom medicine has nothing more to offer, what have you got to lose? I have seen it do the impossible, and where all else has failed. I merely present you with an idea, an opportunity that may turn your life around also.

Now let me be the devil's advocate and take the opposite stand. I'm always reminded of a story about doctrine versus tradition and their roots: Three generations of women in the same family make a special ham dinner for the holidays according to their grandmother's recipe. Because the recipe was so good, they dared not alter a single part.

As the youngest was being instructed by her mother, she was told, "Now first you must cut off both ends of the roast. Then...."

Years later, this younger one was with grandma in the kitchen at holiday time and asked, "Tell me grandmother, why do you always cut the ends off the roast to start? Does it allow more spices to get into the meat, or...?" "No my dear, it is so it would fit in my pan."

The problem with knowing how far you can veer from a recipe is to know the reasons why it works in the first place. Is the reason many foods, for example, are prohibited simply because they didn't have them in Japan, or because there really is a property to them that is not beneficial? I suspect it's a little of both. For example, tomatos are not endemic, and they do cause a lot of arthritis, acne and eczema. So for sure, they should be on the forbidden list while one is healing. But how does that explain generations of healthy Italians?

Likewise, milk is not endemic to Japan and yet we know many allergic people with chronic sinusitis, rhinitis and asthma make much phlegm when they ingest milk products. But how does that explain the gorgeous Swedes, Norwegians and Danes?

So for now, because we do not have all the answers, I suspect it is best to follow the formula that has done the impossible, then once you are well, experiment to find some of the answers you seek. Always maintain a grip on common sense and the appreciation of biochemical individuality. A consultation of all options with your doctor is recommended.

WHAT IF THIS IS STILL TOO DIFFICULT?

You could try working into it slowly, or start with transition foods (like shrimp, oil, vinegar, tamari) that will be eliminated once you get ready for the strict healing phase.

Week one: Cook a whole grain and have a little at every meal, even if it's one scoop. If it is too soggy, bland or tasteless, make the gomashio (roasted sesame salt) or roasted pumpkin seeds or sunflower seeds to sprinkle on top. Cook enough so you only need to cook it 2 or 3 times a week. If you really dislike it, saute it with onions and finely diced carrots and celery. Simmer in shoyu and add to the rice. Or add a hand full of shrimp or next time you cook it, reduce the water. When it is done, uncover and let steam off as you fluff it several times.

-91-

After a week (or longer if needed), now add a green each day to your meals. It steams quickly in 2-4 minutes. Collards are very easy. Just cut out the long central stems. They can be added to your compost bag or finely chopped and steamed prior to adding the leaves. Lay the leaf halves on top of one another, and roll up tightly into a cigar shape. Now make razor thin slices of the cigar and steam your "collard spaghetti" a few minutes. If you need, a dash of umeboshi vinegar, ginger juice, lime juice or tamari will liven them up.

Take a week or two getting used to grains and greens at every meal and gradually lower the volume of your regular food to make room for them. Because they are more bland, you will need to eat them first, as well.

Next, you can make a hearty soup that can last a couple days and have it once or twice a day. It could be broccoli, squash, cabbage or leek base (or all four at once) with just spring water, kombu stock or "green juice" stock (your compost soup bag) as the liquids. If the soups are too bland, again you could go transitional and add herbs like basil, spices like nutmeg, or heavy cream, a dollop of tomato sauce and/or blenderize them as well.

With time, you can experiment with other vegetable, bean and even sea vegetable dishes.

"But, I still don't know what to do with the seaweeds." This is so common a problem that it deserves more attention. If you do not dislike them, then there is no problem. If you do, you'll need to hide them in soups with the help of your blender.

The roasted pumpkin seeds can disguise the taste of nori, or after toasting it, crumple it and mix in with grain. Wakame, the basis of miso soup, can be pre-cooked 15 minutes then added to sweet squash where it becomes lost in the sweetness. Kombu can be cut very fine after the initial boiling and also lost in the cooking. It disintegrates and mixes with the juice of marrow beans, for example and tastes like a meat gravy. The addition of some 2 or 3 year old dark miso can even enhance this property.

Hijiki and arame often require a few drops of ume vinegar, a tofu sauce, or other vegetables to mask them and so you may want to save them for last as you explore a new seaweed weekly. Sea palm has a milder flavor, and you may prefer that first. Just take your time to ease into them.

WHAT'S FOR DINNER?

How many times have we heard that? And the answer? "Steak, your favorite," or "Pot Roast," or "Pork chops," or "Veal ala Oscar," or "Fried chicken," or "Fish." In essence, dinner has come to mean meat!

Or should you go out for dinner, when you order, there is usually no mention of the vegetables, as though they really are unmentionable. If you ask what they are, they are so inconsequential that often the waiter does not even know what they are. Or when the fish arrives, you need a microscope to find the vegetables that accompany it.

But, just persist, for the constant quality of the blood, the substance that battles and heals our cells, is determined by what we eat.

And when you hear the same question at home after a challenging day, don't panic. Your crew can manage nicely on salad, steamed vegetable and their meat. So you just have the vegetable and your grain that is always on stand-by. Don't bother to cook a seaweed now that will stink up the house. Don't worry about an elaborate meal. Do be sure that you have things cooking or soaking for tomorrow, though, for it is a bright new beginning. If you persist, chances are you will succeed in pulling a coordinated meal together sooner or later.

When you might start to get down on yourself for not being perfect, remember from whence you came. I was your average nutrient-ignorant doctor. I never had a turnip in my life before macro. Now I average a half dozen a week. Squash I had at Thanksgiving, now it's weekly. I thought cabbage was something people added to corned beef, which I made maybe once every 2 years. When you consider the volume and diversity of vegetables we now consume on a daily basis versus never having had many of them even once a month, we are doing infinitely better than ever before.

So maybe you won't get 6 veggies in today. Maybe it will be a rushed day and you'll have steamed greens and grain for dinner. Maybe lunch will be in the car on the way to an appointment so you rolled rice balls in gomashio at breakfast for today's lunch. Maybe breakfast was cold leftover Brussel sprouts and/or grain eaten in the car, or only miso soup. That's fine. You are O.K.

The things to bear in mind are (1) to remember how far you have come, (2) how much better even these meals are compared with what you used to have, and (3) these setbacks are probably temporary and you will eventually get more organized so that 5 out of 7 days a week you will eat pretty well. Of course, if you have cancer, it had better be 7 out of 7, initially. But most likely you will be able to get a little assistance from someone else, should you need it temporarily.

Also, there is nothing wrong with simpler meals. Some people do not do well with a hodgepodge of 6-10 vegetables a day. A simple steamed green, grain and one root veggie may be what makes their systems perk along easier. It depends on the individual and the severity of the illness. In the case of fewer foods, just try to get a large variety in every 3-4 days. And bear in mind that should restricted or narrow eating emerge, imbalance, boredom, biochemical deficiencies and cravings will emerge, not to mention failure to improve as fast as you would like. And once boredom does emerge, try to correct it within the realm of macro. You can give a lot of zest to miso soup with just a few drops squeezed from freshly grated ginger and a few drops from the squeeze of a quarter of a lime, for example. Look at some transition recipes for a vast number of ideas. Don't get stuck on rice alone. Vary it with chestnuts (pre-soaked) or other grains, or abandon it entirely for other grains and/or mixtures of grains.

As for the times when you are tempted to eat things because everyone else is having it, is it partly because you feel guilty? Some of us go through a stage where we feel we are killing our families by feeding them what they want. We feel like we are killing them by acquiescing to their requests for bacon and eggs. So what's wrong with a little soup as a prelude? Or what's so crazy about a few Brussel sprouts magically appearing on the scrambled eggs (for color, of course). Never give up hope, for you can most likely figure out more and more ways of improving the health of your loved ones, no matter how much they may resist. The easiest things for them to accept initially are the soups and desserts. MACRO MELLOW is loaded with ideas on how to feed family members healthfully who have no intention of going macro.

THE WORK WEEK

So let's see what your first week might start out like:

Day/Meal   Menu

Sunday/Dinner   1. Miso soup w/garnish
                            2. Rice w/gomashio
                            3. Steamed green
                            4. Aduki/squash/kombu
                            5. Sauerkraut condiment
                            6. Nishimi (root) dish
                            7. Hijiki/carrot/onion
                            8. Pressed salad
                            9. Bancha tea

Time: 2 hours (aside from the hijiki salad, you made this menu your first night)

Monday/   1. Miso soup
  Breakfast   2. Rice porridge
                            3. Steamed green
                            4. Herb Walley
                            5. Kombu tea

Time: 15 minutes. Now is where the fun begins! If you have 30 minutes, cook sweet vegetable drink and/or broccoli soup for the lunch thermos and nori rolls. Or make quinoa salad with rinsed, finely chopped pressed salad.

Monday/Lunch   1. Rice/condiment
                            2. Green
                            3. Hijiki salad
                            4. Nishimi vegetable
                            5. Soup or bean or other vegetables

6. Sweet vegetable drink or tea
7. Pickle

Your choices are to bring leftover dinner and\or additions you made at breakfast. If you can't quite get it together yet, broccoli (miso) soup in a thermos and a little container of grain with gomashio and green will suffice nicely.

Monday/Dinner

1. Soup and/or bean (depending on whether you had bean already today or soup twice already)
2. Millet w/pumpkin seeds
3. Rolled, sliced collards, steamed
4. Baked squash
5. Daikon pickle (bought or homemade
6. Root vegetable dish (like gingered carrots and onions w/kuzu or parsnips and burdock)
7. Arame w/julienned parsnips and/or onions
8. Pressed salad
9. Tea

Time: 1 hour. Now would be a great time to make a soup or nori rolls for tomorrow's lunch. Even if you just cut up the veggies or cook the grain you've done half the work for later.

So if periodically suddenly you feel overwhelmed, you're surrounded by vegetables, exhausted and in tears, relax. And just recite after me: "With G, G and B, how happy I will be." Seriously, just have your grain and green and pack it in for the day. You're not perfect, so what. You are on your way to better health.

Before you turn in, do a hatchet job on some veggies so you can at least cook your soup in the morning while getting dressed, run it through a blender (optional and preferred, *not* to blenderize your food yet), simmer in miso and pour into a thermos. It will be so great at lunch! So you only have grain and green in your container, you will eventually remember to soak those beans and find a time to cook them. And you will eventually find a moment to axe some root veggies for the veggie bag. Then when you go to chop (or don't forget that fast hand held shredder) for nishimi, your work will be half done. Taking lunch admittedly requires more planning than going home for lunch. So be patient with yourself.

But now you can more clearly see the organizational problem. So tonight as you drive home, you start planning: (1) meal for rest of crew, and (2) my macro needs. Timewise, what needs to be started first? Can you enlist any help from any crew members?

Think not only about what your immediate macro needs are for the night, but for the following breakfast, lunch and dinner. Eventually you will stagger things so that, for example, the grain lasts 2-3 days, beans and seaweed dishes 2 days, etc., so that you end up cooking just a few things each day. And, for example, you can work it so the longer cooking items (grains and beans) can be cooking while you are eating a meal. This cuts down on your actual in-kitchen time.

When you get pressed for time and find yourself forgetting to even serve some of the items you have served, remember the little reminder: grains, greens and beans, seeds and weeds, roots and "fruits." It serves to remind you to balance your meal with G, G and B. Of course, the beans need only be once a day and not even every day if you are strong enough.

The seeds are your condiments like gomashio or pumpkin seeds (contain vitamin E oils), the weeds are short for seaweeds (the minerals are necessary to help the body gear up for discharges), root vegetables are self explanatory, and "fruits" are goodies that provide more flavor and help digestion and eventual discharges, like miso.

So ease up, don't panic. If you can only handle grain, green, root and bean, that's terrific. In a few days you'll figure out how to factor in a sea vegetable dish. And as your strength rises, your creativity with vegetable combinations will as well. Keep it interesting, and if it becomes drudgery instead of a fun, challenging game, back off, rest and just do grain and green. If you get too yin (weepy, for example) from doing this too long, you'll know you have come to the time where you had better balance out and learn to cook a root dish, beans and sea vegetables. The whole thing hinges on an optimistic attitude that you <u>will</u> make it work. I've seen a few people who struggled through the diet without a laugh or a smile, angry all the time over having to do this diet in order to get well. It won't surprise you to know that in most of those cases it didn't work.

Okay. Let's try a common scenario--You get home from work, you're tired and hungry and you have to be at a class, concert or dinner meeting in 1 hour, and you forgot to prepare.

Mix a small aliquot of your soup that is in a jar in the refrigerator with miso, add more soup and some of your grain, heat and eat from thermos on way to engagement.

Or if you have more time, steam some chopped kale or collards to go with it.

And, while you change, boil a 3" strip of crumpled wakame with coarsely cut or grated carrots, turnips, cabbage and onion. And there you have it! Miso soup, grain, green and root veggies. That's great.

You'll learn all sorts of tricks, like never, never run out of grain. Always have some greenie and root vegetable bags ready to dip from. Save all your cooking water for soup stocks or for boiling vegetables. For example, kale cooked in cabbage/onion juice is very sweet, and as you get more in tune with your health, you'll see you get much more energy from your own home grown kale than the pesticided stuff in the grocery. You can start a few pots early in the house from seed to put out in the spring. And keep replanting as you use it, because the September-planted crop will grow all through winter. Just dust off the snow and pick. So put some pots by the back door. Also carrots, parsnips, kohlrabi, parsley, Jerusalem artichokes and other foods last well into the winter and some until spring. Even a small plot is worth cultivating.

And start going to the farmers' market. The veggies are fresher, there's a bigger variety, prices are lower, it's fun, you meet organic growers and you avoid the fumigation spraying of two extra middlemen: the wholesaler and retailer.

Remember from whence you came. Myself and many others never bought vegetables that weren't frozen and all cut up for us. I never had a turnip in my life, not to mention a dozen other veggies that are now weekly staples. When visitors rummage my refrigerator for a bottle of wine, they have to fight off mountains of huge green leaves and strange looking plant life they've never seen before. You'll be amazed at the volumes of veggies that will pass through that machine each week. But now you understand why the diet is so healthful. Everything you eat is as utterly high in nutrients (or nutrient dense) and balanced as you can possibly make it at this point in your life. And it can only get better as you strive to improve upon it.

Make a new recipe each week. Use <u>MACRO MELLOW</u> and just omit the ingredients you should not yet have. Use the other books and learn one new recipe a week. As you build your new culinary repertoire, meal planning and cooking become progressively more effortless. It's only when you run out of ideas that it becomes boring and a chore. But that's true for anything. The only difference is that with this hobby your life depends upon it.

There is infinite variety in taste that can be achieved. Here are 3 different meals, all take about 1 hour to prepare and in the course of that time you are also stockpiling items that will be used in future meals.

Meal #1   Broccoli soup
               Pressed salad (cucumber/radish/carrot/onion)
               Lentil/onion/carrot/wakame
               Rice with millet
               Gomashio
               Steamed watercress
               Arame
               Daikon/soy pickle

Meal #2   Miso/daikon soup
               Chickpea/onion
               Rice with hato barley
               Pumpkin seeds, roasted
               Steamed kale
               Squash/turnip
               Hijiki/onion
               Cabbage/tempeh/sauerkraut

Meal #3	Corn soup
	Aduki/kombu/squash
	Rice with chickpea
	Steamed collards
	Cabbage/turnips/onion/daikon with kuzu/shoyu
	Carrot/burdock kinpira with ginger
	Umeboshi red radish pickles

Meal #4	Marrow bean miso soup with kombu, onion and celery
	Millet burger
	Quinoa/carrot/onion/sunflower seed/ume salad
	Steamed bok choy
	Julienned daikon and parsnips
	Brussel sprouts with sea palm
	Sauerkraut
	Cousous "apple cake"

FIGHTING OFF BOREDOM

When you find yourself not satisfied with the food or fighting off boredom, it's time to read and broaden your cooking. We've listed the books to start with and the possibilities are endless.

For example, if you're getting tired of greens, often it's because you're coarse chopping and boiling. You're stuck in a pattern for lack of time. Yet a few simple modifications can perk up the very same greens.

First the cutting changes the taste. For collards, cut out the tough central vein and finely chop. Lay the leaves on top of one another, roll tightly as into a cigar and slice as finely as possible. Finely slice a halved onion and coarse grate or julienne a piece of daikon and steam all three ingredients 3 minutes. Even the quality of your water, such as leftover sweet squash cooking water, will change the taste.

Next dilute 1-3 tsp. kuzu in cold water, add to the stock, add 1/2-1 finely chopped umeboshi "plum" (apricot), and a dash of shoyu. You could also add a few squeezed drops of freshly grated ginger. Once you learn this, it takes no longer but tastes infinitely better than your boring coarsely chopped and boiled greens.

If the grains bore you, combine them in soups and add a little cumin powder. Or water saute with finely diced vegetables. Make some quinoa/barley burgers, or buckwheat/quinoa burgers. Just use no oil and markedly reduce or omit the spices and ingredients that are on your restricted list (if you are on the strict healing phase and have had no chemotherapy/irradiation).

Or say you have become stuck in making broccoli soup each day because you can't bear to eat it (or turnips, or seaweed or whatever else you are hiding in it). Don't despair, you can change it dramatically by blending in some cooked marrow beans or chickpeas and/or some cooked sweet squash. Then a different miso, or a dash of shoyu, and/or ginger can be added and a minced scallion garnish. Be sure to vary the spices, though, or all your dishes will taste the same.

As you get more sophisticated, you can begin to balance meals for the 5 phases as well (see Colbin's The Natural Gourmet). Just bear in mind as you use all these wonderful books that you still need to limit yourself to the ingredients and amounts that are prescribed if you are trying to heal and/or force a discharge.

On the other hand, if you feel great on the program and have good relief from your symptoms, you may be ready for some transition foods and spices. Since your body never lies, it will soon tell you if you were premature. But limit them to once a week.

And when hectic life situations inevitably arrive, it's better to back off to transition than possibly set yourself back to zero by totally abandoning your healthful eating program.

In summary, strive for breakfast, lunch and dinner to contain on average 5, 7 and 9 items respectively. You won't be perfect (or hungry) three times a day, every day. Nor will you be able to pull it off that consistently, but the overall picture is what counts.

Breakfast can be a Herb Walley, miso soup with garnish, steamed greens, porridge with condiment and kombu tea. Lunch can be grain with condiment, green, root vegetable dish, sea vegetable dish, pickle, sweet vegetable drink or tea and bean or other vegetable dish. Then dinner can contain soup with garnish, grain with condiment, green, root veggie, sea veggie, pickle, bean or other vegetable dish, condiments and garnish (perhaps a special one), and a prescribed medicinal drink or regular tea.

Garnish (a raw finely chopped vegetable like grated carrot, chopped scallions, minced parsley) and condiments (like a roasted seed, a roasted ground seaweed powder, cooked scallion/miso condiment, tekka or grated spice) are a last minute, (often prepared ahead of time) but necessary part of every meal. Without them the meals will get very dull and cravings will emerge. Likewise variety in basic ingredients, cooking styles, recipes and menus are crucial to success in order to maximize interest, nutrient content, simulate satiety and avoid boredom and cravings.

And avoid the diet where you have a dozen ingredients in every dish, trying to get all the phases in. Remember to keep most dishes fairly simple with 1-3 ingredients and let one dish be the star performer at your meal.

Remember our purpose with this book has been to fill a gap: to spell out how to get started with the strict healing phase diet. It is not intended to be a recipe or cookbook. So if your cooking is boring, read books on technique. I would suggest in order, MACRO MELLOW by S. Gallinger, The Quick and Natural Macrobiotic Cookbook by A. Kushi and W. Esko, Basic Macrobiotic Cooking by J. Ferre, and the many others we've listed here (all available through N.E.E.D.S.). Just remember to remove oil (substitute water), veggies that are not on you daily list and other ingredients that you should not have in the first few months of strict healing and disease reversal.

In spite of the repetition and detail here, we still hear, "I just don't know how to start." So steam, pressure cook or boil brown rice (1 part rice to 1 1/2 parts of water for fluffier rice and 1 part rice to 2 parts water for softer rice; bring to boil, add pinch of salt, simmer 45 minutes). Later as you get more sophisticated you could pre-roast it for a nuttier flavor and combine other grains. But for starters, simple is best. Or later you can soak it before cooking for an even different quality.

Next wash a cup of sesame seeds or pumpkin seeds. Roast until dry and browned in a dry fry pan. Stir or turn them frequently to avoid burning. Add 1 tsp. pre-roasted salt to the sesame seeds.

In the morning eat rice plain with either seeds on top, or cook the grain first in an equal volume of water for 10-15 minutes as a porridge. Then sprinkle on your seeds.

Breakfast is the one meal with no peer pressure. Certainly you should have more staying power with a whole grain breakfast than some boxed cereal and milk or sweet roll and coffee.

You have seen that there is no lack of macrobiotic cookbooks. But most cooks fly by the seat of their pants and would prefer guiding principles and then to be left to their own creativity rather than be chained to a cookbook. So here are just a few ideas on which you can elaborate, with or without the many cookbooks.

You miss creamy soups? Blend in tofu, or cooked oats, barley, rice, or beans (or nuts as your condition allows).

You made enough aduki/squash/kombu to last until Christmas? Add sweet vegetable juice, miso, blend and simmer. You have a new soup the whole family will enjoy (but for Pete's sake, don't tell them what's in it).

You are sick of rice, want something less chewy? Make millet with cauliflower, and use 3 cups water to 1 cup millet. Or cook 3 grains 1:1:1 together like wheat berries, quinoa and millet or buckwheat or rice.

You need a soup that tastes like there has been meat in it? Cook 2 1/2 hours marrow beans, kombu, onion. Or use kombu water with dark miso, mash in a portion of the beans, add sweet vegetable juice for right consistency and simmer (with a pinch of cumin if your condition allows).

You're going to be on the road all day tomorrow and you'll need food that will not make you want to stop and pick up something "bad?" Steam red radish and collard greens, make carrot/onion/hijiki with a dash of umeboshi vinegar and shoyu. Cook lentils, bring your grain and gomashio, washed sauerkraut and burdock/onion/turnip/lotus in ginger/lemon/shoyu/kuzu sauce. You can make all this in less than an hour and pack it for travel. You'll have so much taste variety that you shouldn't be driven to stop for something non-macro.

Or a friend is coming and you can't think what to make. Does this menu sound so bad?

MENU

Cauliflower Clear Soup with Parsley
Short Brown Rice with Roasted Sunflower Seeds
Aduki Beans and Squash
Nappa Cabbage with Scallions and Wakame with Miso-Ume Sauce

Steamed Carrots, Broccoli and Turnips with Lemon Tamari Sauce
Baked Apples with Kuzu Raisin Sauce
Bancha Tea

MACRO MELLOW is loaded with menus and cooking directions and tips. Just modify and omit what you cannot have. If there is something that would really perk up your cooking but was not recommended, discuss it with your counselor/physician. Perhaps you really can have it. Regardless, within a few months you probably can.

Or say you can't handle whole grain for breakfast yet; your taste buds are still waiting for the old familiar tastes. So back off for a while. Do transition. Put sliced bananas or raisins and cinnamon in the rice porridge. Add yogurt if you need or maple syrup. With your whole grain you are still getting more nutrient density than you would with your boxed granola (baked with oil). So abandon the guilt and enjoy the transition stage. Just don't delude yourself that you are doing the healing phase at this point.

Or you're having guests for dinner and you plan on making "regular" food for them and dovetailing macro for yourself. Everyone will enjoy a broccoli-lemon soup. If in doubt, mix theirs with heavy cream. You could have steamed kale when they have salad. You can have sweet vegetable juice or beet juice (from a juicer or from boiling beets) in your wine glass. Your main course can be cabbage/sauerkraut/caraway seed/tempeh casserole, plus millet with tofu/miso/mushroom gravy, and steamed turnips or carrots. Factor in meat and French bread for them etc. Once you get the hang of it, you're dynamite.

You might say that you're having the same vegetables over and over. But it surpasses the Western diet which has the same devitalized processed bleached white flour over and over again in cereals, muffins, breads, pancakes, waffles, crackers, pasta, sauces, cookies and cakes. The difference is your repetition of vegetables is much more nutritious.

Or you hanker for a salad after too many grains and greens? Try this:

QUINOA TABBOULEH

2 c. cooked Quinoa	1/2 tsp. basil
1 c. chopped parsley	1/2 c. lemon juice
1/2 c. chopped scallions	1/4 c. olive oil
2 tbsp. fresh mint	1/8 c. sliced umeboshi or
1 clove garlic, pressed	toasted sunflower seeds
whole lettuce leaves	
sea salt to taste	

Place all ingredients except lettuce and olives in a mixing bowl and toss together lightly. Chill for 1 hour or more to allow flavors to blend. Wash and dry lettuce leaves and use them to line a salad bowl. Add tabbouleh and garnish with ume or seeds.

Right away you'll say, "Yikes! She's trying to kill me!" Raw veggies, garlic, oil, seeds, lemon, salt not cooked in! But if you have been eating well and crave this sort of thing, once every 2 weeks is not going to hurt you and you'll know if it's wrong for you. And it may just be that you are periodically in need of and ready for these tastes.

You can't stand the gassiness of beans? Soak overnight (except lentils) and discard soak water (except for aduki and black soybean). Bring to a boil and discard again. After they come to a boil a second time, add the rest of the cold water so they are 'shocked' and forced to come to a boil again. This would be the time to add any stock or sweet vegetable juice, or vegetables. Don't add salt until the last 20 minutes, as it toughens them. Also try cooking beans much longer like 2-3 hours. Remember it need not be all at once. They could cook an hour in the morning and another hour while you are preparing dinner. Adding a slice of ginger root to the pot may also soften them. And make sure they are fresh or they will be tough regardless of how long you cook them. I found a wonderful source at the Farmers' Market. They are home grown, hand shucked and organic. They are the best beans I've ever had.

For your occasional pasta dishes, try soba (buckwheat) noodles. Just remember you must shock them (add cold water after they have reached a boil) 3-4 times to get the best texture.

Or say you need a root dish for dinner and your mind is a blank. First put on your list for next week, "check Oriental market for daikon, lotus root and burdock!" This will remind you to get out of your rut and experiment. Also make a date with a friend to hit the local Saturday Farmers's Market. You can go at 6:30 a.m. and not interfere with your day's plans. You'll undoubtedly spot new items that are not at the grocer's, plus they should be fresher.

Meanwhile, you are in need of a root dish (nishimi). Do you have red radish, carrot, parsnip, onion, turnip? You could just steam the radishes with your greens. Or you can make a simple miso soup by first cooking the wakame, grate in some root veggies, cook 2 more minutes then simmer in the dissolved miso. Or maybe it's your day to try and splurge on a sweet potato. Whatever you do, don't panic. If you don't get any roots in your diet today, you'll get around to it.

And don't do what many of us did: You have a whole cauliflower, so you cook the whole thing, for example. Before you know it, you're sick of it. Cut off only what you need and store the rest in a bag that may get used in the compost soup or other dish. It sounds so simple but many of us were driven by the need to not waste. Consequently, our cooking suffered. The foods are your tools to make the best creations possible. Little leftovers are permissible and will probably find a niche.

Or say you want a new taste sensation. Take 1/2 a package of tempeh and finely dice into 1/4 inch cubes or less. Saute in a few drops of oil or water over moderate heat until browned on all sides. Takes about 8 minutes. Add 1/2 inch water to the fry pan, 2 cups chopped cabbage, a tsp. of caraway seeds and 1-4 tbsp. of macro kraut (available at N.E.E.D.S.) or any coarsely cut macrobiotic sauerkraut over the top. Cover and simmer a few minutes until cabbage is just barely cooked.

This will be your green for today with a bright new twist. If the salt was too much, you'll know in the a.m. Of course it all depends on how much of it you eat at a time, and for how long versus how much you share with the rest of the family. You'll learn how to listen to your body and make what is right for you at this stage in your life. Remember, you will be constantly evolving, so nothing is cast in stone.

Or say you are running behind in the morning or are not up for greens. Slice a little Nappa, Chinese, or regular cabbage into your miso soup. Or add your collards or parsley or scallion tops. Normally the morning miso should be a light, delicate, thin, sweet, only barely salty taste, not cluttered with a lot of vegetables. But there is nothing wrong with making it more substantial a few days a week, or even having a thick, heavy, hearty soup for breakfast and save the lighter one for another meal.

If mornings are rushed, you may need a soup that has grain, bean and vegetable that you can sip and chew from a thermos in the car occasionally. Just don't make it a habit to eat under such circumstances. Remember, mealtime should be relaxed.

Or let's say you are bored with the varieties of misos and seaweeds. Squeeze some lime or lemon and/or ginger into the soup. Or a dash of cumin in your bean soups. See what seems right for you without going too far from the strict phase. And then discuss it with your counselor/physician. Remember in a book, we can't factor in your biochemical individuality, the climate where you live, the time or season of the year, your ancestry, your physique and energy needs, nor your taste preferences. And then on top of all this are the particular needs for your condition that you are attempting to clear. But these somewhat universal middle of the road guidelines should get you off to a solid start until your consultation.

I hope we have given you a taste of strict without prison bars, and liberal without going off the deep end. It is a constant, ongoing process to balance the body as nutritiously as possible. When in doubt, eat along the safer recommendations that we have witnessed to do the impossible. But if boredom and/or cravings take hold, trust in your body and constantly growing wisdom to help you eat what is right for you.

CHAPTER 4

BEYOND THE DIET

The macrobiotic program is much more than just food and diet. It involves the whole total lifestyle, for there is much more to healing than just what you eat. For example, if you have a body with too much fat clogging the lymphatics and organ systems, how are you going to dislodge this fat the quickest way possible? The lymphatic is like the circulatory system of blood vessels (veins and arteries) but it carries lymph, not blood cells. Lymph is like the sewage system for cells in that it carries away all the waste. If left to build up, it causes the cells to become sick and malfunction. Another way the lymph system differs from the arteries and veins is that it has no pump like the heart but rather depends on changes in pressure induced by muscle contraction, heat, local massage or change in pressure induced by breath holding. Stimulation of the body's lymphatics can be done in a variety of ways: shiatsu, massage, body scrubs with a hot towel or with a ginger soaked towel, deep breathing exercises with yoga or meditation and exercise like swimming are just some of the ways.

As well as accumulating cell waste products and everyday chemicals in our bodies, we also accumulate electromagnetic energies. Everyone is recommended to walk outside for at least half an hour each day, preferably in bare feet (if the weather permits) to help ground the body with the universe. Also scrub the entire body with a hot towel, morning and night. This is not in the shower; this is a separate entity before the shower. The towel can first be dipped in ginger juice to make it even more stimulating. The body should be scrubbed until it is red. If you are pressed for time, at least do the feet and legs up to the knees, and the hands up to the elbows since these areas have some of the smallest vessels and the poorest circulation, and all meridians go to these areas.

You should sing a happy song several times a day. This opens the chakra, or energy centers in the body. You know what I mean: you feel that energetic or open feeling that you can get when you're singing a happy song. Remember, you're trying to energize and improve the circulation of the body in as many ways as possible. If you can't get in the happy song mood, record music that you hear that makes you feel good. Then play it daily. You'll need a half dozen songs and play a different one each day.

Also you will want to wear only cotton next to the skin and have cotton bedding as well. Do not have polyester touching your skin. Use gas cooking if it is tolerated. Some people can cook on a backyard gas grill. Some severe cancer patients have to get a little camping gas burner to cook on. Others can do well with electricity, especially if they are gas sensitive. Incidentally, some people told me they have portable gas stoves in their suitcases for travel. This is about the dumbest thing I can think of. If it was defective and blew up or caught on fire, you and hundreds of others are dead meat. If you can't afford to buy a gas cartridge at your destination, cooking on electric for a couple of days is not going to kill you. But travelling with a gas canister in your luggage is criminally idiotic.

Remember to eat as much as you want as long as you keep the proportions 50-50 for grains and vegetables and keep the meals down to 2 or 3 a day. Chew 50-100 times for each mouthful and do not eat 3 hours before bed. The gut is one of the first organs that has to heal. If it doesn't get to rest, how can it heal? To heal a broken leg we cast it and rest it. To only eat within 12 hours of a day or less is to allow the gut to rest at least half the day. If you are famished before bed, have as light a snack as possible.

For many, soaking your feet in a pail of hot water with a handful of sea salt is good to stimulate the circulation for five minutes before bed. The following are some of the most common recommendations that should be followed daily:

* Plants in the house to increase the oxygen

* Body scrub upon arising and before bed

* Walking half an hour each day, outdoors, preferably barefoot

* Singing or listening to happy songs 3-5 times a day

* Cotton clothing and bedding next to the skin

* Feet soak before bed

Remember to use any still moments for meditation and positive imagery. Try to reflect on what keeps you ill and imagine how life will be when you are well. Imagine how the inner process of the body works, looks, sounds and feels as it is healing. Indeed, there is a strong psycho-neuro-immune connection and the brain has a tremendous amount of power over healing.

In <u>Tired Or Toxic?</u> we talked about the toxic mental load that many of us carry on a daily basis. This can be more devastating than the toxic chemical load. There are several things that you should keep in mind that will help you reduce this toxic load and help speed healing:

1. Learn to practice thought control and thought selection. You can't be very healthy if you're depressed, cynical, worried, hostile, spiteful, vengeful, jealous, angry, etc. Don't dwell on the negative. It takes practice, sometimes meditation, sometimes professional guidance, affirmations, sometimes spiritual help and many other modalities to keep yourself on the track so that you keep pleasant thoughts in your head and not dwell on things that you can't change, or that have happened or might happen.

It's far healthier to count your blessings, feel a tremendous amount of gratitude for what you DO have, and make optimistic plans for how you are going to bring about your future goals. This planning should fill you with a much happier feeling. Be proud of your decision to make yourself healthier. After all, you could still be living on processed, fast foods and eating in restaurants where it's still, at this point in time, impossible to get whole grains, and where very rarely is there a vegetable that isn't slathered in dressing, cooking oil, heavy cream sauce or butter. So you're far ahead of the rest of the world in terms of healthful eating.

2. Learn to surrender or accept or forgive. Many of us are constantly fighting the need to be perfect. We are slaves to our job or our self imposed "ought to" directives. Surrender to fate and try not to impose such perfection on yourself. Don't try to change others or judge them as well, but accept them and forgive them for what they are. It is worthwhile for your peace of mind and ultimate healing.

3. Let go of the need to find nurturing and love outside of yourself. No friend or spouse or anyone in the world can guarantee to make you happy every moment of the day. You must find your own love and peace within yourself. It is surprising how many people do not love themselves. When you have that type of restriction, how much love are you willing to extend to others? This can be extremely limiting in all areas of your life.

4. Love unconditionally, for real love has no strings attached. If you can love for the sake of it, without expectations that may leave you feeling jilted, you'll have a happier emotional status.

5. Recognize that much of what you notice everywhere is a mirror of yourself. You are the sole actor on your stage. What you see in others is often a reflection of your feelings of yourself. Things that you hate and dislike in others, or mock out, are often things that you fear for yourself. With an awareness of this, you should be able to have more compassion and peace of mind, for in essence, we are all brothers and have a vast amount of similarity among us once the fascades are penetrated and we get to know one another. This is partly what world peace leaders have tried to show for centuries.

6. Next, try not to take yourself so seriously and practice seeing the humor in yourself and all of life. Try letting go a little more. Also, decide what the top three most important things in your life are. If health is not among them, you might as well stop here. If your health is not one of your top three priorities, this endeavor is doomed for failure. Rather than putting yourself and your family through a great deal of aggravation, you might want to sit down instead and decide how you arrived at your priorities before you go through the aggravating business of changing your lifestyle so that you can be healthier. Realistically, someone who really is not happy is doomed for failure when attempting a difficult lifestyle change (even if it will most likely improve their longevity).

7. Have gratitude for all that touches your life, for nothing is without purpose, and it is difficult to have gratitude and anger at the same time. Events may seem like a cruel joke of fate at times, but it's only because we cannot see the "big picture" or opposite side. So try to focus on the positive with everything. Make it an automatic response to find at least one benefit in every adversity. What you focus on and

dwell on in your mind is what multiplies. The same goes for negative people as well as negative events. In actuality, there really is nothing negative in life. You only temporarily perceive it as negative. So be grateful for everything, accepting and non-judgemental. It helps rid you of the harmful emotions that retard healing.

8. Opening the heart is the key; it's our purpose and reason for existence. So forgive yourself, forgive all of your past hurts. Begin to love yourself first like you never have before, and stop constantly looking for love from others. They can't give you all the love that you need. You must first accept yourself, then you can start loving others. There are no negatives, there is only love.

Last, keep vigilant for whether you are really committed to getting well. For many people, the only time in their lives when they got sufficient love and attention was when they were ill. Hence, they crave, albeit unknowingly, being ill, still seeking the much needed love that it used to bring. Once you catch yourself in this trick, you are free.

NEGATIVE ENERGIES

Throughout life, we encounter negative energies. You've experienced it when you've been around someone who makes you feel exhausted and drained afterwards. When you explore something like macrobiotics for healing, you'll bring a number of these negative energy people out of the woodwork, so you'll need to be prepared to protect yourself against them.

First try to understand where each person comes from. Some may just plain unconsciously not want you to get better. Your wellness does not fit into their lifestyle. Others do not want to be bothered with the extra thought and work involved in helping you. They like things the way they are, and your being ill fits in nicely. Try to stay as far away from this type as possible until you can eventually eliminate them entirely from your life. You don't need them.

For others, like some medical people, their ego is so fragile that if they don't know about something, they figure it must not be worth knowing. I was this way. They'll dogmatically assert that they need to at least see the published papers on macrobiotics, proving that it works. They'll insist that if it's so good, surely it's been published so that every doctor would know about it. But even when you offer books such as Mishio Kushi's The Book of Macrobiotics, or Elaine Nussbaum's Recovery, or Dr. Anthony Sattilaro's Recalled by Life, or Tired Or Toxic?, they do not read them. Nor do they talk with the scores of local people who have healed their own cancers and other conditions when medicine had given them up for terminal.

Some people will never be convinced even in the face of published studies, because it's not high-tech, it's not easy to learn, it doesn't heavily depend on physician involvement, nor does it glamourize, mystify and deify the physician and put him on a pedestal. I've actually seen people clear their cancers and then return to the doctor who gave them a maximum of three months to live. Here they were alive two years later and perfectly healthy, and the guy still didn't even want to talk to them about the diet. In having seen them do the impossible, the physician acted as though they had personally affronted him by daring to be alive. For these people, I must say, until medicine can show us something that has a better track record than macro, all that counts are the results. And any physician who belittles your progress in order to maintain his ego is never going to be interested in your health first.

A word about cancer treatment statistics is in order here, for when one carefully studies how they were obtained, you quickly realize you can give anything statistical verification if you manipulate the data enough. But that would entail a whole book to critique how cancer survival statistics can be manipulated to promote the chemotherapy/radiation/surgery business.

ORGANIZING THE DAY

So when you awaken, you'll want to start scrubbing and singing. You can fix one of your medicinal remedies like the shiitake/kombu remedy or your grated carrots/daikon with umeboshi and shoyu.

For work, you can take your sweet vegetable drink in a thermos for mid-morning pickup. You could walk outside in fresh air in place of a coffee break. At home try to have dinner when you arrive so there's no eating three hours before bed. Have a walk after dinner and a song and maybe one of your remedies. At bedtime, remember to snuggle in cottons and have plants that provide more oxygen to the air. Give thanks for all that you have to be thankful for and do your nighttime scrub. Some will have a hip bath or douche to do, while others will have a foot soak or compresses to do.

Do not use electric blankets or waterbeds and have as few electrical devices around you as possible when you sleep. Keep the T.V. time to a maximum of half an hour and physically stay as far away from it as possible when watching it. The same goes for computer time, as you are trying to decrease your amount of time in electromagnetic fields which also retard healing. At least when using the computer try to stay 30 inches away, rather than right on top of it. And beware that even when some items are "off," they still emit fields. For example, the T.V. tube has a warmer that is always on so when you turn the set on you don't have to wait a few minutes for the tube to warm up to show a picture.

NOT ENOUGH TIME

Macrobiotics has had remarkable results with many types of cancers and incurable conditions. Prostate, breast, leukemia and pancreatic cancers come quickly to mind as I have seen people with all of these clear their conditions. But many people with lethal diagnoses will not do macrobiotics. As one man said, "It's not covered by my insurance." In essence, there is an excuse for everything. If you want to bail out with excuses, bon voyage! There is never enough time in life for anything for anyone. I don't have enough time to be writing a book on healing when I prefer to be with my husband and when I myself am well.

Just ask yourself, "Am I the kind of person I would devote my whole life to becoming? Is my lifestyle conducive to my health? Is my life worth the 1-3 hours a day I need to spend to become healthier? Is my health worth restructuring my life to make room for the necessary health hours each day?" If not, why not double your working hours and finish yourself off quicker? Cut down on earth pollution.

-115-

Others will say, well I'll just hire a cook. But personally, I would not put my health in the hands of someone else. And since my health is intimately allied to my foods, I feel it would be foolish delegating such an important matter.

There are many ways you can learn to save time. Make use of telephone time while you're cooking and cleaning the kitchen. There are many people who need you. We all know people who could use a word of love or encouragement, enthusiasm or just someone checking in on them every few days by telephone to let them know that they are loved and cared for. But this telephone time eats up precious hours in the day. To maximize this love-giving time, get a speaker phone in the kitchen or a phone with a long enough cord to reach the refrigerator, stove and cutting board. Get a shoulder rest on it so that your hands will be completely free.

This provides an excellent time for your catch-up cooking:

This is a time to cook any grains that you might want to have for the next meal or a special different grain to add variety.

This is also a good time to soak any beans, seaweeds or dried roots.

This is a good time to make any condiments such as your gomashio (roasted sesame salt) or roasted pumpkin seeds or seaweed salts.

Make sure you have your vegetable bag ready to go with lots of cleaned vegetables in it.

Make sure your greeny bag is also ready.

Make your sweet vegetable drink for the next day (equal parts of pumpkin or hard winter squash, carrots, onions and daikon or cabbage.)

This is a good time to make your pressed salad (where you can use those little veggies that you may miss but are only recommended to have once a week, such as cucumber or celery).

This is a good time to make special remedies that may be prescribed for you such as ume/sho/kuzu, grated carrot/daikon or kombu/shiitake tea.

Last, but not least, this is a good time to make your soup stock. Bring out that extra bag in the refrigerator besides the veggie and greeny bags which we call the compost soup bag. Keep any vegetables in here that would be good to add to your soup stock, but that you would not actually include in your finished soup. For example, the core of a cabbage, tough broccoli stems or cauliflower cores or even clean cauliflower leaves, bok choy stems, celery leaves, parsley leaves or even the cobs of corn. These things have good nutrients that can be extracted from them through boiling and they produce a wonderfully nutritious soup stock, after you have discarded the vegetable matter. Add kombu as well.

Other time savers, of course, can be to cook double when you do beans so that you have other beans to be made into a vegetable dip for the rest of the family or a bean pate (see <u>Macro Mellow</u> for many of these recipes.) Also, why not have a night when you don't cook, but you eat with a macrobiotic friend and vice versa. This way, you will both learn more and have more fun. Likewise, try to get to the local macrobiotic or East/West Center periodically, as this will give you another night of reprieve as well as more creative ideas on food preparation, not to mention the companionship of those in various fascinating stages of healing. In fact, just observing how people eat may give you insight into what may be slowing their progress, or yours.

One last word regarding time: Many women nowadays work plus take care of the home which leaves them doing double duty. We have many male patients whose wives are unable or unwilling to learn macrobiotic cooking in order that their husbands can get well. What is the solution? You're right. The responsibility for wellness lies with the individual. There are no excuses. These men all do their own cooking. And these men include CEO's, physicians, dentists, engineers, salesmen, factory workers and college students. So whether you make over a million dollars a year or are living on borrowed money, when it comes down to health, we are all the same.

TRAVEL TIME

For traveling, you will want to try any of the following and there are many other ideas in the <u>Macro Mellow</u> book as well.

1. Grain/vegetable/bean miso soup in a thermos

2. Nori rolls, and carrot/cabbage rolls

3. Rice balls (rolled in gomashio, nori flakes or naked)

4. Grain-veggie scramble

5. Dinner leftovers in a sectioned T.V. dinner-style travel container.

In your suitcase you will want the following:

A hotplate (less than $20)

A covered metal pot

Lightweight plastic covered storage containers to hold grains while you are cooking your vegetables

Dish, preferrably non-breakable

Bowl

Spoon, fork or chopsticks

A Mac knife and a small cutting board

A hand-held grater

A vegetable peeler

A small colander

In the suitcase you'll also want to pack enough:

grains

greens   (hard greens like kale, or better yet, cabbage or
                kohlrabi travel better)

(forget the beans since they require another pot and long
cooking time, and you'll get enough protein eating out once
or twice anyway and you'll have fish that night.)

vegetables (above and below ground, like squashes, carrots,
                onions)

miso   (Put it in a small, covered container. Don't bring
                the whole tub.)

kuzu

umeboshi(especially good for reactions)

bancha tea bags (for "coffee breaks")

pressed salad in a jar (the salt will help preserve it, so you
                merely wash off portions as you use it)

nori sheets

fresh ginger root

And order ahead of time for a case of glass bottled spring water to be brought to your hotel.

The following is a list that can be used if you go on a long
vacation or camping. It includes all of the macrobiotic foods that you
will need for your healing phase. Just copy the list and store it in the
pantry or your suitcase so it's ready to be filled before you leave.
This list is for a long vacation where you will be setting up housekeeping for a few weeks. You can simplify it for shorter trips.

{Items in brackets are not for the first month of the strict healing phase}

Grains	Beans
Rice	Aduki
Millet	Chickpea
Barley	Lentil
Quinoa	Black soybean
Wheat berries	Dried tofu
{Oats}	
Amaranth	
{Buckwheat}	
Tempeh	

{Flours; whole wheat pastry, corn meal, rice, stone-ground un-enriched white, rolled oats}

Sea Vegetables	Condiments
Nori	Gomashio
Wakame	Umeboshi {vinegar}
Kombu	Umeboshi plums
Arame	
Hijiki	

Other

Miso	{amasake}
Pickles {like sauerkraut}	
	{sunflower oil}
Shoyu	{yinnie rice syrup}
Pumpkin seeds	{tahini}
Mochi	{tempeh}
Noodles {like soba or udon}	
Sea salt	
Bancha tea bags	
Shiitake	
Lotus root	
Kuzu	
Dried Daikon	

So with all my lecturing and traveling during the first 2 stricter years, how did I cook in my hotel room? Not very easily. But when you know your very existence counts on it, you find a way.

Usually start by bringing containers of cooked rice with go-mashio and vegetables (steamed carrots, cabbage and turnip with shoyu) to hold you over on the plane and first night in the hotel room. Then in the morning cook a fast grain like 50:50 buckwheat and quinoa, or teff, or amaranth. Have your pumpkin seeds (that you made at home) and that may suffice for breakfast.

If you are more energetic, boil some veggies like carrot, onion, cabbage, turnip, squash. Then dissolve 1-2 tsp. kuzu in water, add to the pot along with 1/2 tsp. shoyu and grated ginger juice and you have your veggies for breakfast and lunch. Be sure to bring another container to transfer your cooked grain into since you only have one pot. Likewise, you could transfer the vegetable stew and steam some grains or cook a seaweed. I usually try to get lunch all ready before I leave for the morning, since there is often not enough time at the meetings to both cook and eat at lunch time.

If you can't handle all of this, make it easier. Do the hot water/grain in thermos recipe for lunch (merely mix boiling water and grain in thermos and in a few hours it is ready). Or you could have some grain/bean/veggie soup in hot sterile canning jars at home and just heat and serve. Whatever you do, do not be discouraged that you will spend extra time at home cooking before you leave, or in your room when you arrive. Everyone else is having more social time because they are buying their meals. But you are always free to do that and get worse. Again, it takes planning and dedication. You know you will need to clean and prepare veggies sometime, so it may as well be before bed rather than rushing in the morning. And when you walk out the door, proud of what you have accomplished, be it ever so little, don't forget a bancha or mu tea bag for "coffee break."

WHO WILL FILL THE NEED?

Eventually there will be a point where enough of us can approach a health food store, a sandwich shop or restaurant and let them know that there is enough interest in patronizing their establishment if they could provide some macrobiotic relief. Let them know that even if they could have some macrobiotic foods or meals once or twice a week, that would be very helpful to you. You could call the local television and radio to alert them of this novelty, and get some free advertising as well. After all, the more we let our needs be known, the more that people who are in the business of making money by supplying these needs will materialize. And the more successful they become, the easier it will be for us.

They could start by offering some unadulterated, healing phase foods and then dress them up further for the family that is on the transition diet. For example, undressed, cooked chickpeas with parsley garnish for yourself, or they could be put into a miso soup. They could be made into hummus as a vegetable or organic corn chip dip for the rest of the family. You get the idea.

HEALING	FAMILY
undressed chickpeas	hummus w/sliced raw vegetables or organic corn chips
lentils w/carrot, celery, onion, kombu	lentil pate (see Macro Mellow for recipe)
aduki/squash/kombu	they might like this as is or blend it and add kombu or vegetable stock and miso and make a soup
nori rolls (for the next day's lunch)	knishes (escellent for trips)
steamed vegetables	can add spices, sauces, butter and "forbidden" veggies
whole grain like brown rice	can be jazzed up with sauteed vegetables, dried fruits, nuts or sauces
pressed salad	salad dressing can be added
soups	heavy cream, tomato sauce, and/or wine can be added after blending the soup

fish, poached in kombu water with grated ginger juice, shoyu and lime	fish, poached in water, wine, milk, broth or stock with herbs

With these foods available from "take out," you could quickly steam your own greens for 2 minutes if you brought this home and add a baked chicken and squash for the rest of the crew.

Or one of your group could even offer to be the macrobiotic cook for one night a week in the restaurant. Offer a 'Macro Night' and get T.V. and radio promotion and see what happens. Pick a night when the restaurant business is usually slow and when they would appreciate more patronage like Wednesdays or Mondays. I'm sure you can come up with more ideas to stave off the tedium of preparing 21 meals per week.

The bottom line is, it can be and has been and will continue to be done, by those who possess the will to live. Your imagination is as boundless as your energy will be when you eat cleaner and more balanced. It took many of us years to become sick, and then several years to become well. What I have learned through meeting or being directly involved with hundreds of these people, I hope to pass on to you. Then you don't have to reinvent the wheel and can best use your talents and energies in actively adding to the foundations presented here, not to mention adding to your other endeavors.

DON'T FRET! IT'S NOT GOOD FOR THE IMMUNE SYSTEM

When things get ahead of you, calamities arise or you're feeling sorry for yourself, go easy. Rather than destroy weeks or months of work in getting your body detoxed, just back off. Just because you can't get it all together for a few days is no excuse for loading fat and chemicals back into the cell fat storage vacuoles and the detox endoplasmic reticulum. Avoid using a calamity as an excuse to completely blow it by taking a step backward in time. Some indiscretions can wipe out a month of work. Also anxiety, guilt, worry and anger are not good for the immune system.

Get a grip and see what you can handle. Keep it very simple. Do not even attempt elaborate or complex cooking unless the cooking is an escape mechanism for you. Can you just steam some greens with your grain each meal? Or as long as you have to make your grain, why not clean out the refrigerator and make a big soup. Broccoli, cabbage, onion, carrot, sea vegetables, turnips or other vegetables you don't like can be hidden in here. Bring to a boil, and simmer 30-45 minutes. Blend and put in a sterile glass jar in the refrigerator. When you're hungry, simmer in 1/2-1 tsp. of miso in as you heat your individual portion. Avoid storing miso, but instead always add it fresh and simmer in just before serving. If the rest of the family will be sharing this soup, to their pot you could add salt and pepper and heavy cream and/or tomato sauce to jazz it up for adulterated tastes. That and some French bread and a salad might satiate them. More on how to feed the rest of the family in Macro Mellow.

Needless to say, if you have too many of these incomplete or unbalanced meals, you should protect yourself and speed up your progress by having your nutrient (vitamin, mineral, amino acid, fatty acid) levels checked more frequently. And guard against a narrow and monotonous diet for too long as it will invariably foster deficiencies. As you get more organized, you should get more cleaned out. Then you should gradually be able to weather the calamities more calmly and keep your own schedule more together.

Remember, if you don't have time to feed yourself correctly, is anything else worth it? If you use the martyr's excuse ("I'm doing it for the others"), that doesn't hold. After all, if you really love them, you'll give them a gift of the cheeriest, healthiest and most vivacious YOU possible, and that means free of symptoms.

Some will be aghast that we recommend running the soup through the blender, because of the harmful electromagnetic fields. However, worrying about vibrational energies is a bit much for the person new to macrobiotics to handle, especially when they are paddling as fast as they can to keep afloat. Yes, they are a factor, but when compared with whether you're going to have an ice cream or a blended soup, there is no contest.

While we're at it, many will say, "Well, why can't I put garlic in," or "What's wrong with bread or an occasional steak?" Nothing, when you're healthy. All we're attempting here is to spell out how people have achieved the impossible. There are biochemical explanations on how it works, but the hooker is, this was described <u>before</u> the science was ever done! There is something here far greater than our current knowledge, so until we can come up with something better, I would suggest we not muck it up until we achieve the results we want.

Some have expressed anxiety over the macrobiotic diet because they thought it was a religious cult or that it was non-Christian. Please embrace your own religion with all your heart while you enjoy the many facets of macrobiotic healing, which are really just good common sense, and living compatibly with nature. Instead of paying money to go to a health club, you work in your garden and grow chemically cleaner food than you could get in the grocer, as an example. There is no cult or religion associated with this practical approach to the chronic diseases of modern society.

PLAYING WITH A FULL DECK

One more facet beyond the diet is nutrition. In earlier days, it was easier for macro to be successful because people had better nutrient levels. Now with the plethora of processed foods, depleted soils, the government constantly battling to lower the daily nutrient standards of normal, and the constant overwork and nutrient depletion of our detox systems, levels are lower than ever.

Some will possibly never clear without first being able to play with a full deck of nutrients. Some need a nutrient correction first to live long enough to allow macro to heal them. Others may have seemingly minor medical problems which resist clearing, for lack of nutrient repleteness. Let's look at some examples of common medical problems that actually stem from nutrient levels and are being incorrectly approached in "modern" medicine.

THE CHOLESTEROL HOAX

You finally had your fasting cholesterol checked, and as you suspected, it was over 200 mg/dl. You have joined the ranks of the high cholesterol generation and are at high risk of early heart attack, high blood pressure, stroke, and a host of other degenerative diseases.

The next step is a visit to your doctor who tells you to stop eating all your favorite foods: eggs, butter, bacon, cheese, milk, cream sauces, and much more. Instead, you should switch to margarines, corn oil, artificial eggs and bacon, and a host of other "plastic" foods. If that fails to control it, do not worry, for there are prescription medications or drugs that will inhibit the absorption of cholesterol from the gut. What he does not tell you is that this treatment, although it makes your blood cholesterol test look normal, is actually so unhealthy for you that it actually accelerates degenerative disease. In other words, it speeds up the time in which you will get a worse disease. It could be anything: a bad back that does not respond to medication, hypertension, depression, arthritis, an early heart attack, headaches, or just plain accelerated aging or chronic fatigue.

The reason is that he has not sought the cause and corrected it; he has merely masked the symptom of faulty metabolism so that whatever is broken in the chemistry will proceed to worsen and eventually involve other organs. For the most common cause of high blood cholesterol is inability of the body to process or metabolize cholesterol. That is why some people can eat unlimited amounts of the "bad" foods and never have a problem. They are playing with a full deck of nutrients and can turn that cholesterol into good things like testosterone (male hormone), adrenal hormone (the stress hormone), myelin (the lining of nerves), and membranes of brain and other crucial cells; cholesterol is absolutely necessary for the maintenance of these. Now you can begin to appreciate why a diet low in cholesterol can be so deleterious to your health. It can lead to impotence, fatigue, depression and much more.

So what inhibits the body from metabolizing cholesterol properly? A deficiency of any of a number of minerals like chromium, copper, magnesium, manganese, and more. Unfortunately most Americans are no longer playing with a full deck of nutrients (vitamins, minerals, amino acids and essential fatty acids) because they have been removed from most foods so that they will last longer on our shelves. Look at the items in your pantry that last for ages. They are practically bug-proof. But if the bugs don't want them, why should you? As well, vitamins like B6 and E have been destroyed or reduced by processing, but these are crucial for delaying the processes that lead to cancer, heart attacks, and other diseases.

So the solution to high cholesterol is to have your doctor draw blood tests that show why you cannot metabolize your cholesterol. An RBC selenium, zinc, copper, and chromium are a good start. But be sure he requests red blood cell levels (RBC), not worthless serum or plasma levels. Vitamins B1, B6, E and urine magnesium loading tests are also indicated. As for the plastic foods, they also lack these precious nutrients. That is why the sick get sicker. And if you eat a diet stripped of cholesterol, how are you going to make testosterone or (adrenal) stress hormone? Furthermore, the corn oil and margarines have been exposed to temperatures in excess of 1000 degrees in their processing. This makes the molecules twist and become what we call "trans" forms: these actually promote arteriosclerosis.

Obviously medicine has now entered the era of molecular medicine, where the environmental trigger and biochemical defect for many diseases can be found. No longer is a headache a Darvon deficiency. And no longer is hypercholesterolemia a deficiency of drugs and plastic foods.

But when you eat a diet that is predominantly whole grains (like brown rice, millet, barley, whole oats, etc.) and vegetables, you get many more minerals and vitamins than you can from the standard American diet or any vitamin pills. Then you have the machinery working in prime order and it can accept and utilize the cholesterol it needs. For the body is a lot like a car. When the red light goes on, you could ignore it (take pills), smash it with a hammer (surgery), or put oil in (treat the cause). And the quality of oil is no small factor if it's a car you cherish and plan to use for a lifetime.

Modern medicine is full of blunders these days, but they are ever so slowly being exposed. For example, an August 1990 issue of the New England Journal of Medicine finally did an article showing what we began writing about in 1985. That is, that because of trans fatty acids, processed foods with hydrogenated oils, corn oils and corn oil margarines (all recommended today by cardiologists) are worse for your heart than a juicy steak.

In addition, other researchers have shown that groups of patients taking expensive ($1,000-$3,000 a year per person) drugs to lower cholesterol (Questran, Mevacor, Lopid, etc.) do not live any longer nor do they have lower heart attack rates. In other words, doctors follow cholesterol blood levels thinking it's a marker for longevity and cardiac risk because it's easy and doesn't require the sophisticated biochemical knowledge required to interpret and correct nutrient deficiencies.

For more information and scientific references read <u>Tired Or Toxic?</u> and <u>Dr. Dean Ornish's Program for Reversing Heart Disease. The Only System Scientifically Proven to Reverse Heart Disease Without Drugs or Surgery</u> by Dean Ornish, MD, Random House Publishers, NY, 1990. Actually, for those who have serious disease, but who fear they could not do macro, they should consider Dr. Ornish's program. However, having read our 5 books, you will quickly appreciate several points.

Ornish's program is a wonderful giant step into nutritional medicine and has paved the way for many who needed further scientific proof. But as you can see, when compared with the macrobiotic approach, there is no contest:

(1) The Ornish program allows more oil (10%) than macro, so the reversal is not as quick as it could be.

(2) It is equally as difficult a diet, so the effort may as well go into the full throttle program, macrobiotics, especially if time is not on your side.

(3) Ornish allows "plastic" processed foods that promote free radicals, like Butter Buds, egg substitutes, non-stick oil sprays for coating baking pans, and chemical sugar substitutes. Also he fails to stress organic foods. It would be interesting to see if range-fed organic eggs give the cholesterol rise that commercial eggs do. We already know range-fed beef have lower levels of trans fatty acids than commercially raised ones. They are different chemically since the latter have

been reared on antibiotics and chemicals, and restricted in terms of exercise all of their lives.

(4) Ornish allows partitioned (not whole) foods that can jeopardize the body's nutrient balance. Foods recommended were commercial phyllo dough, packaged sauces, boxed cereals, all-purpose (bleached) flour, non-fat milk, fruit juices, egg whites, imported specialty ethnic foods, non-fat yogurt, etc.

(5) Ornish may find a high level of arthritis emerge with all the nightshades allowed: chili peppers, tomatos, potatoes, peppers, eggplant.

(6) He may also find a high degree of adult acne and eczema from the high vinegar, fruit, fruit juice, raisin, cayenne, Jalapeno and lemon recommendations, or severe aggresion and anger from vinegars.

(7) Even though the principles of macro have been used, not one mention of or credit to macrobiotics was given. Miso, soy sauce, tofu, mirin, tempeh, seitan, hijiki, tamari, even nori are in some of the recipes. Unfortunately, so are Teflon coated pans (you gradually eat the coating) and microwaved food, and there is no warning about aluminum cookware, or aluminum in salt and baking powders, etc.

(8) Ornish, a Texan, recommends a very hot, spicy, expansive or yin diet. His patient group seems to have been mostly white collar workers from California. I wonder how Northern snowbelt husky blue collar workers will fare on this fare? Will they become airheads or very depressed and suicidal, or just plain overwhelmed by cravings?

(9) The most glaring omission is lack of nutritional biochemistry assessments. But he is not alone, as the Journal of the American Medical Association (June 13, 1990) showed 90% of the doctors never ordered a magnesium test on over 500 hospitalized patients who were deficient. If a guy is having coronary artery spasm because of a magnesium deficiency, it takes many months or years of brown rice to correct what could be turned off in hours or days. Likewise, copper deficiency, induced high cholesterol may take years to correct with diet, versus months on supplements. And there is no mention of the fact that potassium assays are useless unless RBC potassium is used and likewise, that a loading test is necessary for magnesium assessment since even the RBC assay misses over a third of those low. (For

details see Rogers, SA, Magnesium deficiency masquerades as multiple diverse symptoms. Intern. Clin. Nutr. Rev., 11:3, July 1991.) Furthermore, it is a rare individual with cardiovascular disease of any form to have all of his biochemistry intact.

(10) Most importantly, Dr. Ornish totally ignores the environment as a contributory cause of cardiac disease. Disease is a combination of 6 factors: genetics, diet, nutritional status, psyche (i.e. meditation), lifestyle (i.e. exercise), and environment. He addresses only half of the total load. Just as cholesterol causes damage in blood vessel walls, so do the 400 chemicals we breathe at home and work everyday. These can cause even more potent free radical induced damage and deterioration in blood vessel walls than cholesterol does. The scientific literature is replete with references on how trichloroethylene or toluene, for example, can cause cardiac arrhythmia. And these commonly outgas from dry cleaned suits, carpet and furniture adhesives as well as construction materials in nearly every home and office (references and biochemical mechanisms in Tired Or Toxic?). We have hundreds of patients who had cardiac arrhythmia from xenobiotics. Likewise, food allergy can present with the heart as the allergic target organ.

I recall dining one late evening, after we had been teaching all day, with Drs. Bill Rea and Theron "Ted" Randolph. At that point, Ted was 80 and he related to us that he had just started having cardiac arrhythmia a few months prior. As the founder of chemical ecology, he first went on the rare food diet and found corn, in the slightest amount was the cause. Of course it is ubiquitous as a sweetener, a flour, in alcoholic drinks, a thickener, etc. If he had gone to a cardiologist they would have tried to drug him. And as you may well know, probably killed him, (1) by not identifying the cause, and (2) by giving an 80 year old heart drugs he didn't need. For all the drugs to curb arrhythmias have as their side effects, the potential to also trigger arrhythmias.

But by making sure he eliminated the corn antigen in every source, Ted was free of arrhythmia...and that was several years ago and he is still practicing.

(11) Anyone doing Ornish's diet should have B12 levels drawn if they have lactase deficiency and can't tolerate the recommended yogurt

and 2% milk. If they do take the general vitamins then they had better check an RBC copper, RBC chromium, RBC zinc and magnesium loading test, because most general products are so unbalanced that they further jeopardize the ratios of these minerals. It is unbelievable to me that he has done such a superlative job in one sense with this 600 page excellent book on heart disease, but in the index the words vitamin, homocysteine, magnesium, calcification, detoxication, free radicals, trans fatty acids and minerals do not appear. Biochemical disturbances relating to these are the basis of the patho-physiology of arteriosclerosis and the appropriate assessment of mineral, vitamin, amino acid and essential fatty acid levels, glutathione, and lipid peroxides are infinitely more useful than, say cholesterol levels.

(12) Likewise, there is the failure to appreciate that salt hardens the fats and makes their release from tissues that much slower, as well as several other omissions.

(13) Or how can you have a book about heart disease and heart failure without mentioning testing for taurine and magnesium. The correction of both deficiencies is discussed in many books (Huxtable and Barbeau's <u>Taurine</u>, Seelig and Altura's wonderful books on the cardiovascular effects and rampant undiagnosed deficiencies of magnesium) with regard to their being simple, inexpensive solutions to a problem that otherwise would lead to drugs and surgery. You'll recall, from our other works, the U.S. government reports the average diet provides only 40% of the daily need of magnesium. Yet a deficiency can cause fatal arrhythmia or sudden death by heart attack.

(14) Failure to mention flax oil as the richest source of omega-3 oils (that help decrease rates of cancer, heart and other diseases).

But I won't belabor these, for my goal is not to critique this work, because obviously if I did not have such regard for it, I would not have even mentioned it. For I suspect and hope that it will receive a great deal of deserved attention. So I want to address some of the concerns that the informed macrobiotic person might raise in view of the biochemical evidence that he is aware of from our earlier works.

If you are going to do either program, they require such major lifestyle adjustments that you cannot have too many facts.

So all in all, we owe Dr. Dean Ornish a wealth of appreciation for his tremendous work. His program is a mega-leap for the average doctor and patient, carrying us away from drug-oriented medicine. But if time is not on your side and you need to get well faster and reverse your deterioration the quickest possible, please do the macrobiotics strict healing phase as well as assess all your nutrients and environmental total load. But if all of this is too much at this point, at least fall back onto his program. In fact, it's so great that I recommend you read it regardless of your chosen course.

He also exposed the studies which show that the ideal cholesterol should be 150-180, not 200 as is commonly recommended. So in spite of being very weak in macrobiotics, environmental medicine and nutritional biochemistry, this is still an excellent book that all should read. It marks the furthest point to which conventional medicine has advanced in the current evolution of environmental/nutritional/molecular medicine. And he has advanced the progress of medicine in many other ways.

He has made people aware of the dangers of hydrogenated oils hidden in breads and packaged foods and the dangers of falling for food labels like "low cholesterol" or "no cholesterol" when the foods actually cause more arteriosclerosis than cholesterol does.

Another great service that Ornish's book provided was in demonstrating to people through the case histories that a little bit of chest pain or shortness of breath is an end-stage phenomenon, not early stage. In other words, by the time there is a "minor" symptom, there can be 98% occlusion (plugging or closure) of the major arteries of the heart. This explains why so many die with their first heart attack. And among those who survive their first heart attack, 40% do not even know they had any heart trouble. For others, they have ignored the very subtle or mild warning signals. Remember, there has to be a dangerous amount of occlusion of a vessel before there is any symptom whatsoever. And then there is the unlucky person for whom the silent or painless heart attack occurs. He gets no warning.

Lastly, does it sound too histrionic of Mr. Kushi to say such things as one egg can reverse the progress? Or one piece of candy or one bite of cheese? And look at how some have bad symptoms from prematurely trying meat. But it is easy to understand if you look at the cholesterol and fat content of foods presented in his book.

Remember, the standard American diet has an average of 500 mg. of cholesterol a day. Ornish in his <u>Lancet</u> study allowed 5 mg. cholesterol a day. Macrobiotics is even lower.

But one chocolate chip cookie has 5 mg., while one pat of butter has 12mg. cholesterol. One ounce of cheddar cheese has 30 mg. One 6 ounce steak has 156 mg., and one egg has 274 mg. And if you really want to kill yourself, one cup of whipped cream (hidden in many foods, especially desserts) is 326 mg. of cholesterol.

So 5 mg., the amount one has to limit to daily to get a small amount of reversal of coronary blockage over one year can be exceeded with one paltry pat of butter. Whereas one steak is a month's allotment. It sets you way back and wipes out months of work.

Meanwhile, Dr. Ornish has shown a diet and lifestyle change that reversed arteriosclerosis. Even in cases that had bypass surgery and balloon angioplasty and cholesterol-lowering drugs and the cholesterol plaques still kept building, he was able with the program to reverse the disease and reduce the arterial deposits.

The evidence is now complete. Multiple studies show the dismal facts of how the American public has been lead down the garden path by the drug industry.

Just look at some of the gruesome statistics from Dr. Ornish's book (scientific references in the book).

* 40 million Americans have diagnosed cardiovascular disease.

* 60 million Americans have high blood pressure and 40% over 50 years old have high blood pressure.

* 80 million Americans have high cholesterol.

* 1 1/2 million Americans have a heart attack each year. For 1/3 of these people, the heart attack was their first indication that they had a problem.

* The American Heart Association and National Institutes of Health have rejected medical articles like Ornish's giving the reason that it is impossible to reverse heart disease without drugs or surgery. Of course the diet they recommend is 30% fat!

* Insurance companies pay about $30,000 for bypass surgery, $7,500 for balloon angioplasty and 0-$150 for a year long program to teach people how to reverse their disease by (methods other than drugs and surgery) diet.

* A 1987 study of 200,000 patients who had bypass surgery that year, was published in the Journal of the American Medical Association. It showed that 25% of bypass surgery recipients did not need it.

* 1/3 who had angioplasty will reclog the opened arteries in 4-6 months.

* A $170 million National Heart, Lung and Blood Institute study showed that by taking cholesterol lowering drugs, one decreased the chance of a heart attack by only 1%, but increased the chance of violent or accidental death to above normal.

* In another study, 43,000 patients on blood pressure medication did not have a decreased heart attack rate.

* In another famous study, the group to take medications for high blood pressure and high cholesterol had double the rate of heart disease.

* All drugs to treat arrhythmia also can cause arrhythmia.

* The cut-off for cholesterol is in error. The level that we should seek is less than 150 milligrams. Stamler studied 350,000 people ages 35-55 years old. If the blood cholesterol was 182-202 mg., (considered great today), they have 29% (over 1 in 4) chance of dying from a heart attack. If it was 203-220 mg., a 73% chance, if 221-244 mg., a 121% chance and over 245 mg., a 242% chance.

* Lastly, stress has an adverse effect on arteriosclerosis in that it makes the blood vessel wall store fat more easily (Kaplan showed

stress increased the arterial wall permeability to cholesterol).

* And the most commonly stressful feeling is that of isolation; not feeling loved or respected, and leads to illness. Ironically, there is a paradox here in that as some work to become worthy of others' recognition, love or respect, they work so hard to become special that it makes them more different, thus further setting them apart and isolating them. If they do become successful, the jealousy, envy and resentment perpetuate their isolation.

THE SOLUTION: Eat right to correct your arteriosclerosis, meditate to realize your own unique self-worth, and spread your love among your ever expanding network of friends.

CALCIUM THE KILLER

Hard to believe, but unfortunately true. The way in which many are supplementing their calcium is killing them. They are actually accelerating the arteriosclerotic process. They are speeding up the aging process as well as the occurrence of the many degenerative diseases that accompany it like hypertension, diabetes, heart disease, arthritis, early heart attacks, liver, kidney and heart failure, and yes, don't forget cancer.

"How can this be? I thought we all needed extra calcium to stave off osteoporosis," you say. Unfortunately, we forgot to stop and figure out why people get osteoporotic. But first you need to understand what osteoporosis is.

Calcium and other precious minerals are normally absorbed from our foods and incorporated into the bones. However if any of the minerals like magnesium, boron, zinc, manganese, etc. are missing, the calcium does not get put into the bone. When the bone is deficient in calcium, we have osteoporosis, or weak bones that can fracture so easily that they do so even without a fall, or as we say, spontaneously. Or the bone can slowly collapse or shrink over time, leaving a shorter person in its wake, often with a great deal of bone pain. One of the first bones to show signs of osteoporosis is the jaw bone; this results in the shifting of teeth and eventual premature loss of bone and the teeth it supports.

And so what happens when one is deficient enough in trace minerals to cause osteoporosis and takes extra calcium in attempt to correct the problem? The extra calcium, still not accompanied by the missing trace minerals that allow it to be laid down in the bone has to find a home somewhere else. And it does find a home. It picks areas that are already weak. The weak areas that need this emergency patch of calcium got this way from a combination of effects of inferior diet, undiscovered nutrient deficiencies and chemicals in the bloodstream from everyday homes and offices. The extra calcium lays down in these areas of weakness or inflammation where the body wishes to put a patch to repair chemical damage and stop a leak, namely in the blood vessels of the heart and brain. We call this calcification or patching of blood vessels arteriosclerosis.

Since the government has published the fact that it is estimated that the average American diet supplies only 40% of the recommended daily amount of magnesium, this makes it rather likely that the average person taking calcium will be contributing to his arteriosclerosis rather than to his bones, since he doesn't have enough magnesium to enable the calcium to be put in the bone. Osteoporosis occurs for any of five reasons. Either the person does not ingest enough calcium, he cannot absorb it well, he cannot incorporate it into the bone, he gets rid of too much calcium in the urine, or he actually pulls it out of the bone. Let's look at some common factors that contribute to each of those reasons for osteoporosis.

First, many processed foods do not contain enough calcium. Did you know that 2 cups of greens contain more calcium than even a glass of milk? Plus the greens also have the correct ratio of other minerals so the calcium can actually be incorporated into the bone. In terms of absorbing calcium, medications like antacids, Tagamet or Zantac (ranitidine) are prescribed to decrease the acid in the stomach. But low stomach acid cuts down on the ionization of calcium so that less is absorbed. More importantly, phosphates in processed foods markedly inhibit the absorption of calcium. Where are phosphates found? Hidden in nearly every processed food that comes in a bag, jar, can or box. They are often not even on the label or are disguised as unrecognizable names. They are buffers, stabilizers, inhibitors of phase separation, dough conditioners, acidifiers and much more.

They are particularly high, for example, in soft drinks.

You already know that most people are low in magnesium, in fact leading magnesium authorities suggest that it is such an unrecognized problem that 80% of the population is deficient. And that's not all they are low in. Many are low in zinc, boron, copper, manganese, and many other trace minerals. Why? Because processing of foods to extend their shelf lives removes these minerals. Often the soils on which the foods are grown are also depleted of some of these minerals, and this leads to a further decline.

Some medications can cause the loss of calcium in the urine, like diuretics or high doses of vitamin C. But how do we pull calcium out of the bone once it has already been put there? Calcium is one of the major buffers of the blood. So when the blood gets too acid and has to be buffered, the body steals calcium from the bone to do it. How does the body get too acid? One way is to eat a diet high in meat (amino acids), soft drinks, fruits and sugars.

So a person who likes a lot of meat, eats processed foods or eats out frequently, has a number of soft drinks each day, or takes medications for indigestion and high blood pressure is at a high risk for osteoporosis; and no amount of merely taking calcium is going to help him. In fact it will help him add to his troubles by calcifying his vessels and speeding his development of arteriosclerosis. This could lead to coronary artery disease, senility, hypertension and more.

So how does one stave off osteoporosis? First you need a nutritionally trained physician who will do a magnesium loading test (Rogers, Int. Clin. Nutr. Rev., July 1991) to see if you have enough magnesium to put the calcium in the bone instead of the arteries. This urine test is necessary, because there is no blood test that can rule out a magnesium deficiency at this point in time. He will also check other minerals like an RBC or erythrocyte zinc (again, because a serum zinc test is inadequate for diagnosis), RBC copper, RBC manganese, and other vitamins (like D3 and B6) and minerals commonly found low in the average person and necessary for incorporation of calcium in the bone. A 24 hour urinary calcium loading test may also be needed, and sometimes a dual-photon densitometry. Once your nutrient deficiencies have been identified and corrected, you want to be sure that you will remain in balance and playing with a full deck.

The best way to do this is by eating as organic or chemically less-contaminated foods as possible. And more importantly you want to eat as nutritionally dense foods as possible; in other words, foods that give you the highest nutrient yield (vitamins, minerals, amino acids and essential fatty acids). This is accomplished by eating whole grains and vegetables as the predominant part of your daily meals, with great variety of foods and cooking styles used throughout the week. A macrobiotic diet fills this bill beautifully.

Remember 2 cups of greens give you as much calcium as a glass of milk. Plus you get the added benefit of the other minerals like magnesium, boron, manganese, zinc, etc. that are needed to make sure you lay that calcium down in the bone. Whereas with fatty cheese, or vitamin D enriched homogenized milk, the calcium is more likely to be laid down in the coronary blood vessels or the brain vessels, leading to early heart attack or senility.

So whatever you do, don't let someone sell you the idea that you just need to take calcium and your worries are over. For with calcium as the instigator of degenerative disease, your problems will be just beginning. Remember, when calcium lacks all the companion minerals, it surrenders and lays down in vessels to plug and calcify or harden them: hence, hardening of the arteries. (For more information on how calcium contributes to the degenerative diseases of aging and what tests your physician should order, read Tired Or Toxic?)

THE PSYCHO-NEURO-IMMUNE CONNECTION

All this big fancy word means is what you and your grandmother have known for years: YOU ARE WHAT YOU THINK! And you are doomed for failure if you do not embrace your new challenge with enthusiasm and optimism. The mind has far greater powers over the entire body than we know.

You can change your heart rate, contractile force, autonomic nervous system control your sweating, blood pressure, fainting and much more. There are certain things I could say to you that could trigger those responses and I wouldn't have to touch you or inject you. You have the power to do it to yourself, actually.

Our thoughts, emotions, reactions, feelings and moods are merely chemical reactions that we have created by our thoughts. Medications like mood elevators (anti-depressants) and tranquilizers can alter this chemistry. And mood chemistry can react abnormally if you are missing specific vitamins, minerals, amino acids, hormones, essential fatty acids or neurotransmitter precursors. If you can't get yourself into a happy enough frame of mind to do the diet, don't overlook investigating your brain chemistry. The impetus to make your health better may be lacking because you are missing specific nutrients in the brain necessary to make one feel energetic and creative, and to synthesize the "happy hormones" of the brain.

Also look for brain allergies (Tired Or Toxic?). And also don't overlook the need to re-evaluate how you perceive the world, as well as how supportive your private world is or is not.

What are your top three priorities in life? For this year? For this month? Why? Do they need re-evaluating? Do you have a solid plan for attaining them? If you want to try to get more out of yourself and your life, read Anthony Robbins' Unlimited Power (Ballantine Books, Fawcett Columbine, NY 1986).

Because the body-mind connection is so important, it will have to be the subject of a next book. I apologetically short change it in this volume only because of the demand for a shorter "how-to" book on the actual mechanics of the diet. But make no mistake, that *real healing* involves much more than just diet and body mechanics. I repeat: Macrobiotics is not just a diet. The general attitude or mind-set, including mind exercise and practice, lifestyle changes, gratitude, physical exercise and other body work and much more must be not only factored in but balanced into your life. Environmental assessments of hidden food, mold, Candida, EMF and chemical sensitivities as well as environmental controls and nutritional biochemical corrections are some of the other integral ingredients. There is a wealth of evidence how each is able to overpower the other and that working in harmony can bring untold wellness.

CHAPTER 5

<u>CONSULTATION QUESTIONNAIRE</u>

      Make a copy of, fill out, and bring with you to your consultations with the Physician of your choice, the following sheets (for subsequent consultations you can merely copy page 1 if there are no additions).

Name:_____ Date:_____

Family Doctor:_____ _____

Check one: 1st consultation_____ Subsequent consultation_____

Condition:_____ _____

_____ _____

_____ _____

<u>6 Worst Symptoms Initially</u>	<u>Duration of Symptoms (years)</u>
1._____	_____
2._____	_____
3._____	_____
4._____	_____
5._____	_____
6._____	_____

Prior evaluations for your condition:

	Doctor's Name	Year	Specialty	Type of Treatment	Did it Help?
1.	_____			_____	_____
	_____			_____	_____
2.	_____			_____	_____
	_____			_____	_____
3.	_____			_____	_____
	_____			_____	_____
4.	_____			_____	_____
	_____			_____	_____
5.	_____			_____	_____
	_____			_____	_____
6.	_____			_____	_____

Use extra paper if needed anywhere in this questionnaire.

Indicate food intolerances and specific symptoms that eating this food causes:

	Food	Symptom
1.	_____	_____
2.	_____	_____
3.	_____	_____

4._____ _____

5._____ _____

6._____ _____

Recommended foods for your use will be indicated.

Date of consultation:_____.

_____Grains- brown rice, millet, barley, quinoa, amaranth, buck-
    wheat, corn, wheat, rye, oats, other

_____Other grains or grain substitutes-tapioca, squash, broken grain,
    tempeh, other

_____Cook with water in proportion of_____

Frequency:_____ Crackers, pancakes, muffins, rice,
                            cakes, popcorn , mochi

            _____ Sourdough, unyeasted, whole wheat
                            or rye bread, steamed

            _____ Whole-wheat (udon) noodles and vege-
                            table broth

            _____ Buckwheat (soba) noodles and vegeta-
                            ble broth

            _____ Special

            _____ Other

Vegetables:_____ Raw salad

_____ Pressed salad

_____ Steamed

_____ Boiled

_____ Blanched

_____ Water sauteed

_____ Sauteed (tempura) with sesame oil

_____ Special

_____ Other

GREENS	ABOVE GROUND	BELOW GROUND
Collards	Hard squash	Turnips
Kale	Pumpkin	Onions
Dandelion	Brussel Sprouts	Carrots
Mustard	Cabbage (red or green)	Parsnips
Parsley	Cauliflower	Daikon
Bok choy	Kohlrabi	Ginger
Chinese cabbage	Corn on the cob	Radish
Lotus root		Leeks

DRIED

Daikon
Tofu
Lotus (balls) seeds
Chestnuts
Shiitake mushrooms

Beans:_____ Tofu

_____ Aduki

_____ Lentil

_____ Chickpea

_____ Black soybean

_____ Special

_____ Other (pinto, navy, marrow, great
                     northern, cranberry,
                     mung, turtle, split pea, lima)

Sea vegetable:_____ Nori

_____ Arame, hijiki, 1/4-1/2 cup
                     _____ times/week

_____ Wakame, kombu, daily in soup, grain,
                     vegetable/beans
                     Maximum
                     amount_____

_____ Special

_____ Other (sea palm, kelp, dulse)

Condiments/seeds:_____ Umeboshi plum

_____ Gomashio/salt ratio 1:16, 1:18, 1:20, oth-
                     er (1 tsp. salt or less per cup
                     seeds)

_____ Tekka, maximum
                     amount_____

_____ Sunflower, limit_____

_____ Pumpkin, limit_____

_____ Shiso leaf powder

_____ Sea vegetable powder

_____ Special

_____ Other

Seasoning/ferments:

_____ Miso: barley (mugi), soybean (hato),
                     chickpea

_____ Johsen shoyu

_____ Tamari

_____ Unrefined white sea salt

_____ Shiitake mushroom

_____ Ginger, horseradish, garlic

_____ Mirin, umeboshi vinegar, rice wine
                     vinegar

_____ Tekka

_____ Lemon

_____ Kuzu (kudzu)

_____ Pickles, 1 tbsp. a day

_____ Umeboshi vinegar

_____ Sauerkraut, (salt washed off)
                           maximum amount_____

_____ Quick tamari pickles

_____ Other

Fish:_____ White: cod, flounder, scrod, sole, snap-
                           per, smelt, trout)

_____ Special

_____ Other

Fruit:_____ Cooked (apple, pear, blueberry,
                           cherry, peach, plum, strawber-
                           ry, raspberry, melon)

_____ Dried (raisin, apple, pear, peach, prune,
                           currant, apricot)

_____ Fresh

_____ Other

Nuts:_____ Almond, chestnuts

_____ Nut butters (tahini)

Sweets:_____ Sweet vegetable drink____ times a
                           week

_____ Barley malt

_____ Rice syrup

_____ Amasake

_____ Maple syrup

_____ Apple juice, apple cider

Beverage: _____ Spring water

_____ Bancha

_____ Roasted barley tea

_____ Kombu tea

_____ Safflower tea

_____ Apple juice

_____ Carrot juice, cabbage, juice, other

_____ Mu tea

_____ Grain coffee

_____ Dandelion tea

_____ Beer

_____ Saki

_____ Special items:

_____ Sweet vegetable drink

_____ Kombu powder

_____ Shiitake mushroom tea

_____Ginger compress

_____ Kombu shiitake tea

_____ Carrot/daikon drink

_____ Kombu gomashio

_____ Cabbage/daikon

_____ Shoyu-bancha tea

_____ Ume-sho-bancha

_____ Ume-sho-kuzu (with or without ginger)

_____ Kombu tea

_____ Lotus root tea

_____ Hip bath/douche

_____ 2 tbsp. black, raw sesame seeds

_____ Grated daikon drink

_____ Grated cabbage drink

_____ Potato/cabbage plaster

_____ Ginger soaks

_____ Foot soaks

_____ Special compresses

_____ Other

DIRECTIONS FOR SPECIAL REMEDIES

Some of the following may be prescribed for you to correct an overly yin condition, improve fatigue, digestion, circulation, or acid condition. Modifications will be made for those who need to be ferment-free yet. Tamari without mirin may be substituted for shoyu twice a week.

Shoyu-Bancha Tea
Add 1/2-1 tsp. of shoyu to a cup of hot bancha tea.

Ume-Sho-Bancha Add 1/2-1 umeboshi plum to the above.

Ume-Sho-Kuzu Dilute 1-2 tsp. kuzu in a tablespoon of cold water. Add 1 cup water and 1/2 umeboshi plum cut in small slices, heat and stir until thickens. Add 1/2-1 tsp. shoyu, simmer one minute.

Another variation is to add a few drops of freshly grated ginger at the end.

For dissolving fats or mucous, some of the following may be prescribed:

Daikon Drink Boil 1/2 cup grated daikon in 1 cup water 5 minutes, add 1/2 tsp. shoyu and simmer one minute. Eat and drink. One variation is to do the same with cabbage. Another variation is 1/4 cup grated carrot and 1/4 cup daikon.

Kombu Tea Boil 3" strip of kombu in 4 cups of water until reduced to 2 cups (10-15 minutes).

Shiitake Mushroom Tea 1 cup water with 1 dried shiitake mushroom is brought to a boil and simmered 5 minutes, 2 drops shoyu added, simmer 1 minute. Good for accumulated salt.

Lotus Root Tea Fresh lotus root grated is best, but dried can be used, but not lotus seeds. Use juice of 1/2 cup grated and squeezed fresh lotus root with a pinch of sea salt or 1/4 cup dried lotus. Add 3/4 cup water. Bring to boil, simmer 5 minutes. Good for asthma and lung congestion.

Other remedies may also be prescribed, so always bring pad and pencil. For plasters and compresses, directions will be given.

Carrot/Daikon Drink: Grate 1/2 cup each carrot and daikon, 50/50. Simmer 3 minutes with 1/2 umeboshi and a few drops of shoyu.

Caution must be taken in prescribing the above since they would never all be used. Even if one is used it must be factored into your daily allotment of salt/ferments or you can swing to too yang and worsen. In the case of cancers it can force metastases. Or you can foster a dangerous discharge or exacerbation of symptoms. Often only one at a time is prescribed and then only once every other day.

Rice Cream
To make rice cream for very sick people who cannot chew or digest, one cup of rice, dry roasted in a skillet till golden and nutty, then pressure cook with 10 cups of water and a 1" piece of kombu for 1 1/2 hours. Pour through a cheesecloth. Save the pulp for breads or soup, and give the liquid to the sick patient. It can also be used for baby's milk, in which case you wouldn't roast it, but you would soak it overnight and use 1/4 tsp. rice syrup. It's very soothing for the digestive system as rice cream (without the syrup).

If too much salt, hot baths or shiitake mushroom tea help.

For resistant, accumulated dairy, cook 30% kombu and 70% black soy bean, in 5 times the volume of water 20 minutes with a pinch of sea salt added near the end of cooking, eat 1/2 cup daily for 1 week then every other day for one month.

Aduki Bean and Kombu Juice every other day for a month for kidney pain. Half a cup of beans, a 3" piece of kombu and 3 cups of water cooked 30 minutes. (Put kombu in another dish after).

To strengthen the immune system, 1) roast in the oven 1

part umeboshi, 1 part shiitake. Cook in a fry pan 1 part black soy bean and 3 parts kombu. Crush all in a suribachi. A teaspoon of this condiment every day for a month. 2) Sweet vegetable drink, 1 cup a day. 3) Kombu tea, 3" piece cooked 20 minutes in 3 cups of water. Drink 1 cup a day, if prescribed.

50/50 Potato/Cabbage Plaster can be applied over a tumor to draw it out. This is applied after hot towels have been used to increase the circulation over the tumor.

In the summer to keep grain from going bad too quickly, mix a little umeboshi vinegar in to inhibit bacterial growth.

When you feel good some days and not on others, look at the balance of your foods, the 5 tastes, the amounts of yin versus yang, variety in foods, recipes, menus, cooking and cutting techniques, your attitude, nutrient levels, and environmental load (mold, chemicals, etc.). Balance is the key.

CHAPTER 6

WHAT IF I'M TOO ALLERGIC?

Many people have started out on the macrobiotic diet very allergic to all grains and many other macrobiotic foods. Plus people with Candida and other mold sensitivities often are intolerant of all ferments like miso, shoyu, tamari, tempeh, tofu, pickles, natto and tekka. Don't worry. There are different ways to overcome these problems.

Most grains (rice, millet, corn, oats, barley for example) and even sugar cane are botanical members of the grass family, and you know how antigenic grass can be for some spring hay fever victims. In the beginning, if you need to avoid these antigens, then by all means do so. Often it helps to temporarily reduce your total load by having injections for grass and mold and foods (see The E.I. Syndrome for details).

Milk and wheat and sugar form the backbone of the American diet in the form of yogurt, cheese, ice cream, macaroni and cheese, breads, cakes, cookies, crackers, sandwiches, pancakes, donuts, etc. Obviously, the things eaten more frequently have more of a chance of fostering intolerances. That's why milk and wheat are among the most common foods for people to be allergic to. So avoid any foods that produce symptoms for now.

As one overloads with a substance, one of the ways the body has of alerting you to this overload is to produce a symptom, often labelled as an allergy, or more accurately as an intolerance to that substance. People who claim to have been macrobiotic (to varying degrees) for as much as 18 years were observed to be allergic to rice. Fatigue was the most common symptom.

Fortunately, this is not a big problem. Omit the food for many months and tolerance often reappears. In the meantime, find tolerable grains and even non-grains for a while. Some need to have food injections, others need to rotate a tremendous amount in order to tolerate many foods.

First, forget about any RAST or FAST and other blood,

instrument or kinesiologic test results that you may have had that told you to avoid certain foods. If rice, for example, gives you symptoms then don't eat it (see The E.I. Syndrome on how to test yourself). You can't eat foods that make you worse.

If you have limited foods, you'll need to start with foods that do not cause overt symptoms, regardless of previous test results. Then try in order, organic grains (cooked with twice the volume of water and a pinch of sea salt) beginning with millet, quinoa, amaranth, teff and buckwheat.

If none of those are tolerated, then try barley, rye, wheat, corn, tapioca, mochi, hard winter squash or other squashes: butternut, buttercup, hokkaido, acorn, pumpkin, delicato, or soba noodles, sweet potatoes, aduki beans, lentils, chick peas, black soy beans, sole, chicken, New Zealand lamb.

If none of these are tolerated as the **SOLE FOOD FOR A DAY**, then you definitely should see the doctor and we should consider food injections or other alternatives for reducing your level of sensitivity so that you might be able to eventually eat macrobiotically. If you are not tolerant of the macrobiotic vegetables as listed earlier, try the following vegetables:

celery	Jerusalem artichokes
cucumber	kohlrabi
endive	snow peas
escarole	sprouts
green beans	summer squash
peas	wax beans

If none of those are tolerable, try the following list:

artichokes	okra
avocado	plantain
bamboo shoots	yam
beets	Swiss chard
spinach	zucchini
breadfruit	cassava

Eat whatever you are able, trying to bring yourself to 50% whole grains and 50% vegetables. Definitely omit any of the ferments such as pickles, miso, shoyu, tekka, natto and any aged materials while you are trying to find safe foods. Rotate as much as possible when you do find safe foods. For some people, considerable bio-balancing is needed and there are people who actually have to have steak and potatoes.

You will notice that sometimes people will have to start on veggies that are not recommended in macrobiotics. For example, spinach is high in oxalic acid and can cause kidney stones. So these steps are meant to be temporary to help develop tolerance to better foods. Many people have jubilantly proclaimed after a few months, "Guess what! I can eat rice now with no symptoms," etc. In many cases it is the environmental (home and office, especially) chemical load or internal intestinal Candida overgrowth that contributes to the food intolerance and not the actual food itself. And, of course, in some it is the biochemical imbalance and nutrient deficiencies that contribute.

As you have already discovered, a very tight or close rotation as we were accustomed to in the past (see The E.I. Syndrome), is not easy if one is eating strictly with ingredients allowed with macrobiotics. However, we have found that in hundreds of people who have done this, a looser rotation works very well. For example, a four day rotation might look something like this:

GRAINS

Day 1- Rice

Day 2- Barley

Day 3- Millet with Cauliflower

Day 4- Quinoa

Day 5- Teff

Day 6- Amaranth

Obviously a strict rotation would only allow one grain from the grass family once in 4 days. Since this would leave you with grainless days, we need to modify. Likewise, the beans are all in the same family.

BEANS

Day 1- Chick Peas (in the rice if you wish)

Day 2- Aduki, squash, kombu

Day 3- Lentil

Day 4- Black soy bean

GREENS

	Breakfast	Lunch	Dinner
Day 1	Chinese cabbage	Bok Choy	Cabbage
Day 2	Parsley	Collard	Parsley
Day 3	Watercress	Kale	Carrot Tops
Day 4	Scallions	Leeks	Mustard Greens

OTHER VEGETABLES

	Breakfast	Lunch	Dinner
Day 1	(If you are too limited, omit for here)	Parsnip	Brussel sprouts
Day 2		Onion	Radish

	Breakfast	Lunch	Dinner
Day 3		Carrot	Turnip
Day 4		Squash	Daikon

PRESSED SALAD

Day 1- Celery, Radish, Nappa Cabbage

Day 2- Onion, Cucumber

Day 3- Romaine Lettuce

Day 4- Sprouts/Scallions

Amount, 1/2 to 1 cup daily.

Remember to have greens and vegetables at least 5 or 6 times a day, attempting to have two vegetables at every meal. Obviously there will be days when you don't, but this is something you strive for. There will be meals when you only have one vegetable or breakfasts where you have none. The more serious your condition, obviously, the harder you should try to have 2 vegetables at every meal, or even 3. As your health improves, you may not have to rotate vegetables and will be able to have them at all three meals and accelerate your healing. Fortunately, people don't usually have to rotate vegetables nearly as much as they do the grains. Also remember that after 100 chews, you change the structure and antigenicity of the molecules so much that they are no longer seen as allergenic ("allergy producing") to the body.

THE MODIFIED MACROBIOTIC DIET

People with longstanding food allergies will readily realize that an absolute four day strict rotation (The E.I. Syndrome) and the strict phase macrobiotic diet are not 100% compatible. Hence we have had to individualize and modify one or both diets for many.

Fortunately, it works for the majority. Some need food injections, most need nutrient corrections and tighter environmental (including electromagnetic) controls to increase their food tolerance.

As an example, the macro grains are all in the same family, except for buckwheat, and if potato, tapioca and Jerusalem artichoke were substituted for days 2, 3 and 4, then it would violate the strict phase macro food recommendation.

Likewise, the mustard family contains the majority of the macro vegetables: mustard greens, cabbage, cauliflower, broccoli, Brussel sprouts, turnip, rutabaga, kale, collards, Chinese cabbage, kohlrabi, radish, horseradish, watercress, bok choy, rappi.

For people not requiring a strict 1 in 4 days rotation, on every other day you could have a different member of the same family. But for a person requiring a strict four day rotation, only on one day of every four could any of these be eaten. This leaves dandelion (Composite family), squashes (Gourd family), onions and leeks (Lily family), parsley, parsnips and carrots (Parsley family), beans (legumes) as vegetables for the other days. Hence, the individualized modifications for special cases.

Then combine this with the fact that many allergic people do not tolerate 50% grains, sometimes not even 30% (because it encourages yeast growth, especially if nutrient deficiencies have not yet been sought and corrected and/or if they are not chewing enough). These same people are frequently intolerant of ferments like miso, shoyu, tekka, etc.

Fortunately through improving their total load (biochemical corrections, mold injections, environmental controls, etc.), most are able to eventually tolerate the macrobiotic diet foods enough to start improving with it. For example, often someone becomes more food tolerant after correcting a hidden magnesium deficiency or removing the bedroom carpet and installing a mold reducing air cleaner.

Rejoice, because you are probably immobilizing stored chemicals from the fat. However, when in doubt, see the doctor. Remember when you start losing weight, the chemicals come out of the fat to be discharged into the bowel, urine and sweat. Since the lipids or fats are what the chemicals were bound or attached to in the cell, the chemicals are also mobilized as they move from the fat to the blood stream. And when chemicals are in the blood stream you (1) have chemically induced symptoms, plus (2) other chemical exposures that were previously harmless now produce symptoms. This is because the detox pathways are already nearly full to capacity and working as fast as they can to process and get rid of these chemicals that are being brought out of hiding from fat storage.

So now when you are exposed to a certain food or chemical that uses that same detox pathway, it is already busy and overloaded; so the chemical backs up and produces a symptom. Since this leaves you reacting to chemicals you didn't react to before macro, it makes you think you are getting worse or more chemically sensitive. But it is self-limited and disappears after you have dieted off all the chemicals stored in the fat. Then you are rid of them once and for all!

So the period of weight loss and increased chemical sensitivity is a time when it is crucial to (1) not "cheat," (2) keep meticulous environmental controls (The E.I. Syndrome) and (3) be especially mindful of the continued health of the detox chemistry and be sure the nutrient levels are optimal.

What do I mean by that? You'll recall that for every molecule of chemical that you detox, you lose forever a molecule of glutathione and other precious detox nutrients. So this is a crucial time when your nutrient levels should be checked (especially if the heightened sensitivity persists more than 2 months or you are steadily getting worse over a month. Detox uses up precious nutrients. So it is also a time to tighten up the nutrient belt. Be sure you have soup twice a day plus vegetable broths (green juice) twice a day. A kombu tea once a day would add even more nutrients.

Obviously gas sensitive and otherwise chemically sensitive people cannot cook in the beginning with natural gas. Common gas induced symptoms are muscle and joint aches. And often a place of old injury is the target organ since it is especially weakened and vulnerable. Because of this, it is common for one to blame the pain on "the old injury," even if it was 20 years ago.

Depression, mood swings, and crying for no reason are other common gas induced symptoms. Of course, one's vulnerability depends on several factors (the total load). So if you are premenstrual, had a bad day at the office and got overloaded with traffic fumes on the way home, it's easy to see why gas induced tears or witchiness could be blamed on other events. Brain fog, or confusion, inability to concentrate and dizziness are also common gas induced symptoms.

Even though most of us now tolerate gas after a year or two of macro, I would not recommend switching back to gas unless cancer is a problem. The world is just too chemically overloaded and none of us ever wants to go back to the nightmare of E.I. (environmental illness).

Some people are very salt intolerant and do not do well with macro because of the salt. For starters, reduce the seaweeds, condiments, pickles and ferments to control this. Also read the salt chapter for the quality of your salt may be the problem.

Some abhor seaweeds. To overcome this, try a Herb Walley. Or put different seaweeds in the soups or beans and blenderize the whole thing to hide the seaweed. Some dislike specific vegetables like turnips or Brussel sprouts. These too can be hidden in a blenderized soup after masking the taste with a predominance of sweet squash or other vegetable.

Last but not least, remember food sensitivity is rarely an isolated phenomenon. Instead it reflects a general overload of chemicals, overgrowth of intestinal and other area organisms and nutrient deficiencies. For example, many were less food sensitive after doing the magnesium loading test. It can also be part of a hormonal deficiency like thyroid or adrenal (see cortrosyn stimulation test in Tired Or Toxic? for the test of a lazy adrenal that won't show up any other way). Often a person is less food sensitive after doing the yeast program, as a gut inflamed by Candida allows larger, more allergenic food particles to get into the bloodstream.

So if food allergy holds you back from doing strict macro, look at the total load (described in The E.I. Syndrome).

MYCOTOXINS

A word about mycotoxins. They are invisible, tasteless chemicals made by molds. They are some of the most potent carcinogens known, more so than many pesticides. There are no easily available tests for them. Therefore, be sure to keep your grains dry. Moist grains grow mold easily and where there is mold there are mycotoxins. Likewise, wash grain and beans thoroughly before cooking and always discard any oddly colored ones. Although this does not get rid of all mycotoxins, it is somewhat beneficial and the most that can be recommended at present.

The reason mycotoxins are so lethal is that they form epoxides. As you recall, these are the very chemicals that attach to DNA (genetic material) and start the machinery rolling for cancer. Likewise, these epoxides block and paralyze some of the detox pathways, thereby making one more chemically sensitive.

DON'T BE FOOLED
BY WHAT APPEARS TO BE FOOD ALLERGY

All is not food allergy that appears to be. For example, many people react to a variety of foods because they have intestinal dysbiosis. Through years of wrong eating, antibiotics here and there for annual sinus problems and/or lots of sweets, it is easy to get an overgrowth of organisms in the gut that normally do not cause problems if their numbers are controlled.

But if they grow too prolifically (because they thrive on the sweets you feed them, for example) several things can happen. (1) You can become allergic to them, especially the fungi like Candida albicans. This allergic reaction can inflame the gut lining. (2) They can infect or irritate the intestinal lining, or (3) they can produce secondary metabolites like acetaldehyde, which also inflames the gut lining and destroys important protective enzymes. These are only three of about a dozen mechanisms by which overgrowth of normally harmless intestinal bugs can create disease and symptoms that baffle doctors unfamiliar with them (or worse yet, there is a group of egocentric docs who have heard of it yet refuse to learn about it but nevertheless, have the arrogance to tell patients that it's all hogwash).

Anyway, when the intestinal lining is damaged by inflammation, it allows large molecules to pass through that normally are filtered out. Once large food molecules pass this lax intestinal barrier, they are recognized as foreign invaders by the body. Antibodies are made in defense and hence, food allergies crop up out of the blue. But treatment of the Candida (The E.I. Syndrome) can reverse all this.

Lastly, many nutrient deficiencies can masquerade as food allergy. For example, magnesium is in over 300 enzymes in the body. Government surveys show the average American diet only provides 40% (less than half!) of the daily requirement. This means (and studies bear it out) that the majority of people are low in it. In fact, it can be part of or the sole cause of many problems from relentless back pain, unwarranted depression, chronic fatigue, angina and hypertension to high cholesterol, nightmares, cystitis, asthma, migraines, spastic colon, leg cramps or sudden death.

In a study we did, over 10% of the people lost their food allergies once their magnesium deficiencies were corrected. Since magnesium is only one of about 4 dozen possible nutrient deficiencies, if one looks for other potential deficiencies, even more food sensitivity bites the dust.

So just because it may appear to be food allergy, remember it may be nutrient deficiency in disguise. Because nutrient deficiencies are so rampant, allow me to show you just a few random articles from our Newsletter:

(1) Starving To Death In The Hospital

In a recent study published in the highly respected journal,

LANCET, it was clearly demonstrated that insurance companies that do not insist upon nutritional workups are foolishly losing money. Studied were 59 patients with a mean age of 82 years all of whom had been admitted with hip fractures. The patients were divided into 2 groups, both of which were treated the same way except for one thing.

One group was tested and treated for a small number of nutrient deficiencies and the other group was not (as normally occurs in medicine today). Of the group that had their vitamin and mineral levels assessed, all were deficient in one or another. The patients were put on some unsophisticated nutrients to correct the few deficiencies that were looked for and discovered, and 56% had a favorable outcome. While in the group that was treated as patients are ordinarily treated, that is without benefit of nutrient assessment, only 13% had a favorable outcome. So there is a four times greater chance of good outcome if nutrients are corrected.

The rate of complication and death for the treated group was 44% while for the standard treated group it was 87%. The mean duration of hospital stay for the nutrient treated group was 24 days, while for the regularly treated group it was 40 days. The death rate in this highly fragile, aged and injured group was 24% for those with nutrient treatment, and 37% for those with standard care. And this study of just a couple of nutrient levels was nowhere near the complete study that we recommend in Tired Or Toxic?

In summary, without biochemical assessment, one can count on spending at least double the amount of time in the hospital and having double the risk of complication as well as 1 1/2 times the increased chance of dying. Older people obviously have worse statistics on the whole than younger persons, since they often have poorer dentition for chewing, many are on fixed incomes and cannot afford the food they need, they have had more nutrient depleting medications, and they have a longer life span over which to have accumulated these deficiencies. And now with the new Medicare regulations, these assessments will be even more strongly curtailed.

(Delmi M., Rapin C. H., Bengoa J. M., Delmas P. D., Vasey H., et al. Dietary supplementation in elderly patients with fractured neck of the femur. LANCET 1990; 335: 1013-1016).

(2) Eat Your Wakame For Vitamin B12

The scientific literature bears out the fact that vegetarians have a lower incidence of heart disease, diabetes, cancer, kidney stones, and osteoporosis than meat and dairy eaters. But they frequently become depleted in vitamin B12 because eggs, dairy and animal foods are the primary source of vitamin B12. Analysis of vegetarian foods revealed that sea vegetables, especially wakame contained significant B12.

Food	Micrograms of B12 per gram of wet weight
tempeh	0.5
arame	1.4
kombu	19.0
wakame	43.0

(Speckler BL, Miller D, Norman EJ, Greene H, Hayes KC. Increased urinary methylmalonic acid excretion in breastfed infants of vegetarian mothers and identification of an acceptable dietary source of vitamin B12. AM J CLIN NUTR 1988; 47: 89-92)

Also, since B12 is synthesized from micro-organisms, we get it from food fermented by fungi or bacteria like shoyu sauce, sauerkraut, miso, etc. (Goldberg, S., Clinical Biochemistry, MedMaster Inc., PO Box 640028, Miami, FL 33169, 1988.

This data is even more important for macrobiotic people when one is aware of a recent NEW ENGLAND JOURNAL OF MEDICINE article that demonstrated several important points: (1) that B12 deficiency can produce a variety of symptoms from peculiar numbness and tingling to fatigue, depression, or even psychosis. And (2) that the usual macrocytosis that most physicians relay on seeing before they will consider checking for a B12 deficiency is missing. So in summary, anyone with fatigue, paresthesia (numbness and tingling), depression or any other psychiatric condition should have a B12 level done to be sure that the symptoms are not merely from a deficiency that is totally curable.

Lindenbaum J, Healton EB, Savage DG, Brust JCM, Garrett TJ, Podell ER, Marcell PD, Stabler SP, Allen RH, Neuropsychiatric disorders caused by cobalamin deficiency in the absence of anemia or macrocytosis. NEW ENGLAND JOURNAL OF MEDICINE, 318, 26: 1720-1728, June 30, 1988.

(3) How Do You Know Whom To Believe?

One of the problems these days is that just when you think you have all the rules for a healthy life down pat, somebody announces that the rules have been changed.

For example, it is a well known scientifically proven fact that anti-oxidants such as vitamins A, C and E definitely help to reduce the risk of cancer. However, studies have been done using vitamin A only to see if the group taking it had a reduced rate of cancer compared with the group that did not take it. The problem with this type of research is that the researchers try to use vitamins as though they were drugs and not one of hundreds of important parts of the whole body and it's chemistry.

Apparently, they were unaware until long after this expensive study was completed that administering beta carotene (vitamin A precursor) to normal subjects leads to a 40% decline in the alpha tocopherol (vitamin E) level after 8 months. In other words, it is near sighted to use only one nutrient at a time and fail to balance it with the rest of the body chemistry. No wonder their conclusion was that beta carotene did not help to control the cancer rate!

(NEW ENGLAND JOURNAL OF MEDICINE, September 20, 1990, Vol. 323, #12, 825-827)

You can't take huge amounts of nutrients as though they were a drug. They must be balanced in harmony with the rest of the body chemistry. So when you hear a report that does not fit with what you believe, there may well be further information that was necessary that was either suppressed (due to the desire to discredit something that interferes with one's vested interest), or that the researchers were just plain ignorant of.

(4) How Often Is Magnesium Deficiency Missed?

In a recent scientific publication in the JOURNAL OF THE AMERICAN MEDICAL ASSOCIATION, a study was done on 1033 patients who were in the hospital for various reasons and whose doctors had ordered electrolyte tests from the laboratory to see if the patients had abnormalities of the sodium, potassium, etc. The study also included a free serum magnesium test to see if this was also abnor-mal and was being missed. Indeed, their suspicions were correct, for over 51% (546) of these patients had abnormal magnesium levels. And in only one out of 10 of these patients did their doctors order a magnesium test. That means that 90% of the patients who had a magnesium deficiency were missed. And don't forget a serum magnesium has been shown by other studies to be the worst assay of magnesium status, as it misses over half those who are deficient. The best test is a magnesium loading or challenge test. (Journal of the American Medical Association 1990; 263: 3063-3064)

So you can appreciate from these articles, chosen at random from my quarterly Newsletter that medicine in general is in deep trouble. It knows nothing and teaches nothing about nutrition (except for some small groups like the American Academy of Environmental Medicine) while the country is getting progressively more depleted. But this sells a lot of drugs. And as people get sicker they tend to eat more "time-saving" processed foods. So the sick get sicker. And oftentimes the mere correction of simple deficiencies solves baffling and serious medical problems.

NEVER FORGET THE TOTAL LOAD

For some people who are just too allergic to do macro, for example those who can't tolerate any grains without vicious symptoms or a merciless flare of Candida, be sure you have looked at your total load. *For failure to address the total load is the most common reason for failure.* If you have headaches, depression, ear and jaw pain, back pain or total body aches from natural gas at home, for example, you may be so chemically overloaded that food allergies will persist indefinitely. Whereas once the load is addressed (see The E.I. Syndrome) within a month we hear, "Guess what!" I can tolerate rice now."

And of course, if you are just too pooped to pop, you won't have the energy to do macro. It becomes a vicious cycle that only you can break with knowledge of the total load:

CHRONIC FATIGUE SOLVED

Chronic fatigue syndrome (CFS) is a catch-all term for "a virus," which often means that conventional medicine just doesn't have any answers as to how to treat it. But there are ways to treat people diagnosed as having CFS. Let's look at some of its causes.

We are the first generation of man to ever eat so many processed foods, and processed foods often have a lower nutritional value. For example, brown rice or whole wheat has five times the magnesium that white rice or wheat bread does. The United States government did a survey which showed that the average diet provides only 40% of the RDA for magnesium. And you guessed it...many people who have CFS are deficient in magnesium. The problem is that there is no blood test to diagnose this deficiency, but there is a before and after urine test, called a magnesium loading test, that will.

Likewise, many people complaining of chronic fatigue are deficient in other vitamins and minerals, but it is not in vogue in conventional medicine to check these since correction doesn't involve prescription drugs. The most common ones that we see are low red blood cell (RBC) zinc, RBC copper, RBC chromium, RBC selenium, and B1. But the assayed levels must be intracellular or inside the RBC because the plasma and serum values are deceptively worthless when they look normal, as they are too insensitive.

Aside from hidden nutrient deficiencies, many people complaining of chronic fatigue have unsuspected mold sensitivities. Mold is inescapable; if you put a piece of bread on your desk for two weeks, it will become moldy. Mold is everywhere, and when you inhale it, symptoms such as chronic headaches, eczema, asthma, sinusitis, or fatigue can result.

Furthermore, some people eat a diet rich in mold antigens (such as yeasted breads, cheese, alcohol, vinegar, and pickles) that can aggravate a mold allergy. But more importantly, because of anti-biotics or a diet high in sweets, some people have Candida, a yeast that manufactures acetaldehyde, which makes them feel depressed and exhausted.

As if this were not enough, there is another culprit that causes even more unexplained exhaustion: everyday chemicals. You know, we are also the first generation to ever be exposed to so many chemicals. This puts a tremendous burden on our detoxification system. Add to this the fact that many of the detoxification pathways are deficient in certain nutrients, and you begin to understand why so many people are actually toxic from everyday chemicals, not tired from CFS. These improperly metabolized or incompletely degraded chemicals back up in the blood and poison the energy pathways of the body.

CLUES TO SUSPECTING YOU ARE CHEMICALLY SENSITIVE

You can smell things better than most people.

You cannot tolerate alcohol well.

Perfumes and strong cleansers bother you.

You feel worse in certain stores or malls.

There are many medications you cannot take.

Vitamins often make you feel worse.

Your reaction time when driving is poorer in city traffic than in the country.

HOW THE SICK GET SICKER

Chemicals back up in the bloodstream when the detoxification system is ailing.

This can result in:

*Chemicals stored in fat, the brain, and other lipid tissues such as regulatory membranes.

*Chemicals poisoning or damaging enzymes and other parts of the detoxification system.

*Chemicals are recycled in the detoxification path and overload it so new chemicals cannot be metabolized.

*Metabolites or secondary chemicals form that are more dangerous than the original or parent compound; these generate free radicals that eat holes in regulatory membranes (nucleus, mitochondria, endoplasmic reticulum, and cell body membranes). When metabolites from chemicals damage the nucleus where the genetic material is housed, cancer can arise. When they damage the mitochondria (where the body makes energy molecules), chronic fatigue occurs; if it's the endoplasmic reticulum (where chemicals are detoxified), then chemical sensitivity occurs, and when it damages the membranes (which is like the computer keyboard), you can get all sorts of problems from allergies to arthritis or diabetes. Some of us had multiply damaged cell areas.

*Chemicals and their metabolites can then get shuttled into new pathways and produce new symptoms.

*Backlogged chemicals can poison or damage parts of the energy systems that are supposed to perform detoxification of all chemicals.

*Backlogged chemicals damage the endocrine (thyroid, adrenal, pancreatic, etc.), nervous, and immune systems, so that any symptom imaginable can result.

Now you can begin to appreciate that without assessing the environmental and nutrient status, a patient who is on a downhill course, has only one way to go...the sick get sicker.

Treatment consists of correcting the nutrient deficiencies and teaching people how to change their environment to lessen the effect of molds and chemicals. But most importantly, people must eat nutritious foods. They must stop eating sugar and processed foods, and begin eating whole grains and vegetables that allow the body to heal.

No two people experience the same causes of their symptoms. For one person, 80% of the problem causing chronic fatigue or other symptoms could be a mineral deficiency: for another, it could be a mold allergy; and for another, it could be a chemical sensitivity. For some people, like myself, it was all these things and more. Those with resistant cases, although it sounds unbelievable, can clear all of these problems by specifically altering their diet, home environment and attitude.

Medicine is in the midst of an evolution. It's evolving from an era of high-tech procedures and drugs to cover up or mask every symptom, to one of molecular medicine, where we can now uncover the biochemical defects and environmental causes for most symptoms. Medicine is just starting to emerge from the era where a headache is a Darvon deficiency and evolve into using the tools we now have with which to find the cause and get rid of symptoms rather than just covering them up with drugs. In hundreds of patients, it is a rare person whose condition is not significantly improved by uncovering and treating some of these 21st century causes.

Reprinted with kind permission from my article in Let's Live magazine, July 1990, 444 N. Larchmont Blvd., Los Angeles, CA.

****

Also, avoid letting yourself fall back into the medicine trap where biochemical individuality takes a back seat. That is one way that drugging all symptoms is justified, by assuming we are all the same. And that is one reason the mysterious causes of many diseases, like rheumatoid arthritis have not been found. They are looking for a cause that is the same in all people and it doesn't exist.

As Lino Stanchich has said, "Just because this coat is good for me, doesn't mean it is good for you." Five people with R.A. may have between them thirty different causes for their arthritis, and they may all require different dietary modifications.

Lastly, a word about a frequently asked question, "Should I have my amalgams removed?" Much of the evidence of the profound damage that mercury/silver dental amalgams can do is in Tired Or Toxic? However, for every person who has had remarkable improvement by having them removed, another person has had no benefit. Also, some were worse with the adhesives necessary to fix the new restorations in place. So it is best to discuss your individual problem first with the doctor. For there is more than one way to detox mercury. Next we can do a test to determine if you have an excessive body burden of mercury. You merely take a medication that flushes mercury from your body for a couple of days and collect a 24 hour urine for mercury. If the level is up, you do need to reduce your burden and there are many ways in which to do it.

We will keep you abreast of these and related issues in environmental and nutritional medicine when you subscribe to the newsletter, Health Letter.

CHAPTER 7

THE DISCHARGE

A discharge is quite different from illness symptoms or from an allergic reaction. A discharge is one of the healing crises; it's a body cleanse or purge; a time when the body can get rid of materials that it has been struggling to get rid of for some time. But it can only do so when it has reached a certain state of wellness.

When the machinery is finally healthy enough to rip into gear and get rid of long time stored materials that it just didn't have the capacity to get rid of long ago, you'll know the difference from a discharge versus symptoms by many ways. First of all, you'll have a feeling of well being. Second, the symptom will not be provoked by any particular event (and you will usually have an overall feeling of wellness while it is going on). If in doubt, you should see the doctor because the reactions can be quite severe and you want to differentiate it from an illness that requires medical intervention. Perhaps we can collect some of the fluid and have it analyzed for pesticides or chemicals to find out what the body is discharging. Also, sometimes the liver enzymes are elevated and this helps us know how hard the liver has had to work to discharge this chemical and when it has fully recovered again.

For example, one gal suddenly had diarrhea and uncontrollable depression and body aches for several days. Her liver enzymes were elevated during this time. There was no precipitating event that would explain the sudden onset of these symptoms, and her previous eczema that was cleared on the macrobiotic diet had returned. A macrobiotic remedy quickly simmered down her symptoms.

Oftentimes asthmatics will have periodic discharges with a great deal of phlegm and chest mucous, but they know they have not done anything that would have triggered their asthma, and that they are not sick. Furthermore, they don't have the feeling that they need the medications that they normally needed in the past; they often feel that they can handle this. There are, again, remedies that can be used to speed this up, or turn it off. Sometimes potent prescribed medications are needed to bail us out. Normally most discharges will pass within two weeks.

One lady developed 4-6" large, erythematous, water filled blisters all down the side of one arm and one leg during the ninth month of macrobiotics. After two weeks, these disappeared. During the two weeks, however, they drained night and day, a clear fluid which we had saved in hopes that we could find a way to inexpensively analyze it for the chemicals that we suspected it contained. This scenario was repeated again one year later.

One gal presented with purple palms. She also brought her bedding and showed me that her skin had been oozing purple the last couple of weeks. Her sheets and pillow cases were stained purple and her eczema that had cleared on macrobiotics, had returned and was oozing purple. Purple was the color of the permanent wave solution that she had used on patrons for 18 years as a hairdresser without wearing gloves. Her body was finally able to depurate it or get rid of it.

One reason I suspect as the cause of the sometimes faster and more dramatic discharges that we have seen is that in all of these people we had drawn blood tests to identify and correct their vitamin and mineral deficiencies. So their detox systems were really primed and performed much more dramatically. Likewise, for people who never discharge and think they are on a good program, they may have some as yet unidentified deficiencies. Remember, we rarely see anyone with normal nutrient levels anymore. And when we correct the deficiencies it takes three to six months often to correct the minor ones. And this is with large doses of specifically balanced supplements of known high quality. The alternative would be to allow the individual to correct naturally which could take much longer.

Discharges should not be confused with the symptoms that one gets from cheating on the diet. These are merely symptoms and in no way mean that the body is healthy enough to now extrude or get rid of chemicals that it has acquired over the years that have been damaging its metabolism. Sometimes people are eating incorrectly. For example, one case at the Kushi Institute started clearing her breast cancer and then developed metastases. In reviewing the diet, she was eating incorrectly and having far too yang a program. You know the bit; if a little is good for you, then a lot should be great. She thought she was doing the diet well, but had far too much miso and seaweeds and was actually forcing the cancer into the bone. By correcting the diet she cleared the metastases.

I had been extremely magnesium deficient for years and knew I was getting low again when the arches in my feet would cramp at night. Taking oral magnesium didn't correct it, so I gave myself occasional magnesium injections in the thigh which did. However, after having been on macro for a year and a half, 2 days after one of the injections, I developed a flaming red, very hot swollen mass that felt like someone was trying to rip my thigh off. I foolishly applied a ginger compress which, of course, made it worse. When it got to the size of a grapefruit, 2 cups of totally non-odorous, white cheesy material oozed out of it over the next week. For a few days I couldn't even walk. I cultured it, had the magnesium cultured and analyzed for preservative or contaminant and all studies were negative. It was so painful I resorted to the highest dose of steroids I had ever taken in my life to turn down the reaction. In retrospect, I believe it was a discharge representing the 15 years of abnormally high amounts of pain medication I had taken daily for my back. In fact, a year later I gave myself several magnesium injections in the same spot from the same batch of magnesium sulfate that I had saved and nothing happened.

If I had been smart enough when it occurred, (1) I would not have used a ginger compress which actually exacerbates abscesses (and cancers), (2) I would have had the sterile material that was discharged analyzed for chemical composition. For I must add that in 21 years of doing medicine, I never saw a mass that large produce material with absolutely no odor and no organisms.

One nurse who cleared an inoperable stage IV abdominal lymphoma had 4 discharges of intense abdominal pain and intestinal obstruction. The first episode she was hospitalized for, but after she saw how little was done outside of observation, she stayed home for the next three and did fine. She was given a 6 month life sentence and is alive and well 5 1/2 years later. But most discharges, if they occur at all, will not be anything to worry about. I have heard from many persons who healed cancers on how they urinated black, or black appeared to ooze from the skin after use of compresses and thereafter the cancer was gone by x-ray examination. We need doc-

-174-

umentation of this kind of occurrence with x-rays, blood tests, urinalyses, photographs, and whatever we can get to increase the awareness of these phenomenon and decrease the anxiety many have about going through one.

If a discharge is too severe, you may need help with it, as I did. And of course medical verification is always helpful, since medicine is riddled with exceptions, rule breakers and surprises.

Rule #1---WHEN IN DOUBT, CHECK IT OUT.

I am very interested in discharges and particularly in the proof they can provide that the body first heals itself and then starts its own housekeeping. I would someday like to produce a book of case histories of various types of discharges and of the proof that could be gathered to support the fact.

A common discharge which is embarrassing is the unusually bad odors that many of us had from our skin, sweat, breath and intestines. There's no way around it that I know of except to grin and bear it.

Happily, the outcome of most discharges is that the person, having mobilized and disposed of further chemicals is subsequently at a new level of wellness and happier for it.

But don't confuse a discharge with symptoms from "cheating."

IS MACRO A LIFE SENTENCE?

We hear stories of people going off the diet and getting bad reactions (The Kamakazi Cowboy by Dirk Benedict, the handsome actor on the "A-Team" television series). Are these true? Yes, but not always necessary. And remember the goal of macro is to get so well, that once in a while, you can eat anything. That's real health.

After the first six months of macro, I was out of the country and went off for one meal of fish and fried rice. I had diarrhea all night and day. After one year, again I was out of the country and decided to pretend I was "Mrs. Normal." I ate "regular" food for four days. Then suddenly with no physical provocation, the severest back pain of my life was duplicated. I was flat out in bed, only to be painfully carried to the bathroom. I recall lying in bed encased in pain, hearing my husband say, "*#@*#@! Sherry, how could you be so *#@*#@! stupid? If I had been through all that you had, you couldn't pay me to go off that diet!" These words were spoken by a man who hates macro for himself, but has great respect for what he has seen it accomplish time and time again.

After a year and a half, I was infinitely stronger and for 3 weeks in Australia managed to have the finest French wine and foods every night, as long as I ate macro for breakfast and lunch. A year later in England/France, I was even more tolerant: two and a half weeks of no macro!

For me, this is a heavenly bonus. Not only did I lose every symptom I ever had and am healthier now than I have ever been in my life, but I can periodically go out with my husband and fake it off as though I were normal, as well as enjoy a yearly vacation. This is heaven for me. The rest of the time, the majority of my life, is 3 great macro meals a day. Not a bad deal for the best energy, outlook and health I've ever known, and 2 years away from being 50.

Yes at 2 1/2 years, I went to England to lecture for the British Society of Allergy and Environmental Medicine. My husband and I went two weeks early to celebrate our 20th anniversary. Since we were traveling throughout France and England I decided to give macrobiotics the supreme test. I had been on now for 2 1/2 years and I was curious just how much healing I had accomplished.

For 2 1/2 weeks I ate continental breakfasts with croissants and jams, romantic lunches of French bread, Camembert, pate, wine and fruit and gourmet 7 course French dinners each night. These included a whole bottle of wine for myself at dinner, sinfully delicious desserts and wonderful goat cheeses encased in grey-blue coverings of fuzzy mold. I was perfectly fine. I did not even have one symptom when we were caught in a mile long tunnel in a traffic jam, or in a room full of smokers, or in a store that was doing some toxic renovations. Nor did I react to the more than 50 foods that I had not been able to touch for years. In fact, I had never in my life eaten so lavishly for such a long time.

An interesting occurrence was that each night, I had profuse sweats that drenched my body: the body's way of discharging or getting rid of excess when it is healthy enough to do so.

Of course, when I arrived home, I went straight to the kitchen and made all my macro back-ups and a meal. After all, if macro is this healing, I'd be a fool to go off. Instead I prefer to see just how healthy I can get, and save my indiscretions for when I am traveling with my husband. I have observed too many people reverse their progress after years of accomplishing the impossible. In addition, the horrid memories of being a universal reactor are too strong. This is a gal who in 1985 had to use 4 tanks of oxygen just to give lectures in a hotel. Even with the oxygen it was a nightmare of symptoms I had endured for over 15 years and never want to experience again.

Over the years now, we have observed two major reasons why some people do not improve with macrobiotics: they have too much of an environmental overload in their daily environment, and they have nutrient deficiencies that have not been discovered. I hope this will be an inspiration to those who consider themselves hopeless, and we will persist in trying to figure out why some people just cannot do the diet at all.

The ironic part was that the last time I lectured in England was in 1986. About 10 different doctors who remembered me from then, came up to me this year and remarked on how healthy I looked. They were also surprised that I was able to eat so many foods that even they could not eat, and that I no longer reacted to chemicals. I had been the object of pity 5 years ago and now I was infinitely healthier than anyone they knew.

Several of them said "Boy, I wish I could get rid of my chemical allergies. They are making my life miserable." When I suggested to them that all they had to do was go on the macrobiotic diet and check their nutrient levels, and get their chemistry squared around, they answered, "Oh, I'm not ready for anything that drastic yet." To me, the translation is that they are just plain not ready to get well, because the macrobiotic diet certainly isn't nearly the handicap that going through life chemically sensitive is.

After 3 years of macro I started to get pretty sloppy in that weekends I would eat what I had prepared for my husband for breakfast and dinner, plus we would go out once a week. I still never got so much as a flu or cold, but did start a half year succession of monthly tennis injuries: severely torn muscles in lower extremities. To me this could only mean one thing: I needed to be consistently good again. Every symptom is a warning and to ignore it is to ask for a stronger warning down the road.

Now some people will immediately ask, what is the use of macro if you are always a prisoner of it? Some have even admitted that they are afraid to start macrobiotics because they (1) fear a worsening discharge, (2) fear worse symptoms if they stray, (3) fear they can't get off without bad symptoms, once they get on macrobiotics.

But don't you see what they really fear? Total control over their health. They don't want to acknowledge that what and how they eat determines their health. Remember the multitude of health problems and unexplainable injuries I had prior to macro? Now I am in control. I can have them or not. The only difference now is I'm unloaded and healthy enough to see the cause and effect. Before it was like some mysterious uncontrollable, unpredictable fate. In contrast, now I am in control and fully responsible.

WHAT IF I GET MACRO YELLOW?

There are several skin colors that people on macrobiotics develop. The sickest who present with end-stage cancers often have a greenish hue to them, others a very dusky grey or sometimes almost purplish grey. Some are so anemic that they are very pale or nearly white. Of course the eczemas, alcoholics, chemically sensitive and other yin skin disorders enter with ruddy skin, being pink to red to cranberry or purple, complete with dilated blood vessels (telangiectasias).

As they begin macrobiotics, most people just get continually healthier looking and begin to glow. But for others, there are two major color changes that I have observed.

The first is the person who is not doing well and just plain looks greyish and sickly. Usually there is an adjustment to be made, the most common being to check the cooking and proportions, assess chewing, check loving/nurturing and the support system in general, and find the environmental chemical overload and detoxification system nutrient deficiencies.

The second is the macro yellowness which can have two causes. One cause of yellow skin is ceroid pigmentation, a yellow-brown discoloration of tissue that accumulates over time in the presence of increased polyunsaturated fats and decreased anti-oxidant vitamin E. If it occurs as a new finding, the vitamin E level may not be sufficient to handle the discharge of fats back into the system as the person loses weight and years of fat stored chemicals. If it has been present a long while, also check pancreatic function since this is necessary for this fat soluble vitamin to be absorbed. Also necessary is bile which means check taurine levels as well as decreasing the environmental chemical overload.

The solutions to this are many. Sometimes increased body work, as in shiatsu or other massage can get the lymphatics open to improve circulation and complete the discharge. Increasing the vitamin E containing seeds would take a long time to effect change and you might want to have a blood level drawn and supplement it temporarily. Of course it should be balanced with complementary nutrients and other nutrient levels should be checked as well since it's unlikely to have just a solo deficiency. Of course, slowing down the weight loss retards the progression, but does nothing for the overall progress, nor the pigmentation that already exists.

A second cause of yellow skin is noted first in the nasolabial folds (cheek folds between sides of nostrils and corner of lips). The soles and palms are often next to become obviously yellowed. This is carotenemia from too much carotene, the yellow pigment of yellow and orange vegetables. Cutting back on squash and carrots (and especially no carrot juice) helps this, but there is still an underlying problem in that the body is unable to handle the pigment as well as others do who ingest the same amount. It may be another signal of blocked lymphatics or incomplete discharge.

Biochemistry textbooks and a review of the scientific litera-ture reveal no problem from carotenemia. Still, my gut level feeling is it is an abnormal phenomenon and until the body can handle this pigment, we should not overload with it. I suspect carotenemia rep-resents a detox deficiency somewhere, since not everyone gets it.

For the pale people, please do not fall into the medical trap of using iron unless you have an RBC (red blood cell) copper level drawn as well as iron. You see, copper deficiency can cause an ane-mia just like iron, complete with small red blood cells (hypochromic microcytic anemia). The problem is that the RBC copper level is more often low than is the iron. But if one sees the anemia and assumes it is due to iron (as is often done), the extra iron serves to lower the copper even more, making the condition worse.

So whether it's an undesirable color or symptom, if it persists too long, check it out; there should be a biochemical solution.

WHAT IF I DON'T HAVE A DISCHARGE?

If after 2 years you have not had one discharge, then you need to reevaluate your program, environmental load, and your biochemical balance (nutrient levels). The lack of discharge is usually either errors in the program, too much of a chemical environmental overload, or hidden persistent deficiencies, especially in the detox system. As I came out of a consultation with Mr. Kushi involving another end stage cancer ridden young gentleman, I couldn't help wonder if he would live long enough for the macro to work. It is my firm belief that for many we need to check every nutrient level avail-able to correct the most seriously abnormal ones aggressively, in or-der to "buy" time for the macrobiotic program to bring about healing.

Here's an example from the recent literature (American Jour-nal of Cardiology, Schecter, M., et al, Beneficial effects of magnesium sulfate in acute myocadial infarction. 66: 271-274, August 1, 1990):

Of 103 patients who showed up at an emergency room with a heart attack, all were given the same treatment. But, half were given I.V. magnesium for 2 days while the other half just had I.V.s with no added magnesium. In the magnesium group, 48% had complications versus 95% of the non-magnesium group, or double. But most importantly, 2% of the magnesium group died, while 17% of the non-magnesium group died. Eight times what the magnesium death rate was!

And this is naively giving <u>one</u> nutrient, one of a possible 40 plus and not even verifying how much to give by measuring the level. So this is the most primitive form of nutrient medicine, and yet look how powerful it is. Just imagine the mortality rate if they had actually measured and corrected *many* nutrient levels. You can appreciate that diet and lifestyle changes are necessary, but almost powerless in the first few days or weeks when the peak of mortality occurs. Whereas nutrient biochemistry is paramount.

You might say, "Well, this study is 1990, so the news isn't out yet. Give them a chance." But this is an example of the sad truth that permeates medical progress. This study is not alone, nor is it the first. The earliest one I found was 1956! The authors (Parsons, R. S., Butler, T., Sellars, E. P., The treatment of coronary artery disease with parenteral magnesium sulfate, <u>Med. Proc.</u> 5; 487, 1959) found a 1% death rate in the magnesium treated group versus a 30% death rate in the group that received none. I could fill a whole book just with other papers with similar results that were published between 1956 and 1990. Yet not only is it not standard therapy, but as you learned earlier, it still is not even <u>looked</u> for in 90% of cases.

That is why you have to learn as much about real but natural remedies as you can. First, because they are in the long run more potent and produce results that drugs are incapable of and second, because they are not patentable and so make no money.

Meanwhile, it stands to reason that to get in as good biochemical shape as possible is to anyone's advantage so they can improve faster. Furthermore, there are reports emerging now in the scientific literature showing that the addition of nutrients can reverse cancers and pre-cancerous conditions. For example, in several studies, folic acid has reversed cervical dysplasia, a cell change in the uterine cervix that precedes cancer of the cervix. Whereas others have actually caused already formed cancers to regress (Shklar, G., Schwartz, J., Trickler, D., Reid, S.; Regression of experimental cancer by administration of combined alpha-tocopherol and beta-carotene, <u>Nutr. Can-</u>

<u>cer</u>, 12, 321-325, 1989). Thus, it need not be stressed any further: the worse or more severe the condition, the more imperative it should be to check and correct the biochemical balance.

And in the meantime, when you discharge, rejoice. Relish in each discharge, for it is a feat to be happy with. For it serves to slow up or even reverse the process of degeneration that eventually takes us all.

CHAPTER 8

DON'T SOAK THE NORI

Throughout the course of my macrobiotic journey, I've learned a great many things through my mistakes and the mistakes of many others and we would like to share them with you so that you needn't duplicate them. Other items here are merely things that we often have needed reminding or repetition on. Dog-ear the page, underline, attach a paper clip, or insert a piece of paper in pages that you need to remind yourself to do. The best tool for learning is repetition.

First, don't ever soak the nori and don't peel the shiny covering off the mochi nor skin the burdock. Simple light scrubbing of the burdock will suffice.

Likewise, there are a number of facts that people should know if they are trying to eat as though their lives depended upon it. So let's roll!

The sweet vegetable drink is good for reducing hypoglycemia as well as many years of dairy fats, and to soften other fats. Boiled grated carrot/daikon with umeboshi and shoyu is also good for this.

People on chemotherapy often need fish oils, fried rice and/or cooked fruits with a pinch of salt because the chemo has been so stressful to the body.

If you're not able to sweat, you should consider shiatsu massage. As well, make sure you do your nightly foot soaks, plus body scrubs twice daily and consider some exercise. See your doctor or macrobiotic counselor for the macrobiotic remedies to help remove fats faster from the clogged glands.

Do not wear digital watches; the electromagnetic fields can interfere with your body's own electrical flow.

If you're tender between the scapulae, most likely the pancreas is tight, weak and fatty. Another clue is if you're tender in the acupuncture point, about 4" above the medial knee joint (about where someone would squeeze your knee if you were seated in order to tickle you).

Rice can be varied in a number of ways. You can mix it 30% with millet or 30% with barley or 10% with one of the (pre-soaked) beans or chestnuts. Or just simply rotate and avoid it 3 days out of 4 (rice, millet, barley, quinoa, etc.).

A strict diet does not mean a narrow diet, and in fact, it's counterproductive (not healing) to be on a narrow (monotonous) diet. If it is not varied and interesting you will become unbalanced and go off because of cravings.

Grains should be eaten with each meal.

Each day you can arrange on a plate the amount of seaweeds that you would eat so that you will make sure to use up your daily allotment. One or two strips of wakame about 3" long for your miso soup, a sheet or two of nori, a 2" piece of kombu to be used in each: kombu tea, the grains and the beans, and be sure to have a quarter cup of arame or hijiki, eaten as a side dish.

For each meal, try for as much variety as possible. Before you serve your meal, go over the reminder: grains, greens & beans, seeds & weeds, roots & fruits. Do you have 50% grain? Did you remember a fresh dish of greens, is it time for some beans? Did you remember some condiments for your rice and garnish for the soup? Seaweeds rich in minerals? Root vegetables? And last the "fruits" or goodies that make things taste good like the miso, shoyu, ginger, etc.?

Trout and carrot can be used in place of carp/burdock soup for special medicinal needs, especially weakness or after chemo.

The vegetable drink can be refrigerated for several days and used daily, 1 cup. The millet sweet vegetable soup likewise can be refrigerated and eaten 3 times a week.

Just one cheat with some conditions, and it will be like starting over. For some people, starting over will be too late. You must be strict for 3-4 months or until your condition is cleared.

The life-span of the red blood cell is 120 days. So in 4 months of good eating you have begun to change the quality of your cells. Other cell types have varying turn-over times.

As people cheat, their conditions come back faster and worse. So learn quickly how to correct your craving/imbalance or see your doctor/counselor.

The biochemistry of the body is amazingly complex. It clearly did not arise as a quirk of nature. There is a power responsible that is beyond our earth realm. That power has given you life. Trusting in that power to guide you further in life can provide a background of serenity that you have never before experienced. A spiritual awakening may be a necessary part of your healing.

Don't have grated daikon/carrot/umeboshi/tamari on the same day that you have ume/sho/kuzu. One umeboshi plum a day total is sufficient, and two would be too much for most people and make them worse.

In the first 1-3 months at least, for most serious conditions, no oven baked foods, even a squash. Eat nothing dry, like rice cakes. No dried crackers, rice cakes, corn chips, rice crackers, baking powder, nuts, popcorn, no crunchy-crispy items, and no baked flour products should be used and salt should be kept to a minimum as well as the miso. Too much salt or shoyu or miso makes one contracted, tight, angry, irritable, aggressive and unable to discharge. When in doubt, stop eating for a day, then return but use no salt or ferments.

For those who are distressed with our emphasis on environmental medicine and nutrient biochemistry assessments, bear in mind these are for the difficult cases that have been unsuccessful with a solely macrobiotic program. Our chemically overloaded generation has changed many of the rules of medicine and macro.

The only raw foods permissible in the healing diet will be grated daikon, finely chopped raw scallion, red radish, or parsley or a tablespoon of finely grated celery or carrot for garnish.

Do not have tofu (unless dried, and then it's only twice a week); also no tempeh or seitan for the healing phase. After 1-6 months it can be enjoyed every 1-2 weeks, depending on the individual's condition and rate of improvement.

Nori, can be eaten 1-5 sheets a day, but only 1 cup of seeds per week (or roughly 1-3 tsp. a day, depending on your condition).

You can't have miso yet? Have miso-less miso soup: wakame and vegetable with garnish. You can't tolerate seeds because of diverticuli? Grind them in a blender.

Dry roast seaweed in oven or pan and grind in suribachi or blender for seaweed powder condiment.

You don't feel well when you awaken? Move the bed and learn about geopathic stress zones and electromagnetic fields. An inexpensive experiment is to put your bed in the opposite part of the room, head facing north for one month. Have no electrical appliances within 6 feet of your head (no clock radios, no electric blankets, unplug the T.V. at night). Is there a difference? If not, put it back. If there is, you'll probably want to learn why.

Hot apple juice, if it's allowed for your condition, is limited to 2 cups a week.

Barley malt, if allowed for your condition is 1 tbsp. a week.

Carrot juice, if allowed for your condition, is limited to 1/2 cup twice a week.

Make sure your sleeping, appetite and bowel movements are good (and that you're getting enough love each day). If these things are deficient, see the doctor for how this might be rectified.

Do not take long baths or showers and don't do the body scrub in the shower. You will wash away too many minerals. However, if one is too tight and irritable, a 10 minute bath with a fist full of sea salt thrown in is soothing.

If you're allowed whole wheat noodles or corn, only have them once or twice a week.

Oatmeal and dairy can make you worse, as they are too fatty.

Use hato mugi (hato barley) 2 times a week, either alone or 50/50 with rice or another grain when available.

Have greens steamed, blanched, water-sauteed or pressed, but make sure they are eaten at least 3 times a day. Six times a day is preferable if your condition is serious.

For the "occasional use" vegetables, choose any two and each one can be eaten in a small portion once a week. A good way to use the occasional vegetables would be 1 cucumber in the pressed salad one day a week and a couple stalks of celery in the pressed salad another day, or cooked in a bean dish.

Dried daikon cooked with kombu and shoyu (tamari without mirin) can be had twice a week. Other vegetables may be added to it.

Whole wheat noodles (if allowed) with broth and vegetables, can be enjoyed two meals a week maximum. And mind the proportion does not exceed 30% of the meal. It's best to still have a whole grain at the meal as well, to make up the other 20%.

Boiled vegetables daily, 3 times; pressed salad, 1/2 cup daily, and steamed greens every day, three times. On days or weeks when this just doesn't fit your schedule, don't worry. Do the best you can while working toward your goal.

Consider aduki bean tea or ume/sho/kuzu every three days to strengthen kidneys and blood.

If too much abdominal gas, usually you're not chewing or you're drinking with meals, leading to improper digestion. Also consider treating for Candida; cut out grains and ferments for 1-2 days and determine if improved.

It takes about 6 months to get rid of dairy. For accumulated dairy that stays, 30% kombu, 70% black soy bean can be eaten every day for three days a week for one month. Just 1/4-1/2 a cup is all that is necessary.

Do not use transition foods at the East/West (Wellspring) centers for the first 6 months. Eat strictly from the special table for people on healing diets. Volunteer to work in the kitchen so you'll (1) learn how to cook, (2) learn how many of the foods that you should not yet be eating are in the meals.

When you take your walk, go whether it's raining or shining, whether it's a blizzard or not. You need the exercise each day and to appreciate Nature in her many phases.

Before your consultation, ask yourself: Are you scrubbing, singing, walking, wearing cotton, etc. so that you can see if you're doing the maximum for yourself.

Try to avoid putting grains in soups very often because you'll not chew as much as you should.

Maximum 2 desserts per week, but less is better, none is best, especially if in a hurry to get well or your condition is fatal. Remember, cancer cases have to play "beat the clock." And since healing via macro takes time, you cannot afford to backslide. And when you do have a dessert, it is a cooked organic apple with a pinch of sea salt.

May have 2 cups of chestnuts per week (in grains or alone, or cooked and blended into a dessert sauce, etc.).

Maximum 4 rice cakes a week, if you must have them, or 2 per day. Also maximum one bottle of amasake per week, and only if you must have it.

No Perrier or other sparkling or carbonated waters or beverages, since these remove minerals from the body. Also, no garlic, no lemon (except on fish), no herb teas, no spices, since these stimulate tumors to grow faster.

For coffee withdrawal headaches, must tough it out. It usually lasts about four days.

Ginger accelerates cancers, so no ginger compresses and minimize it in cooking.

Roast kombu in a dry skillet and then crush it. Then it can be added to dry roasted sesame seeds for kombu-gomashio.

The daily proportion of kombu can be 50% of the total seaweeds ingested; the rest of the sea vegetables make up 50% of the total and are in equal quantities.

For kombu tea, use 2-3" strip, reduce by boiling 4 cups of spring water to 2.

May add leftover dinner vegetables to porridge in morning.

No soy milk.

No Ramen noodles, bread, powdered miso mixes. Avoid noodles the first 1-3 months if you do not crave them.

Be sure to mix and match to rejuvenate. Variety is important.

I recall the first time I went to New Orleans, my husband bought me Antoine's Cookbook. When I got home I was disillusioned that every wonderful recipe contained a sauce that usually was a combination of two other sauces, each of which took about 8 hours to make. Obviously, one does not make these things from scratch for the sole purpose of making one dish. First you make one sauce from scratch for one particular dish, you make another for another dish later on, and when you have a little of each leftover, the combination is new and exciting for a third dish. This is what you can do with your macro meals. You will make some interesting combinations from small amounts of things leftover that can be put into soups and other dishes, like squash or beans added to soups whole or blended for a new taste. Shoyu, scallions, ginger, parsley, condiments are still necessary to be used, and a few leftover roasted seeds or beans, or a dash of a sauce can dress up another dish. For example, the aduki/kombu/squash dish can be blended with "green juice" and simmered with miso or shoyu for a new sweet soup.

Prepare the greens fresh before each meal, and prepare as the last item before serving.

Remember, no eating for three hours before bed. You must heal the gut to get healthy. Like a broken arm, if you don't let it rest, how will it heal? And since it is the only way your nutrients can enter, you must heal the gut first. Before macro, I showed my plasma amino acids to a biochemist who specializes in interpreting deficiencies. It was sandwiched in among a bunch of other patient results I was consulting him on. When he saw how low they were, he asked, "Is this patient still alive?" After 1 year of macro, I redrew them and they were perfect, as contrasted to earlier ones showing severe malabsorption. My gut had healed, bloody painful colitis and all.

Fish can be eaten once a week, steamed or poached. Some conditions can have it twice a week, others should have none for a month or more. But the portion is a small 3x3" piece or 1/9th of meal.

Make sure to have a hanging rack for storing pots and pans in the kitchen. They're expensive, but well worth the money in time and energy saved in having the pots handy overhead and not having to bend, stoop, clang and rummage through pots and pans stored in a cupboard.

Old beans will not cook soft regardless of how many hours you cook them. When you have beans that are tough, even though you cooked them for the recommended time, usually it's because they're old. So don't get down on yourself for not having cooked them correctly when you have followed the directions.

A red face and nose often designate an alcoholic to Americans. Likewise, more subtle symptoms can be seen. Very shiny skin on the back of the hands with tendons showing easily are sometimes from too much chicken. Cancer of the throat or prostate accompanying that chicken-type neck fold is often from too much chicken with sugar, alcohol and stimulants. White, doughy palms often designate too much dairy, and a greenish cast, especially at base of thumb or on forearms can indicate cancer. In fact the very greenest forearms I ever saw were in a woman with active breast cancer.

To make onion pickles, only use one onion per week per person. It helps make the intestines stronger. Too much and you will crave sweets.

Stress a variety of cooking styles and ingredients or you'll get into trouble. Also, what is good for you now may not be good for you in a year. As the cure is in the kitchen, the key is in the cooking. Long term maintenance must be adapted to the season and your current state of health. Take cooking lessons and read, read, read. Compare notes with macro friends and constantly fuel your knowledge.

Wash vegetables always in cold water. But wait until the cooking water is boiling before putting in them.

For kale and collards, cook the stems longer than the greens. Cut the thick parts of stems out away from the greens. Chop them and cook them while you're chopping the rest of the greens, which are added in just for the last minute.

Gas cooked foods have more vitality, energy and taste. I doubted this for a long while. But as you get well and more unloaded, you'll be able to appreciate these subtle changes. I now often use the barbecue grill on the back yard patio for my grains, in a cast iron pot.

Don't peel vegetables if possible, even if not organic. Just wash vigorously.

Don't worry about keeping dishes hot. When you eat meat, if it's cold the fat solidifies and the taste decreases. In macro, there is minimal fat, so meals taste good at room temperature.

Never eat straight from the refrigerator. Food should be room temperature or warmer.

A handful of steamed parsley is great for breakfast. It cooks in 30 seconds without a lid on it.

Mustard greens and watercress are usually too bitter for soups or green juice.

When blanching vegetables, blanch only one cup at a time and start with the least strong. Otherwise, all the veggies will taste the same.

Make your soup stock, condiments, pickles and other added attractions at times other than mealtime so they will be ready.

Your water needs to be alive. Taste different waters so you can know what "dead" water tastes like. Check your source and try to periodically get it from a fresh spring, well or stream.

Don't put the pressure cooker under water to cool. It forces the steam into the rice.

Chewing less than 50 times is a waste of time.

You need a different breakfast every morning. Don't ever let yourself get bored. If so, start reading the cookbooks in the Resources or see your counselor/doctor.

Miso helps clean the blood.

Garnish is necessary for all soups; use a teaspoon of finely chopped scallion, parsley, celery or finely grated or shaved carrot, radish, etc.

Heavy facial lines are often due to too much salt and meat (yang food).

If you're hungry by 10:00 a. m., omit the breakfast miso. If you are always hungry, something is out of balance or you are low in a particular nutrient. It's the only way your body has to tell you it lacks something. The same goes for a craving.

To decrease animal fat from the body and accumulated fat from around organs like the prostate glands and ovaries, there are 3 remedies: (1) the sweet vegetable drink can be used (grated cabbage, carrots, squash, onion with 4 times the amount of water cooked 20 min.) 1 cup a day for a month. If you are too orange (carotenemia), substitute daikon and parsnip. (2) kombu/shiitake cooked until 4 cups of water reduces to 2, take 1/2 cup a day for 7 days then every other day for a month, then every third day for a month. You can use

the leftover mushroom and seaweed in soups, (3) grate 1/2 cup daikon and carrot each. Boil 3 min., then add 1 umeboshi and several
drops of shoyu sauce and simmer 2-3 minutes. Have 1 cup every 3
days for 5 weeks.

Grains are usually cooked 1 to 1 1/2 or 2 with water for the
healing phase and gomashio is usually 1 to 18 which will make it 2
tsp. salt per cup of seed since a cup has 16 tbsp. in it. Ask what your
specific ratio should be.

Always simmer miso and shoyu for about 3 min. It's more
relaxing, less tightening. Never just add it and serve.

Cabbage and daikon, 50/50 with very little water, can have
twice a week.

1 tbsp. washed pickles a day (wash the salt off for the healing
phase).

No fruit unless it's craved, then cook 1 cup of it with a pinch
of salt, maximum once a week.
No meat. It's tightening and can cause cancer to go (metasta-
size) to the bones.

A tight feeling in the epigastrium is usually pancreatic stress.
This is right under the end of the breast bone where many people
think their stomach is. Sweets, too much food, too salty food and
many other errors can cause it. Also discomfort in the upper back
(pain between the shoulders) can indicate too many sweets, ice
cream, poor chewing and pancreatic stress in general.

If there's green discoloration at the base of the thumb, this is
often a sign of trouble in the colon or a lung.

For patients that are dying and have no energy, immediate
change to gas cooking is recommended.

Sweet vegetable drinks can decrease worry and fear.

Ume/sho/kuzu can lift spirits and depression.

Kombu tea, 1 cup every other day for a month helps dissolve fats by supplying minerals. Cigarette smoking and other chemicals help to keep the fat solid (and loaded with chemicals), thus delaying discharges and healing.

No meat, dairy, sweets or stimulants.

Weekly fried rice with oil for radiation patients plus trout with carrots three days every other week times four.

Sour dough bread and mochi to decrease depression, but only once a week, if allowed. Also good to help keep weight on.

No sunflower seeds for six months for many (too fatty), but chestnuts and pumpkin seeds are OK.

10-15% beans equals the proportion for the whole day, not a meal. However it can constitute the proportion of the meal if it is once a day, usually 1/2-1 cup a day, maximum.

Hot towels to palms and soles to stimulate meridians, minimum once daily.

Cook the quickly cooked vegetables just before you eat and eventually try to avoid storing them. Longer cooked root vegetables (nishimi and beans) can be cooked every 2-3 days.

Limit the umeboshi plum to 1/2 or one whole plum every day maximum (total all forms, for example in tea, salad dressing, nori rolls, etc.).

Fruit causes melancholy and depression.

At each meal strive for two freshly cooked strong and crispy vegetables, and one longer cooked (stored) one. You should at least achieve this at dinner time.

For cancer, no ginger compresses, no long baths and no cheating. But strict does not mean narrow eating. Variety and making the meals delicious is important.

Beware of any foot lesions, disease, discolored toenails, warts, corns, callouses. These can designate blocked meridians. For example, warts, corns and other lesions of the fourth or fifth toes, because they are in the gall bladder meridian can indicate early problems there and the need to restrict oils.

Arame or hiziki, one cup three times a week or 1/4 to 1/2 cup daily is preferable, but always well-chewed.

Try putting the steamer basket for greens over your seaweed when you pre-boil it for miso soup. This way you use one burner to accomplish 2 tasks.

Medically terminal does not mean macrobiotically terminal. Never before were you treating the cause. Now you are finally doing something in an attempt to remedy the cause rather than just poison the cancer (and the rest of the body).

White patches, freckles and moles on the skin can indicate excess dairy. It's interesting to see them disappear on the diet, as we have observed.

Leg cramps and pain are often due to too much fruits and drinks, or deficient minerals like magnesium or calcium, or deficient fat soluble vitamins like E.

Headaches are often due to increased fruit and dairy.

One bowl of chopped, boiled cabbage every day for one month to relax.

No vinegar, as it's tightening.

Ginger compresses to areas that need chiropractic manipulation. Also do magnesium loading test, as people who need constant adjustments are often magnesium deficient (as well as deficient in other nutrients.

An oily nose usually suggests heart and intestines are in trouble since they are on the same meridians.

Raw black sesame seeds, 2 tsps. a day for 3 weeks. They are preferred over white since they have more minerals, especially iron.

Be thankful for symptoms and disease. They have prevented you from dying by alerting you to a problem before it advances.

Chewing also pumps the meridians which all come through the teeth. Without teeth, just mix food with saliva for three minutes.

Chew every mouthful 100 times even if the food is bad (off your macro) and especially if there is very little food available as you will get more nutrition from it.

The head and sexual organs are two major areas where energy enters the body chakras. So hairsprays and pantyhose interfere with this. Plastics and synthetics inhibit energy transfer. Cotton is already known to be indicated for women with recurrent vaginal discharge. A study in Clinical Ecology from India showed that putting people in all cotton decreased their blood pressure. Obviously cottons help the energy transfers from the body.

A shopping mall is a totally isolated place from the universe and exhausting. It has artificial light, water, air and food. Yet many people spend the majority of their free time there. Don't YOU if you're interested in healing.

An orderly house, especially kitchen and dining area, aids in digestion.

Do not microwave foods. The energy is not good for food or your body. Just look at what it does to a piece of French bread.

Mustard footbath for sweating out colds.

Nurture yourself daily. If you wanted to take the best care possible of a precious small child or animal, you would lavish nurturing in many forms on it. You need to do this to yourself. Likewise nurture others, for you get what you give.

Cotton only for compresses; never use polyester or other synthetic fabrics.

The lymphatic system does not have a pump (heart) as does the arterial system, so stagnation occurs more easily. When fats plug them, disease begins. Hence, decreasing fats and increasing physical stimulation (massage, exercise) to the lymphatics helps organs to re-establish a good nutrient flow to begin healing.

Scrub at least the hands and feet to the first major joint (knee and elbow) twice daily, using a hot, moist (using water, or better yet, ginger water) washcloth to stimulate meridians.

Remember to keep a starter bag with an assortment of clean vegetables in the refrigerator, as well as a greenie bag and a soup bag for your "compost soup" stock.

Headaches almost always come from the intestines, so think in terms of what is wrong with the intestine.

Raw foods are hard on the intestines. Baked foods tighten the intestines even when one is healthy.

Daikon and carrot drink helps break down and dissolve animal and cheese fat.

Tamari/bancha/ginger tea for a pick-me-up. Omit the ginger, though, if there's a headache present.

Never use a ginger compress for a cyst, tumor, cancer, headache or diarrhea, as they can become worse.

If there is no liquid in the pressed salad in 1/2 hour, add more salt.

Longer, slow cooking is necessary with larger chunks or nishimi root vegetables.

Learn how to cut carrot wedges by rolling the carrot over 1/2 a turn so you don't have to change the angle of the knife. Are you craving something? Stop and figure out what you're having too much of. Usually this is the case rather than too little. For example, the cause of sugar craving can be too much salt or oil.

Dietary restrictions are always temporary, for as you get progressively healthier, you should reach a point where you can eat whatever you want, at least once in a while.

If your diet is too yang, you may be thin and always very hungry. You need a gentler course, less salt, no fish (temporarily).

If you're afraid of using too much shoyu (tamari), dilute the bottle with water as you'll get too yang, hungry, thin, never feel satisfied, eat all the time and still lose weight.

As soon as the rice is cooked, use a wooden spatula to separate it from the sides of the pot (around the edges and then at the bottom) to let the steam out and aerate it; and then transfer it to a wooden or glass bowl. This makes it fluffier and less soggy or sticky.

Rice balls retard spoilage better in brown paper than Saran Wrap, and better if you have a piece of an umeboshi plum inside.

Most common reasons for failure: 1) eating processed foods or poor quality foods (including poor quality salt and water), 2) digestive and liver functions have been destroyed, 3) no family support, 4) failure to do the program accurately, 5) poor habits; lack of chewing. All of these are reversible. If you can manage your food, you can manage your life, for food is the essence of life, so that you can change your destiny with how you eat. If you don't choose to re-prioritize your life for a year or two to cook and eat more healthfully, disease will win out. So why not take control of your life and your health now?

If you awaken cold in the night, you probably have low blood sugar which is a sign of pancreatic stress. Check the third and fourth toes for any lesions, poor nails, fungus, infection, corns, etc.

Cook beans 80%, then add the salt and the pot cover for the last 20 minutes.

Urinary urgency is usually too much fruits. Ume/sho/kuzu

helps.

Osteoporosis is usually too much sugar, dairy and acid (like fruits) since the acid pulls calcium out of the bon es because it requires so much buffer and this buffer is available from the bone. This is why extreme eating such as balancing beef with fruits is not healing, even though it's balanced, because it's still draining the buffer system and precious minerals necessary for healing.

If you have cough and colds all the time, that's usually too much fruits (yin foods produce yin symptoms).

You must do the program honestly and happily, chew well and have gratitude daily for friends, people you meet, people you don't even know but are responsible for your food, etc. The person who angrily says, "Well, I'm doing everything by the book and I hate this stuff. How come I'm not better yet?!" rarely does get better.

You know you're in trouble when the doctor keeps changing your prescription medicines. You're on a downward course at that time and it's time to start healing yourself.

Purple blotched hands and purple fingertips often are due to too much chocolate.

Red palms are often due to too much fruit (or alcohol).

Yellow palms and soles can be liver troubles or too much yellow vegetables. Likewise, the nasolabial folds (crease from cheeks between sides of nose and corners of mouth) will take on a yellow hue. Cut back on yellow foods, do body scrubs.

The worse your condition, the more important it is to be strict 3-4 months after you have totally cleared your symptoms. If you feel like a splurge, do it with sensible moderation. If you feel pressured to be good and are miserable due to cravings, you should see the doctor: something may be missing.

Sweet vegetable drink is good for abdominal gathering tendency where the weight gain tends to be right in the abdomen. This is often a sign of an ailing pancreas as well.

No grain coffee because it's dark and roasted and too yang.

Dark tongue edges and tenderness just above the medial knee, epigastric tenderness and lesions on the third and fourth toes often suggest pancreatic problems.

Herbal teas and garlic can stimulate the heart and blood pressure. They are too stimulating for a healing phase.

Most conditions could benefit from ume/sho/kuzu every three days for a month.

Always on the table: tekka

black sesame (gomashio)

nori flakes

Eyes tearing frequently can be too much fruit. Need ginger to the kidney and black soy beans in the diet.

If a lung problem exists, there's also usually an intestinal problem (it may be as yet undiagnosable) because they are in the same meridians and are paired. Likewise, the weakened and plugged intestines also effect the lungs because they share the same meridian.

If you're weak, it can be too much miso, not enough variety, not enough beans or fish.

If you're losing too much weight, increase the oil, have mochi for snacks and broken grains.

Sweets are expansive and weakening, then dairy comes in and makes too much mucous, plugging up the swollen, expanded tissues with mucous. Congested tissues lack good nutrient circulation and disease sets in as degeneration proceeds. Other foods are too acidic and pull out the minerals, thus further weakening the area. The result is organ disease.

Some people actually need steak and eggs and home fries, or

they feel awful. But this type of chemistry requires more monitoring due to the dangers of hypercholesterolemia, and I've never seen anyone heal their cancers on it.

Not even 5 raisins would be allowed in the porridge until healing has occurred in dangerously "terminal" conditions. But you can add sweet vegetables, miso, shoyu, condiments or scallions.

A medical report card is necessary to fill out periodically, so you have a more objective measure of your progress. People tend to forget very quickly how awful they felt once they get well. Once they feel great for a while, it's easy to fall off and reverse all the good you've done by prematurely broadening the diet. Also with the slow subtle progress of macro you can use this report card to be sure you are on a steady uphill course. When you stop making progress, or reach a plateau, it's time to reassess. Perhaps you even have an undiagnosed nutrient deficiency or too much of an environmental overload.

Biological stressers are the following:

> microbiologic contamination (bacterial or yeast infection, for example)
>
> physical over-exhaustion
>
> allergenic overload (food, chemical, dust, pollen, animal, mold, etc.)
>
> extreme temperature variation
>
> drug side effect
>
> psychological stress
>
> environmental pollutants
>
> nutritional deficiencies
>
> low level radiation

electromagnetic pollution

geopathic stress

negative thought energies, worry, depressive
people in your life

Medicine tends to devote itself to the top few, whereas macrobiotics tends to address all of these, for that is what the attainment of health often requires.

The quality of the blood is the most important thing for healing. It must be brimming with nutrients at all times. That's why you work so hard at cramming so many vegetables into your daily diet.

A Nobel Prize winning scientist discovered years ago that he could keep a fish or chicken heart alive in a beaker of water for years if he just put in the correct nutrients. There was no blood, no special oxygen pumped in, just salt water with the necessary nutrients.

Michio Kushi says that 50% of the people who are terminally ill want to change, but do not develop the proper understanding of cooking or they improvise and add other things to it. It behooves any of us to change a method that is unsurpassed in doing the impossible, or at least until we are well. 25% have no support or approval or encouragement to go macrobiotic and so they soon return to their old way of life. 15-20% will improve with macrobiotics; many of the rest do not do it correctly. We have tried to help you improve your odds by 1) helping you organize and teaching you throughout this manual, 2) by buoying you up from the indecisive stage with case histories and biochemical evidence and helping you relieve your psychological stumbling blocks and to learn from the mistakes of others.

Do not use wheat-free, yeast-free tamari. It usually contains byproducts of the shoyu manufacturing that are undesirable, and always check the ingredients. Many contain mirin which is an alcohol and is not for healing. Mr. Kushi says when macrobiotics was first brought to the U.S., in order that people would not confuse shoyu with grocery store soy sauce containing corn syrup and carmelized coloring, the word tamari was used. Then the nature of tamari changed but all the texts were already written. Likewise, an umeboshi "plum" was mistakenly translated in error. It is an apricot.

Learn how to test pancreatic function with applied kinesiology. Ask at your counseling session or read books on it.

Be sure you are not overloading your body with harmful, electromagnetic fields. Never use a waterbed or electric blanket. This is swaddling your body in electromagnetic fields which are harmful and have even caused psychological disturbances and cancers.

Remember that no one is perfect; not you, not me, not macro counselors. Several well known macrobiotic leaders in fact are smokers. So don't get down on yourself for not doing things perfectly every day. Macrobiotics is time consuming and difficult. I have never done it perfectly week in and week out. However, no one knows what level of near perfection each of us has to attain or strive for in order to accomplish the impossible that many have done. You will notice that the harder you work at it, the better you get. I would suggest you read The E. I. Syndrome, You Are What You Ate, Tired or Toxic? and Macro Mellow as well, since the more information you have, the better off you'll be. I also suggest you read many of the other macrobiotic books in the bibliography. If you are sick enough, you need to get as much knowledge as possible.

So what if you can't orchestrate all of this? Remember, it took many of us several years. No one is perfect, including yourself. But because this has had such a marvelous track record, it certainly is worth attempting to do for one year out of your life. Remember, there are different bio-types and a consultation may reveal that you are a person who just cannot do macrobiotics, and in fact shouldn't do it. Also remember, the body is in constant change and needs to adapt. You may not be able to handle the diet every day, so what if you do it every other or every third day to completion, eating simpler on the "off" days. Breakfast could just be soft grain, gomashio, nori and steamed green. That takes 15 minutes. Lunch could be left overs: pressed salad, breakfast greens, grain, soup, root dish, and maybe a bean. Just don't depend on eating leftovers too often as they have lower nutrient value. And if you need a break periodically (providing you do not have cancer), switch into the Macro Mellow book.

Or say you just find all of this utterly overwhelming. Let's start even easier. What do you have for breakfast usually? Nothing? Cereal, toast, donuts, eggs, pop-ups? This weekend make some brown rice (45 minutes cooking time during which you can do other things). Also some roasted pumpkin seeds or sesame seeds (gomashio) with salt.

Now you have brown rice and a sprinkling of seeds for breakfast. You can warm it up, cook into a porridge consistency with an equal volume of water, or eat at room temperature. Or you could switch off to precooked breakfast millet, oats, barley, quinoa, etc. The whole grain and seeds provides you with about 5 times more minerals like magnesium, chromium, manganese, copper and zinc than any of your regular items. If you can't handle the blandness, go transition and perk up your porridge with nuts, dried or fresh fruits, nut milk, soy milk, or yogurt, etc.

When you get ready in a week or two to advance, you can take 5 minutes while you are heating your grain, make a Herb Walley and steam some greens. And there you have it! Next on a weekend, take 2 hours and make a couple dozen knishes from the <u>Macro Mellow</u> book. They freeze well and are great for lunch. They are a transition food, not healing, but you may need to ease into healing a lot slower.

In essence, it's exciting to know that the power of health really belongs to each individual. What more power can you have than health? When your mind and body are vibrantly healthy, then everything is possible.

A note about reactions to this book. Some macro counselors will denigrate it and say it is too rigid. You can say that about everything because there is no standard way for everyone for anything in the world. But having seen what scores of near death seriously ill patients were prescribed, and what people have followed who healed the impossible, has provided us with a pretty fair starting point. Some may denigrate it because they are worried that a book will replace the need for their services. But for any counselor worth his salt, this can never happen, because there is need for too much individualization.

Remember, too, there is a small subset of people who will actually be worse on this diet. Some will be worse because they have become unmasked (see Tired Or Toxic?) too fast; others because they are allergic or their bio-type actually requires meat, at least for now. And remember also, there are people who are not ready to get well. It would not fit into their life, or the lives of those closest to them.

Physicians, of course, who denigrate it will do so for a variety of reasons: Many suffer from "If I didn't read it in The New England Journal Of Medicine, it doesn't work" syndrome. First, remember that this journal is heavily subsidized by the drug industry. For example, they published a report by Jewett et al, in August 1990 "proving" that provocation-neutralization testing (used for diagnosing food and chemical sensitivity) does not work. Yet in the very first paragraph on procedures, they spelled out in no uncertain terms the fact that they had the entire protocol absolutely wrong ("a neutralizing dose shall be defined as one that produces a 2mm. increase in size"). They were actually using the dose that turns on symptoms to try to turn them off. You can imagine how many other errors there were if they had the basic premise wrong! And that journal is supposedly renowned for being peer reviewed and a leader in medicine. They were so dishonest that they did not publish one rebuttal pointing out their errors. For example, the study was done 7 years prior to publication and none of the studies in the last 7 years supporting the technique were referenced. This is unheard of in the medical world, but not in dirty medical politics. And for their guest editorial, they picked some foreign doctor none of us ever heard of who was not a specialist in food allergy, when the normal choice would have been a famous immunologist (J. Brostoff) who authored a huge medical text on food allergy. But their intent was to destroy, so they couldn't. After all, why did they break all protocol by publishing a 7 year old erroneous study and alert all the news media nationwide 3 days prior to release when it had no marked bearing on national health? Furthermore, in that same issue, there was a study worthy of national attention but it received none. Because to do so would jeopardize the food industry, drug industry and credibility of thousands of doctors. So for physicians too insecure in their knowledge to make their own unbiased decisions, there is no hope. They will forever rely on dishonest sources other than their own innate abilities to judge, never seeking out the real facts. They are incapable of making honest decisions for themselves.

You could copy and use the following arguments to attempt to interest your doctor in considering your diet. If he understands a little about it, it will not be so foreign, and therefore threatening to him. If he is intelligent and honest, he will see that it fits today's most healthful recommendations and eating guidelines and that you have nothing to lose by trying it, once he has determined that you do not have hidden renal disease, heart failure, etc., and have had a good physical.

WHY THE PHYSICIAN SHOULD CONSIDER RECOMMENDING A MACROBIOTIC DIET

Sherry A. Rogers, M. D.

Since most patients with chronic or terminal diseases or environmental illness have exhausted all that medicine can offer, it is especially frustrating when these patients fail to respond to last resort environmentally oriented management. A treatment failure is someone who has exhausted all that conventional modern medicine has to offer. Furthermore, he also has resisted all that environmental medicine has to offer by having tested inhalants, foods, chemicals, had appropriate injections, carried out environmental controls, evaluated the Candida program, had hormonal and nutrient levels assessed and corrected, and has a loving and supportive family. In spite of all this, the person is sick, unable to tolerate stores and offices and unable to be employed.

Goal: To introduce a variation on a diet that has cleared many symptoms resistant to all that medicine has to offer and made many people less food, chemically, mold and EMF sensitive. As well, with this program many have cleared cancers, chronic conditions (like colitis, rheumatoid arthritis, optic degeneration, lupus, multiple sclerosis, chronic fatigue, diabetes, hypertension, high cholesterol, etc.) and corrected nutritional deficiencies that have resisted supplementation programs for over two years.

Macrobiotics has become known as a Japanese diet of rice, vegetables, beans and seaweed for which documented cases (several of whom are physicians who had incurable cancers) exist where people have cleared end stage cancers. It is more than a diet, however, and involves eating and living within the laws or balance of nature. We decided to explore this diet for use with our resistant cases. We found, however, that we had to modify it for our allergic patients.

Case examples have been given in our three macrobiotic books of many people who were diagnostically or treatment-wise, over a barrel and there was nothing left for them. These people cleared their conditions totally and when they went off the diet, the conditions started to recur.

The discharge phenomenon occurs when healing has reached a point where old toxins or chemicals are able to be mobilized and discharged through the body and examples of this are also given.

The basis of the diet is 50% whole grains which can be rotated, 20-30% greens, ground and root vegetables, 5-10% beans and the rest in seaweeds, nuts, seeds, fishes and soups. The diet purposely avoids processed foods and meats and other foods that are on the extreme pH end of the scale. It also avoids foods that are nutrient poor and high in sugars. Because it is high in vegetables it is an alkaline diet and therefore does not stress the pH buffering system which is already stressed with daily chemical detoxication.

There are multiple mechanisms through which the diet is so healing. (In fact, there are over 40 and many of these are described and referenced in Tired Or Toxic?). Brown rice, for example, contains five fold more magnesium than white bleached rice. The same goes for whole wheat versus bleached enriched white wheat flour.

The causes of all disease are easily broken down into (1) genetic (many of which can be overcome with biochemical manipulation and dietary manipulations such as PKU, diabetes mellitus, etc.), (2) environmental (trauma, infection, chemical, pollen, dust, mold, physical factors like temperature or EMF), (3) psychogenic factors, and (4) diet/nutritional. Sugar, for example is a negative nutrient, and dairy is known for its mucous producing capability. In fact, in the newborn calf, that is exactly what it's purpose is. It is to protect the infant calf from the stomach acids as it is learning to be a regurgitating ruminant.

Fat has been shown throughout the literature to be the precursor to not only cardiovascular disease, but most cancers as well. And grocery store cooking oils like polyunsaturated corn oils and margarines are now known to cause more arteriosclerosis than saturated oils of steaks (NEJM 8/16/90). Meat is well known to putrify in the gut and disturb the bacterial flora as well as increase the beta glucuronidase enzyme that in turn removes glucuronic acid (GA) from conjugated chemicals that have been discharged into the bowel, thereby allowing for the reabsorption of that very chemical. Therefore, the energy of conjugation is also wasted along with a molecule of GA for every molecule of a chemical that the body attempts to detoxify when one eats meat regularly.

It is well documented that due to food processing, at least 50% of the U.S. population has one or more nutrient deficiencies. These have been proven to contribute to the pathogenesis of a vast number of diseases.

As well, food allergy inflames the gut leading to malabsorption, and when the gut is inflamed there is, of course, compromise of the xenobiotic detoxication system that lines the gut and is so crucial in this target organ.

For the psychological causes, macrobiotics stresses the importance of daily laughter, hugs, singing, dancing, exercise, meditation, and other aspects of a healthy psyche.

Phosphatidyl choline is lost in the detox process but is crucial in determining the endoplasmic reticulum membrane function (xenobiotic detoxication). Membranes determine the fluidity, stability, permeability, binding, neurotransmitters, and many more functions. For example, it is known to be able to stop and in early cases, reverse Alzheimer's presenile dementia. Likewise, for every molecule of daily office and home chemical detoxified through glutathione (GSH), a molecule of ATP (energy) and GSH is lost. So our modern chemical world also adds to nutrient loss.

When one looks at the biochemical bottlenecks of detoxication and their nutrient requirements, it is readily appreciated why a macrobiotic diet is so healing on many levels.

(1) Being a low meat diet is low in beta glucuronidase so there is less loss of glucuronic acid and glutathione and energy in daily detoxication. A low meat diet also unloads xanthine oxidase which can pinch-hit for alcohol dehydrogenase in the detox scheme. Most importantly it is low in fat, which has been proven to be the most crucial variable in reversing cardiac occlusive disease without drugs or surgery (Ornish, Lancet, 336:129, 1990).

(2) It is low in sugars. Sugars through non-enzymatic glycosylation can do all the damage that chemicals can such as gene mutation, create faulty messengers and damage enzymes. Also a high fructose diet (corn, fruit) causes swelling of the endoplasmic reticulum, thereby compromising detoxication; also it augments copper deficiency (copper is necessary in super oxide dismutase which scavenges free radicals resulting from chemical overload. When these free radicals are not quenched, they proceed to destroy sulf-hydryl groups of regulatory enzymes and lipid membranes of the energy producing mitochondria, for example). A low sugar diet also unloads the aldehyde bottleneck, thereby helping to reduce a person's allergies, especially reactions to foods and chemicals.

(3) An increase in whole grains increases the minerals necessary for detox and regeneration as do all the vegetables, seaweeds and soups. On average, whole grains have at least 3.5 times more minerals than processed grains and flour products.

(4) Beans give more lecithin for the endoplasmic reticulum as well as other membranes, plus provide molybdenum for the aldehyde oxidase enzyme which is one of the biochemical bottlenecks of the chemical detoxication scheme.

(5) It is an alkaline diet so it decreases the exhaustion of the buffers and increases detox enzyme functions (which function better under alkaline conditions).

(6) It is high in cruciferous vegetables which provide more sulfur for phase II detoxication via glutathione, PAPS, cysteine and taurine.

(7) It is also pretty much oil free for the first one to three months, as excessive lipids have been documented to accumulate in the endo-

plasmic reticulum and disturb its function (Feuer, <u>Molecular Biochemistry of Human Disease</u>, volume 3, page 113, CRC Press, Boca, Raton, 1990).

It must be remembered that airborne chemicals overload and deplete nutrients. For example, glutathione is lost in the bile as chemicals are conjugated; also phosphatidyl choline is lost from membranes including the endoplasmic reticulum where detoxication actually occurs. Case examples and the "how to" for the beginning patient are in <u>You Are What You Ate</u>; then proceed to the sequel, <u>The Cure is in the Kitchen</u>. <u>Tired or Toxic?</u> provides referenced evidence and should be the starting book for physicians.

Even the American Heart Association and the American Diabetic Association and the American Medical Association are slowly coming to the realization that whole grains and vegetables should predominate in the diet, and that processed foods and sugars should be down-played and meats should begin to take a back seat instead of being the primary focus of meals. But the trend is slow and those who are very ill need an intensive, guided program. Ornish's program that has reversed heart disease, proven by PET and other techniques (publ. <u>Lancet, JAMA, Circulation</u>) is the second best (and most restrictive) lifestyle change proven to reverse disease.

And the medical and other scientific literature (references further on in this book) are now full of evidence that many chronic degenerative diseases, including cancers, are caused in part by dietary fat, arteriosclerosis being a prime example, and are reversible through diet and lifestyle changes.

For some patients a transition diet is necessary, as described in <u>Macro Mellow</u>. One must always remember for the ecology or highly allergic patients to never violate good ecologic principles, rotate foods, especially the grains, always adapt the diet to the individuality of the patient and the climate, avoid natural gas, avoid ferments initially and keep close follow-up with the patient, especially with biochemical nutrient assessments.

Conclusion

The macrobiotic diet modified for chronic cases and E.I. patients is a practical and extremely nutritious whole foods diet that has enabled over 350 patients in 5 years in my practice to markedly decrease their food, chemical, Candida, EMF and inhalant sensitivities and correct resistant cancers, reverse crippling rheumatoid arthritis, chronic fatigue syndrome, and nutritional deficiencies, and certainly should be one of the tools with which the specialist in environmental medicine and internal medicine as well as all specialties is familiar. For that matter, it should be investigated by anyone who does not enjoy completely good health. It is especially useful for patients who can no longer tolerate injections or who do not have any money to do further investigations.

Bibliography

Rogers, S. A., Tired Or Toxic?, Prestige Publishing,
P. O. Box 3161, Syracuse, NY   13220, 1990

Rogers, S. A., You Are What You Ate, Prestige Publishing,
P. O. Box 3161, Syracuse, NY   13220

Rogers, S. A., Zinc deficiency as a model for developing chemical sensitivity, Intern. Clin. Nutr. Rev., 10, 1, 253-259, January 1990

Rogers, S. A., Magnesium deficiency masquerades as diverse medical conditions. Evaluation of a magnesium loading test, ibid, 11, 3, 117-125 July 1991.

Klaassen, C. D., Amdur, M. O., Doull, T. (ed), Casarett & Doull's Toxicology, Macmillan Publ. Co., NY   (1986)

Jakoby, W. B., Enzymatic Basis of Detoxication, Vol. I & II, Academic Press, NY   (1980)

Kushi, M., The Book of Macrobiotics, Japan Publ., NY (1986)

Kushi, M., A Natural Approach to Allergies, Japan Publ., NY (1985)

Halstead, C.H., Rucker, R.B., Nutrition and the Origins of Disease, Academic Press, NY (1989)

Ornish, D., Dr. Dean Ornish's Program for Reversing Heart Disease; The Only System Scientifically Proven to Reverse Heart Disease Without Drugs or Surgery, Random House, NY, 1990.

Ornish, D., et al, Can Life-Style Changes Reverse Coronary Heart Disease? Lancet, 1990, 336:129-133).

Taken from The Cure Is In the Kitchen: The Strict Healing Phase for the Macrobiotic Diet, by Sherry A. Rogers, M. D., Prestige Publishing, 3502 Brewerton Rd., P. O. Box 3161, Syracuse, NY 13220.

PLAY IT AGAIN, SAM!

Other tips and questions that frequently come up: (I apologize for some that are repetitious as well as my digressions, but they reflect those points that keep re-surfacing).

Kombu cooked with beans helps to soften them and increase their digestibility, whereas salt contracts them and it takes longer for them to cook and soften. Use a 2-3" piece of kombu for each cup of beans and hold off adding salt (if needed) until the last 20 minutes when they are 80% cooked. "Shocking" technique of adding cold water also softens.

Avoid misos in plastic bags as they have been pasteurized so that they will not continue metabolizing and put out gas that will rupture the bag. In essence, they are no longer living cultures; they are dead. Long term misos aged two to three years, such as barley and hatcho, are better for healing and sold in tubs.

Aduki beans and lentils are the lowest in fat and are recommended for serious illness. In good health you can enjoy any bean. For aduki and black soy beans, save the soak water, but for chick peas, kidney, pinto, lima and soy, discard the soak water.

Black soy bean juice from cooking is good for dissolving fats, especially in the reproductive area. When cooking beans, they should be simmered for an hour and a half until 80% done, then the salt added and cooked 10-30 minutes longer. Keep checking the water to see that they do not need more to prevent burning.

When you eat too much oil then you crave salt which then leads to the craving of sweets.

When you're lacking sweets in the diet, use more yin cooking such as quick pressed salad and quick steaming to decrease the craving for sweets. These foods must necessarily be sliced very thinly. This is where your Mac knife is handy.

Yin cancers, such as skin, breast and brain are generally from too much sugar, cream, cheese, ice cream.

Raw foods are more difficult to digest. They're more yin. They add more stress to the body. Pressed pickles help strengthen and relax the body.

Nappa cabbage, radishes, onions, cucumbers, celery are good for raw salads. If you have cancer or a serious health problem, blanch sliced onions for 30 seconds and omit cucumber and celery until better.

Never use cucumber if the patient is cold or weak.

Wild plants such as some herbs like lovage have strong energies, are bitter, make people thirsty, may get rid of oils too quickly and the person may crave oil or proteins.

Garlic is appropriate only if eating meat. Ginger, horseradish and daikon are better.

For dairy craving, substitute tempeh, sauteed vegetables, beans, natto, or have what you're craving in a small amount. It may stop the craving, in which case a small amount may have been harmless and actually necessary.

To dry roast anything, such as rice, seeds for gomashio or grains for grain tea, such as roasted barley tea, wash it first and roast it damp in a skillet until it is dry. Be very careful not to burn it. Do your affirmations while stirring. Then proceed to cook the rice or steep the barley tea as needed.

If you're camping, one trick is to dry roast your grain, add one and a half cups of boiling hot water in a thermos and leave it all day. When you come back, it should be ready to eat!

Have a variety of seaweeds every day: nori, wakame, kombu and arame or hijiki.

If using salt in place of kombu in the grains, put it in after it boils ten minutes. If you put it in at the beginning, it tightens the outer shell of the grain so it can't open up to adequately cook, unless it has been presoaked overnight.

-214-

Burdock helps discharge old oils and fats and strengthens the reproductive organs. Dried daikon also helps pull out old fats.

Arame only gets rinsed. Hijiki, however, should be soaked for several hours.

Patients losing weight too fast often have too much salt, miso and too little variety.

When preparing to use kombu, you can merely wipe it off with a damp, clean cloth. Some just use it as is. You are not trying to remove the white powdery dust which is good for you.

For indigestion, rice cream and long-cooked beans (3 hours), mashed.

To gain weight, bulk up and increase strength and endurance, use sweet rice, mochi, tofu, nuts, soy products, fish. But these are after healing has occurred.

Be sure to massage whatever hurts, as with arthritic joints massage right to the end of that acupuncture meridian for that particular problem. You want to get the energies flowing. Stress eating the foods that help heal the organs that are companions to that meridian. The Kushi books will guide you.

By decreasing grains and increasing greens you can slow down the discharge and moderate it.

The more threatened someone is, the more rigid they generally become.

Of the cancer modalities that are damaging to the body, surgery is the least, then radiation and then chemo being the most, since it poisons every cell.

People new to macrobiotics eat huge meals, too much food and too many beans. If you're in a rush for a healing phase, watch your proportions right away and keep the beans to 10-15% total for the day. Some days it's fine if you don't even have any.

Macrobiotics involves a lifestyle change, and sometimes even a career change. The food helps to change the spirit and enhances the endorphin release and decreases tension. If you're hostile toward the food, consider psychotherapy or don't waste your time. And consider learning how to love yourself.

The macrobiotic approach forces you to slow down and to hear the birds, smell the roses and rediscover the quality of life. Ironically, many are even more productive because they are more focused.

Shiitake mushroom helps mobilize old oil and salt, while hijiki, rice and miso help with old chemicals.

Making people too yang so they can't discharge, can come from overeating salt or seaweeds.

Side dishes of seaweeds (hiziki or arame) at lunch and dinner should be about 3-4 tablespoons or 1/4 cup a day maximum.

When people get tight, they overeat, have mood swings and crave sweets.

Put leftover raw corncobs in stews for extra nutrition.

Depression can come from being too yang, too contracted, overeating.

Only leave food in a plastic pickle press for a few hours. Other-wise use a ceramic crock for longer pickles.

Hatto mugi is a wild grass, not a true barley. It's the most medicinal of the barleys and helps discharge animal fats and protein.

Cold, yin foods tend to go to the lungs which is why ice cream and milk often cause congestion.

Dry roast grains if you want fluffier, nuttier flavor and lighter rice, or if you've had too much liquid and yin, or if you are weak and need more energy.

For tight kidneys, ginger compresses and hot towel scrubs and soaking of the feet, plus shiatsu helps. Also avoiding oils and nuts, and eating a clean, standard diet and 1/4-1/2 cup aduki beans 3 times a week and kombu tea daily, for one month.

When the kidneys are tight, the face will erupt. Asthma and other mucous conditions will occur.

To discharge salt, have 1/2 c. grated steamed daikon. Also shiitake tea is helpful.

Yelling and aggression are more yang. Whining and insecure complaining and a "Woe is me!" attitude are more yin.

If urine smells of ammonia, there can be too much seaweed. If it's too clear, it's too yin.

Pain in the top of the shoulder can signify trouble beginning in the gall bladder or the small intestine, whereas between the shoulder blades is often pancreas.

For anger, check out the liver, not enough greens. Fasting a day or two often helps and when eating is resumed, reduce salt.

Mood swings can be due to low blood sugar or hypoglycemia. The pancreas gets harder by accumulating fats. Cookies, baked things, bread all make it tighter, plus cheese, seafood, chicken and eggs increase the protein and the fat. It gets harder and harder and can't secrete digestive hormones, but yin insulin is able to be secreted and you get hypoglycemia. Eventually excess fat can start to create a tumor.

All aspects of life depend on a modest diet.

Major message: LESS IS MORE.

Can change physical and mental vibrations of a person through eating and thinking (prayer, meditation, positive imagery).

Sugar and spices stimulate tumors to grow bigger and attract yin, and expand and spread (and certainly the biochemistry supports this).

Greenish hue about mouth can suggest uterine or ovarian cancer.

Osteoporosis or weak bones comes from eating too much acids from meat, sugar or fruit that require alkali buffering from the bones and pulls calcium from the bones along with other minerals.

Liver meridian starts on big toe, goes up inside leg. Gall bladder starts at the outside corner of the eye and down the outside of the leg to the fourth toe. So beware of lesions in these areas and modify diet accordingly.

Hatto mugi barley gets rid of extreme protein and oil.

Daikon helps digestion and to get rid of hard animal fat. It is good grated and eaten raw after too much food or meat. Good to use for excess water, fat and protein.

When you don't discharge every day, that's the beginning of a problem.

If constipated, use grated radish. Have a teaspoon of grated radish with every breakfast. Standard Japanese diet at breakfast is rice with miso, grated radish, toasted nori and pickles.

Ume/sho/bancha for over acid condition and insomnia.

Umeboshi helps digestion, promotes saliva, helps yin frontal headache. Remember to limit to one a day in total diet.

Deep neck headache with tired eyes needs sweets. Sweet vegetable drink is good.

Remember to always simmer misos, tamaris and shoyu for 2-4 minutes. Salt requires longer cooking.

Purplish or milky color along lateral aspect of lower foot can signify beginning of prostatic cancer.

Check for callouses as signs of stagnation in meridians.

No nuts for strict healing phase. Maximum one cup total of all seeds a week.

Quality of foods (including salt and water) makes a major difference.

Never use plastic or polyester with compresses.

Signs suggestive of intestinal parasites: biting fingernails, gritting teeth, overeating, cross ridges in nails.

We are constantly discharging any excess foods through many routes, but if we take in very fatty foods, they plug the pores and lymphatics, stagnation occurs and diseased organs arise as circulation is compromised.

Approaches to improving health include skin brushing with hot towels to open the pores, exercise to sweat, singing songs to make better breathing and discharge for CO_2 and reduce eating of high energy foods and simple sugars. High energy foods in stagnated organs can eventually erupt into cancer. Avoid mustard, pepper, curry, alcohol. All are high energy. Must reduce volume and chew very, very, very well.

If skin brushing is not done, shiatsu and other body work is not effective.

Fear of cancer is a bad thought. A negative picture goes through the chakras and through every cell and it inhibits one from getting better. Therefore, especially the cancer patient needs a happy, positive, optimistic, loving mind.

No synthetic clothes, only cotton since you can only discharge through cotton.

Fat is the cause of cancer. Sugars, alcohols, fruits and spices stimulate it, but fat blocks the flow of nutrients so that the organ begins degenerating. The government is just now starting to realize that some cancers are already proven to be correlated with fat intake, such

such as breast cancers.

Each person is the only person who can change his destiny.

Macrobiotics can clear cellulite. It's merely stagnation of fat and poor circulation in an area. You need to diet it off and rebuild with chemical-free fats.

Soaking feet in hot ginger water or hot sea salt water for five minutes every night helps meridians balance quicker.

Dizziness may mean lack of minerals, needing more salt.

If liver is stagnated (contracted), needs yin energy, so need lots of green leafy vegetables, low salt, short cooking.

All the meridians are connected, so when you do something to one, you automatically affect the others. That's partly why when a medication is taken to suppress one symptom, some other body organ acts up. In the medical system you go to a completely different type of doctor for a condition in another organ, so the correlation is often missed. Besides it takes months to years to happen.

When doing exercises, tingling means energy is being released. Burning means you're stretching it too much.

If the back is tense, try sitting with your legs out straight on the floor, and walk forward by sliding one leg forward alternately on your butt.

Energy vibration can be healing, which is why chanting and singing are important.

Tender spots usually mean stagnated mucous or inflammation. Try to work out the meridian through massage.

Yang diseases, such as cancer of the pancreas (not all cancers are yang), are very fast, violent and dangerous. Acute pancreatitis attracts strong yin such as alcohol (a known precursor as well as exposure to yin chemicals like pesticides) and swells.

If eating too yang, you are predisposed to a slipped disc and arthritis. The body is so tight that the disc is extruded from between the vertebral bodies. To treat a ruptured disc must discontinue eggs, meat, chicken. It takes a long time to clear (but nutrient corrections can more than halve the time of healing). Chicken is very tightening to the back. In fact, chicken is more tightening than meat, especially to the neck. If orthopedic injuries (tears, sprains) occur, learn yoga stretches and cut out animal products including fish.

Colitis and cancer are a mixture of yin and yang, as are most diseases including many forms of arthritis. If arthritis involves the fingers, it's usually in fruit eaters and quick to heal. If it's in the hips and spine, it's yang and slow to reverse.

Be sure to ask yourself when something is bothering you, is your stomach bothering you or are you bothering your stomach? Do you have a pain or are you a pain? Likewise, if you can't do the diet, is there a reason you need to still be ill? Was it the only time you got attention and loving as a child?

A good rule of thumb is if something is too yin, don't give straight yang but give a mixture of yin and yang. If something is more yin, you need more caution regarding treating it with strong yang because it may be damaging. Moderate.

Some patients have gone to 80 pounds to clear their cancers.

Some very beautiful people are rotting inside.

A tumor is a good guy. It's trying to clean up the body before it falls apart. It's the garbage can of the body. Metastases are departmentalizations of the garbage for survival. Sometimes surgery and/or chemotherapy is necessary.

Worry causes heavy stagnation.

Sickness is our saviour.

Never do macrobiotics if you hate it.

Medication does not cure, it postpones.

Destroy or build, day by day. The choice is yours.

All study about food is useless unless you practice.

The mind cures, not the diet. Change the food to cure the mind and spirit. Thereafter, you can eat freely.

If you've had a lot of cheese, sometimes it takes 3 years to lose the weight. Must chew well and decrease the salt.

With binging, you lose the original macro glow, become swollen and dark.

Glass lids on pots so you can see what's happening.

Morning ritual could be scrubbing, exercise, showering, singing.

Grated daikon raw twice a week, minimum.

Three seaweeds a day, minimum.

No Chinese herbs, they're too stimulating, especially for cancers.

A little soup or grain before bed if you're really hungry. Otherwise, no eating 3 hours before bed.

No ginger compresses for cancer or head areas.

Always hear a light hiss from the pressure cooker throughout the 45 minutes of cooking or the rice will be soggy.

Keep adding cold water as needed to the aduki/squash and other bean dishes. This is the shocking method to expand and contract repeatedly, to soften the bean. They should be 80% cooked before salt is added for the final contraction and then covered.

Quickly blanch pickles (like red radish) in order to marinate them for a few hours.

Quick pickles can be anything as simple as half an onion in 1 tsp. soy sauce. Mix, let marinate 2 hours.

Boil or blanch vegetables one minute, have a portion every day, plus steamed greens and 4 other vegetables dishes.

Vinegar is tightening.

3" piece of wakame for miso soup for 1-2 people. May chop the wakame very fine after it has soaked.

Use shiitake if you get too tight, but caution: you'll get weak if you eat too many fat dissolvers.

Use daikon and cabbage daily, if able.

For kinpira (burdock and carrot matchstick pieces, water sauteed) for 4 people, use 1 tsp. soy. It should taste sweet, not salty or you'll get too tight. Should be lighter, happy feeling.

An evening meal should be a grain and condiment, soup and garnish, bean, green, vegetables (can be an above ground or root vegetable or preferably both), a sea vegetable dish, pickles and the medicinals which could be kombu/shiitake tea, carrot/daikon drink or sweet vegetable drink.

Variety and freshness are stressed. If it's a choice between a wilted old discolored organic veggie versus a fresh, crisp, non-organic, opt for the latter, especially if eating organic in your locale limits your variety severely. Use the older one in a soup.

When cooking, always add the vegetables to hot water, not to cold water. It minimizes their nutrient loss.

Try not to use carrot or burdock for miso soups. They're too strong.

Keep one of the daily soups light and uncrowded. Daikon and/or greens (cabbage, collards, watercress) are good for soup.

Once tofu is open, put it in a dish with fresh water and renew the water every couple of days.

The use of tofu should be about a 1 1/2" cube per week per person. That's why it's important to read <u>Macro Mellow</u> and learn how to use it in the rest of the family's recipes. Many people who think they are on the healing phase, are using a whole package for themselves a week, since they don't want to waste the remaining 3/4 of a pound of it. (* Tofu turtles are a great treat.)

Use the roots of scallions when you have them and try to use the whole of any vegetable when possible, like carrots and their leaves, and daikons and their leaves.

If you're cooking small quantities of rice, or you don't like it because it's too sticky, put a metal bowl or a glass measuring cup with the rice and the water inside the pressure cooker. Add 2 cups of water to the pressure cooker itself to surround the secondary vessel that holds the grain and proceed with your cooking directions.

For gomashio, remember to roast and grind the salt first, then the seeds and make it fresh at least every week. Black sesame seeds are preferred.

Maximum 1/2-1 flat tsp. miso per person in most dishes.

The most healing misos are the barley or hatcho soy aged 2-3 years, not the lighter ones.

Kuzu is good for sweet cravings and G.I. upset. For sweet craving, mix it with amasake or rice syrup, barley malt or cider. It neutralizes excess acidity of foods.

Can often see in the nails, white lines or dark areas which show sugar ingestion several months ago at holiday time.

Number 1 cause of asthma is dairy. The next is simple sugars. The next is fruit juices and fruits. The next is cold, icy drinks and the 5th is stimulants such as mustard, tomato sauce, pepper, potatoes.

Causes of asthma are the opposite of causes of colitis, which is why it is necessary to treat someone who has both conditions with a middle of the road treatment.

For someone whose face breaks out with seaweeds, don't stop eating them. It will stop when they're done discharging.

Wild rice is too oily. It's used only occasionally.

Exercise is okay as long as it's not exhausting, and as long as it feels great.

Weight loss is okay, and in fact necessary. You should get too skinny before you clear and normalize.

If all garments are not cotton, at least have cotton next to the skin.

For hypoglycemia, 1-2 cups daily of sweet vegetable drink.

To get rid of meat and fat, grated daikon and carrot daily and shiitake/kombu, 1/2 cup every other day.

Dried tofu preferable over fresh in early strict phase.

Eat as though your life depends on it.

Tamari/bancha for a pick-me-up. 1/2 tsp. tamari in a cup of tea. If it doesn't pick you up, you may be too salty. Umeboshi neutralizes acidity of the stomach. It's the antacid of macrobiotics.

Use steamer basket for leftovers. Can use a Chinese steamer basket over the pot that you're cooking grains in while you're traveling and put the vegetables in the steamer. Thus, you can cook two things at once.

Be sure to clean out the steam escape of the pressure cooker periodically, for if it plugs it can explode.

Use a soapstone or a whetstone to sharpen the Mac knife.

The less bean and vegetables in rice balls, the longer they'll last. Just put a piece of an umeboshi "plum" inside. Wrap them in waxed paper and a brown bag and they'll last almost a week.

Undersalting beans or rice can give gas. For each cup of dried beans add 2 pinches of salt.

When adding shoyu or miso to soups, only add it to the aliquot you are eating at that meal. And add it fresh to each aliquot as you heat it later for another meal, either as is or with a new twist.

You should be able to complete the cooking of a full macrobiotic lunch or dinner in the time that it takes to cook the rice (45-60 minutes).

Cause of most cancer of the prostate, is meat first, chicken and eggs second, and cheese. Heavy animal fats cause stagnation. Then it's accelerated by the expansive things; sugars, stimulant spices, alcohol and baked goods. Should have no salty taste to the cooking. No buckwheat or oatmeal for many serious conditions for the first 3 months. Soups twice a day. Blanched vegetables every day. Pressed salad 1/2 cup every day. Steamed vegetables every day. Variety is important. Maximum 1 fish a week, the less the better. Try to hold off for 2nd or 3rd month. If you feel good, you do not need it. If you need it, keep portion small (10% total daily volume or about a 3x3" piece). Poached is best, or in soup. White meat fish is harmless to prostate cancer, but first need 2-6 months to get all animal protein fat out. No fruit, no nuts, no sunflower seeds, no grain coffee. Lemon only on salad or fish. Chew 100 times. No eating 3 hours before bed. Eat as much as you want, but chew and check your proportions. If you don't have gas, get a little portable camping stove (Coleman) for severe cancer. Have sweet vegetable drink every day, daikon/carrot drink every three days, shiitake every other day as a tea, grated daikon fresh (1 cup with a few drops of shoyu), three times a week for a month to reduce egg, milk, chicken and fat that has caused cancer. No baked flour products. If you crave fruit, cook green apples with a pinch of salt. If feeling good, ignore the weight loss. Shiitake is very yin and helps move the meat excess out. These would be basic recommendations for prostatic problems.

A 70 year old had his first discharge in three weeks. He was depressed for a week so bad that he couldn't get out of bed for two days. Then it oscillated with shorter periods and less severe periods. At first he felt great for 1 hour a day, then the good periods got longer. Then it went backwards for a few days. The important point was that someone could have quit macrobiotics at that point if they didn't understand that the severe depression was a discharge. In fact unknowing relatives would have probably forced him to eat, saying, "You had better get off this diet. It's no good for you, it's making you worse."

CHAPTER 9

ANECDOTAL CASE HISTORIES

One of the greatest tools many of us have found that helped us in our macrobiotic sojourn, was hearing directly from others of how they struggled to successfully heal the impossible. I hope the following cases of mine and other doctors will be as helpful to you as they were to me. I am extremely grateful to each of these "winners" for sharing their pain, their trials and their victories with us. I have a deep love and admiration for each of them, for they have shared their private pain with us so that we might grow.

RHEUMATOID ARTHRITIS

As I limped into the doctor's office, I was desperate at this point to find relief from all the pain and discomfort I had been experiencing for the past 7 1/2 years.

I didn't realize until talking to the doctor that my rheumatologist was offering me cancer drugs (methotrexate) to relieve the pain and swelling, since I was beyond everything else.

After my operation (joint surgery) in 1987, he told me that the gold salt injections that had relieved my pain for almost 3 years would probably stop working.

He was right. About 2 months after my surgery, the pain started coming back: pain in both hips, pain in the knees, swelling and pain in the wrists and hands, swelling and pain in the feet and ankles. By April of the following year, the shots were discontinued; before that time I was taking 2400 mg. of Motrin and 4500 mg. of Tylenol daily in addition to the gold shots, and it only relieved about 50% of the pain from my 7 1/2 years of rheumatoid arthritis.

By this time, the pain started to get unbearable. Strangely enough, the pain was worse and more joints were affected than before I took the gold shots. The idea that I had to live in pain all over again after having been out of pain for almost 3 years, psychologically, was difficult for me to stand.

Now I had to live my life again having the simplest functions in life, like brushing my teeth or combing my hair, even getting dressed, take a great deal of time and effort.

Extreme fatigue set in. I felt I spent most of my life sleeping. Ten to twelve hours a night was my required amount of sleep, needing two to three naps a day lasting anywhere from two to three hours. When I had the desire to do a cleaning job in the home such as clean out a closet, I had to take a nap first. By the time I woke up, I was either too tired or lost the desire to perform the task. This was very discouraging for me. When a friend of mine asked me at the time how old I was, I told him 36 going on 80, because that's what I felt like at the time.

By June of 1988, I had the decision to make whether to take the cancer drug with all its possible serious side effects or consider some other treatment. My alternative treatment came when a friend of mine told me about another doctor and her success in treating people with various types of illnesses.

So I said to myself, "What have I got to lose. If this doesn't work, then I'll go back to my rheumatologist."

After talking to the doctor, she assured me of the success she had in treating people with rheumatoid arthritis so she encouraged me to undergo her treatment.

I was very skeptical at first and found it difficult to believe that allergies to food, chemicals, and my outdoor environment could actually cause pain, swelling, and stiffness in arthritis. But as I started to bring each one of these factors under control, the pain slowly started to diminish until it was gone completely.

Of course, if I expose myself to wrong foods or one of the other factors, the pain would return, only temporarily until I got it under control again. The macrobiotic way of eating though, has left me less sensitive to some of the above factors.

After being on allergy injections for one year, doing environmental controls in my home, correcting my mineral deficiencies, and eating a restricted diet, to my surprise, a year and a half later the pain was gone. Not only that, the fatigue was gone also. No longer did I require 10 to 12 hours sleep a night. Eight to nine hours was sufficient and I woke up refreshed. I no longer need a nap during the day and have the energy to function and accomplish many things and be satisfied at the end of the day.

I'm no longer sensitive to weather changes. At one time I could predict a rainfall or would be very achy on damp days; this is no longer the case. At one time our daily house temperature would have been over 80 degrees, now it's about 70 degrees. In the winter months, I no longer have to pile on the clothing as heavily as I used to. Some of my friends who do not have arthritis now get cold sooner than I do.

Of course, it wasn't easy, but all the effort was worth it. I'm able to live without pain, using no medication of any kind. As long as I control my eating of foods I am allergic to and avoid exposure to chemicals that trigger my pain, I stay pain free.

I would have never imagined that allergies could actually cause joint pain, but I have to believe it because it worked for me, and I'm so grateful.

-Contributed by Gloria

A WORD FROM GLORIA'S DOCTOR

Gloria's case also reaffirms something else that macrobiotics espouses: that symptoms leave in the reverse order that they came in. When her rheumatoid arthritis began 7 1/2 years prior to when I saw her, she merely awakened one day with a sore ankle. Within a few weeks both ankles were painful and swollen. Shortly it progressed to her knees. By the time I saw her, she was a very pretty face on a stiffened body, shuffling into the room like the Tin Man in the "Wizard of Oz." She was a prisoner encased in an immobile body in constant pain.

As she lost her arthritic pain and swelling, it first left the hands, then her shoulders and progressed downward until only her ankles were left in pain.

Another tenet of macrobiotics that her case demonstrated was the need to get rid of all the body's excess toxins or poisons before healing could occur. Since they are stored in the fat, this means she had to lose nearly all her fat, which can be dangerous and requires medical supervision. She went from 135 pounds to 86 pounds within the first year. Whenever we tried to put her weight back on, the arthritis would flare, telling us we were too premature.

The ironic part was that for years, she had been a prisoner trapped in a painful suit of armor and was now pain free. But instead of sharing her joy, friends and relatives could only concern themselves with her weight loss. Mind you, they could not concern themselves enough to learn how to cook when she visited or read about why the weight loss is necessary so they could support her. This is an important aspect of macrobiotics which has led to the failure of those with less fortitude and not blessed with the loving and devoted husband that Gloria possesses.

A third point that makes this a case from which we can all learn is that she had multiple nutrient deficiencies that had to be identified and corrected. This gave her the increased energy with which to learn, cook and heal faster.

****

A very sharp young mother with rheumatoid arthritis recently presented because she realized she wanted to find the causes of her arthritis and get rid of it, not merely mask or cover it up with drugs.

When she told her family doctor she was coming, there was the usual pregnant pause followed by "Well, that program is rather eccentric: it will place a lot of restrictions on your life......" To which the young mother replied, "You don't think being a mother of two with rheumatoid arthritis has restrictions?!?" Even though there are over two dozen scientific papers showing that food sensitivity is part of the cause of arthritis for many sufferers, the average rheumatologist still resists the notion. Thus, the general docs cannot allow themselves to even think for themselves, much less believe the patient when she tells them she is better with certain food avoidances.

MULTIPLE CHEMICAL SENSITIVITIES WITH CHRONIC DIZZINESS AND EXHAUSTION
or
Bats in Her Belfry

M. S. is a lovely 28 year old housewife and mother of two who presented with a very difficult problem.

In 1989, she began having severe headaches, dizziness, nausea, vomiting, confusion and says that she walked around like a robot. She was tired all the time and even had black out spells. She had EEG's, CAT scans and even psychiatric consultations. She had been to chiropractors, neurosurgeons, had arteriograms and had multiple other symptoms including constant headaches and wavering vision in the right eye. She would spend a lot of time just lying at home on the couch and would have to hang onto it because she felt so dizzy. Sinus x-rays showed that there was some evidence of sinusitis. She went to a large medical school teaching hospital where she was examined by a neurologist and had a spinal tap. She was subsequently rehospitalized after the spinal tap because of severe disorientation, headache, vomiting and the feeling that the room was spinning and she had more ENT (ear, nose and throat) specialists and neurologic consultations. She described herself as feeling as though she were brain dead. Fortunately for her she wasn't totally brain dead because she made her own diagnosis when all the doctors were baffled and began to doubt her sanity, and started herself on the road to recovery.

She noticed that while in the hospital, she started improving. But her poor sister who had stayed home to watch her children and household for her, began developing the very symptoms that she had complained of. Together they started putting 2 and 2 together and realized that in January of 1989, the house was exterminated for bats in the attic, plus there was a gas leak in the heater that had to be fixed. So doctors who thought she had bats in her belfry were actually right, but for the wrong reason.

She consulted an occupational medicine specialist and was disturbed that he did not recognize her chemical sensitivity and urge her to reduce her chemical overload in her environment. She then saw a doctor who specializes in environmental medicine and allergy. He sent her to a detoxification program in California for 3 weeks which did not help her. She then went to another famous clinic in another state, also without benefit.

When we saw her she complained of having many food, chemical and environmental triggers such as dust and mold that would give her sudden throat swelling and closing.

We took an environmental history and environmental controls were explained. Labs were done to check the efficiency of her xenobiotic detoxication system, (as described in Tired Or Toxic?). Her magnesium loading test showed 74% retention, whereas normal should be 50% or less. Since magnesium is in over 300 enzymes, it is of course, very prevalent throughout the detoxication pathway. She had a vitamin B1 deficiency of 9 (normal 10-64) as well. Her RBC folate was 237 which is rock bottom of normal (235-725), but she had a normal iron, RBC copper, B2, formic acid, B6, vitamin A, RBC selenium, RBC zinc, B12 and an elevated IgE, or allergic antibody count of 321 (normal 14-100).

Testing revealed she was quite sensitive to a variety of trees, grasses, weeds, house dust, house dust mite and several genera of fungi. Although she didn't test out positive to glycerine, when we gave her glycerinated extracts, we absolutely made her worse with throat swelling, headache, dizziness, breathing problems. We used phenol-free, glycerine-free injections. She reports now that she is markedly improved and rates herself as 75% better in terms of all of her symptoms. Many of them are even better than 75%. The toxic brain symptoms and confusion are 75% improved and she never thought she would get this good again. She attributes most of this to the injections. She has much more energy, less dizziness, less muscle soreness, congestion, eye swelling and throat spasms. The nausea and vomiting are gone, the eczema is clear, the paresthesias (numbness and tingling) are gone, the fatigue is much improved and the abdominal pain is fine unless she eats some of the wrong foods.

She is on the macrobiotic diet which also had and continues to have very positive effects on the detoxication pathways. She can feel she gets stronger the longer she is on it. And one of the major factors in her improvement, I am sure, is her loving family, since it always makes these very difficult endeavors easier.

She is an excellent example of many factors in typical E.I. cases:

1. The victims have stumped all doctors and usually through reading and constantly seeking, they actually figure out the diagnosis themselves.

2. Even E.I. programs are often without effect until the underlying biochemical defects in the machinery are fixed: nutrient levels must be checked and corrected. Then the macrobiotic diet helps bring them to undreamed of levels of wellness.

3. Injections serve to unload the person from sensitivities so they can have enough energy to do the macrobiotic diet.

4. A supportive spouse is crucial and never to be overlooked.

5. The more severe the case, the more crucial is the total load (see The E.I. Syndrome): dust/mold injections, nutrient corrections, addressing hidden food allergies, Candida program, environmental controls, patient reading, a supportive spouse, and much more as well as the macrobiotic diet. The macrobiotic diet is wonderful, but a thorough ecological program can speed up the process immensely, even in seemingly hopeless end-of-the-road cases that have done everything and been everywhere and no one even knows what's wrong with them, much less how to make them better. Remember the best diet in the world can't compensate for a toxic environment. Likewise, the best environment in the world can't compensate for a lousy diet.

6. When medical doctors get stuck, their ego is sometimes so strong that they figure if they don't know how to fix it, you must need a psychiatrist. If they can't figure out what you have then you must be imagining it!

LEARNING DISORDER, CHRONIC FATIGUE, ELECTRICAL SENSITIVITY AND MULTIPLE CHEMICAL SENSITIVITY

I can recall realizing that I was suffering from something resembling E.I. in the summer of 1988. At this time suddenly I was experiencing many cerebral symptoms including intense fatigue, slurred speech, and slowing of thought if I ventured into certain buildings, rode in the car, or ate certain foods. Even though this may sound horrible, I am fortunate such a precipitous decline finally occurred. This is because for most of my life I can remember experiencing constant less severe related symptoms, but could not relate them to any particular cause. But finally I have, and the cause was allergy.

Before I tell of my travels on the road to recovery, I feel I must tell of my travels on the road to sickness. My first recollections that my health was far from normal occurred when I was about six years old. At this time my first grade teacher advised that I be held back the next year since she felt that I was suffering from a maturation lag, due to my being almost a year younger than the other children. My parents went along with this recommendation convinced that all would be well. I would no longer be ridiculed by my peers for mispronouncing when counting one, two, tree.

This did not happen, thus within two years I was placed in the school speech therapy program. My problems did not end here since I was also placed in and out of school programs in which my intense problems with fine motor control were worked on, for example, my very poor handwriting. Despite having received no more formal help after the fifth grade, this did not mean these problems were resolved.

My handwriting remained atrocious throughout all my years of high school, and my coordination was so horrible that I was constantly ridiculed in gym class or at any physical activity. Despite these persistent handicaps, I wanted to appear as normal as my peers and achieve as much as they did. I was able to accomplish this with severe strain on my health and well-being. I coped with attention and learning problems by copying all that was written on the black-

that my peers were able to learn in class. Remarkably, I usually did much better than most of my classmates, allowing my induction into the National Honor Society in my junior year.

Despite the appearance of scholarly achievement, I felt very stupid, as many of my peers accused me of not being able to solve problems at the blackboard as the related material was being taught and almost immediately forgetting material as soon as I was tested on it.

The next blow came to my self esteem when my driving instructor accused me of having a learning disability because try as he might, he could not teach me the hand over hand motion needed to drive.

Despite all these problems, I was coping and was happy overall, but this soon changed as a result of treatment for acne, consisting of antibiotics and the drug accutane. Immediately, my health sharply declined, necessitating a two hour nap every day to keep up my energy level.

Despite all of my previously mentioned difficulties, I achieved my goal of attending a prestigious college. My stay didn't last long because my energy level and concentration plummeted to the point that I became incapable of doing any college work, even unable to read and comprehend the newspaper. Consequently, I left college three months later to solve my fatigue problem.

At home, I saw an internist who was unable to come up with anything medically wrong. Finally I realized that my intense brain fog must somehow be related to the learning problems I was helped with when I was younger. Thus I went to a neuropsychologist to check out my theory. Tests did indeed diagnose me with a visual processing problem, which he explained meant that I did in fact have a learning disability and he said with shock, "You must have busted your ass to make it through school (pardon my French)."

At this point my story winds back to August of 1988 at which time I realized that allergies were the causative agent of all my difficulties. Immediately I had my mother find an allergist who could treat my problem so I could once and for all be free of it. She found a clinical ecologist who determined I was allergic to dust, molds, and foods.

With his treatment I became much clearer in thought and could now read the newspaper, though my reading speed was almost a snail's pace. Within a few months with much effort, I took a college accounting course.

Even though I had more mental clarity, I was quickly worsening allergy-wise. I became allergic to almost every known food and chemical, so in order to be able to slightly function, I had to limit what I ate to almost purely meat, since this was one of the few foods I had been treated for. Also my entire family had to stop wearing hairsprays, make-up, aftershaves, etc.

This situation finally started to change when I saw a second ecologists in September of 1989 when I was given my first allergy injection to neutralize my inhalant allergies. I felt much better than I did with my previous treatment. The reason was that this program was comprehensive in testing for and treating for many more molds and pollens that could cause a reaction. This thoroughness resulted in my allergic load being lowered enough to start the macrobiotic diet and not requiring food shots.

Despite being given more freedom diet-wise, I still had most of my allergies to chemicals. Also during my visit to the doctor, it was found I reacted to the fluorescent lights in the office. I had many more symptoms and more difficulty thinking and speaking under the lights than when I was removed from them. She explained that this meant that I was electromagnetically sensitive. So this meant that I had to stay away from the television, fluorescent lights, and computers. This made sense as I had recognized I was worse watching T.V. or working on the computer (but didn't relate to the cause). At the same time, I had to learn other environmental controls needed to lessen my allergy load.

After my visit to the doctor, I began the macrobiotic diet. I did it simply by boiling carrots, daikon, squash, onions in water for twenty minutes, along with eating boiled kale and pot boiled rice. Even with this semi-macro diet, I was given enough improvement to tolerate newspaper ink and cigarette smoke picked up on clothing.

Within one month, the doctor recommended I go to the Way of Life Seminar at the Kushi Institute where I tasted and learned how macrobiotic food should be prepared. By eating the food this weekend, I had improved enough to be able to eat corn, wheat and fermented foods. This was exciting because there were probably over one hundred foods I could now eat on the diet compared to about thirty that I had on my old rotation diet, plus I was learning how to eat nutritiously rather than eating maybe frozen corn and hamburg for supper.

Also at the seminar I had a consultation with Michio Kushi who gave me special diet guidelines to recover from my E. I. When I arrived home I started these guidelines, but because of my very low energy, I had a lot of trouble carrying them out. My cooking almost took me six hours a day, so many days my parents could not even get near the stove to cook their own food, so they went out to eat. With time, I became a little more adept at cooking and could do the cooking for two days in three hours. Also my parents began eating my leftover food, so I had the kitchen to myself.

With my new way of eating I was slowly improving. My energy level improved to the point that I didn't need a two hour nap every day. I also noticed I could now handle car exhaust without wearing a special mask.

During this entire time, the doctor continuously gave me her advice and encouragement, comforting me in my inability to fully carry out all my guidelines from the start. She frequently checked my vitamin levels to determine my progress on the diet which was exciting to me since I saw how the diet alone had corrected a zinc deficiency in six months. The only supplement that she did give me initially was magnesium which turned out to be very important for me. This alone had corrected the problem of my hands turning bright red, chapping and finally bleeding every winter.

Despite the progress that I had made, I felt that I should be making more, feeling that my house was the cause of the handicap to my recovery. The reasons were that when I left the oasis of my clean room, I felt more tired and less clear in thinking in the rest of the house. Also we had the local power company come to our house and they felt that we had an intense mold situation since black mold could be seen growing on all the ceilings, a problem that had persisted and been there since I was an infant. The representative from the power company felt that this was because the house was built too tight, which trapped high humidity in the house. Even though he recommended that we install vents, I was still suspicious of the amount of mold present. I used a specialized mold service and cultured both the living room and kitchen and my suspicions were found to be correct, finding an excessively high amount of mold in the house.

Because of this persistent mold problem, I moved out to an apartment which had very little mold. In my new environment I made steady progress to the point that I had virtually no chemical sensitivities. This allowed me to attend the residential program at the Kushi Institute in Beckett, Massachusetts, since I could tolerate the gas cooking used there. During the week, I learned how to properly cook the most important dishes on the macro diet. Thus, when I returned home, my cooking had improved to the point that my parents actually liked it. Since my energy level was now better, I was able to cook a fresh macro meal every night in about three hours.

Presently I am recovering more and more every day and am better in some ways than I have ever been in my life. For example, a persistent problem of toeing in while I walked which I have had since I was an infant has disappeared. My concentration has improved to the point that I was able to write this personal history with ease. Even more exciting is the fact that now I am able to drive a car once again.

As I look to the future, I hope to resume college and slowly forget about the sickness and pain E. I. caused me, and think of the macrobiotic diet as a diet to stay healthy, rather than something I need to recover my health. By doing this, my parents will no longer have to unselfishly devote all their time to getting me well, whether it be driving miles to find macrobiotic foods, organic produce, cleaning, giving me ginger compresses, all without which I would never have recovered my health. All in all, I am glad that they are also on the macro diet, because I very much wish I could give back to them the support that they have given to me, in their old age. I am glad I will never have the opportunity, as they will be able to avoid most of the debilitating diseases of old age on the diet.

-Contributed by Gary

A WORD FROM GARY'S DOCTOR

Gary's parents were amazing in their profound love and support for their son, went on the diet to help him and look 10 years younger for it. I have had the opportunity to watch them also grow into healthier, more energetic and handsome people and cast off a number of annoying physical ailments. I agree with Gary that he most likely will not have to worry about their getting debilitating diseases when they reach old age.

Gary's case teaches us a great deal. He is a perfect example of a person with a gifted intellect who appears to barely make it through life and has to struggle for each accomplishment due to the fact that most children with E.I. are not diagnosed. They must grow up and diagnose themselves.

As for Gary, when his adoring parents first brought him from New Hampshire, I was struck by their devotion and commitment to his wellness, which I agree has materialized only through their efforts. For Gary really, truly was helpless when he came. And it was interesting to watch him deteriorate as he was brought into a small exam room with fluorescent lights and 4 close walls of electro-magnetic fields. His voice pitch would rise and his speech rate would double. He couldn't think and verbalize what he wanted and it was extremely frustrating for a young man with his brilliance. And his face would swell, his lids would droop and his muscles became weak and asymmetrical, as he looked more like an old man.

If I then walked him out of the electromagnetic field, he metamorphosed. He began within minutes to stand taller, his face was more alert and youthful, and his speech and thought processes became more controlled.

He is unique in that when you were around him, he kept a steady verbal account running of his mental and body reactions. In other words, he would rattle off all the bizarre symptoms and feelings he was having every second, as fast as he could talk. To a physician untrained in environmental medicine, it would have made him appear fully psychotic. But to us, it was extremely helpful because it showed even a dumb doc like me that he actually was reacting to electromagnetic fields. Otherwise, I might never have picked up on it. He had great intuition as well as intellect and sensed that he should remove the T.V., computer and other appliances from his room even before I picked up on this. You see, electromagnetic sensitivity can be thought of as an extension of chemical sensitivity. And as Gary demonstrates, it, too can be reversed with enough attention paid to the total load. Also, correcting the mineral imbalances seems to be particularly important to getting well for the EMF sensitive person. But because he was doing so well with his macro, we decided to watch his zinc deficiency and see how long it would take to correct it. However, the magnesium deficiency was so much worse (and jeopardizes so many other enzymes) that we did not dare. We corrected that one plus an extremely resistant copper deficiency. And I'm glad we did, for it provided another giant step forward. You'll recall, for example, that copper is in superoxide dismutase which is necessary to fight the free radicals generated by chemicals.

No, I have no doubt that Gary will continue to progress and I await with fascination to see what this young man will accomplish next. As for his parents, I feel privileged to have witnessed such intensely loyal devotion. Any other young man with the symptoms that Gary, had would have probably been institutionalized. But they believed, persevered, and helped him return to an even more accomplished young man than before.

CHRONIC FATIGUE AND ANAPHYLACTIC THROAT SPASMS:

Dance, Ballerina, Dance

This is a long medical history for someone only twenty-one years old, but it has a happy ending. I was fortunate enough to find a wonderful doctor who helped me become macrobiotic. This is my story of how macrobiotics has changed my life.

I think I was born with allergies. As a baby I had severe colic for three months. This was later diagnosed as a milk allergy. I had all the typical hayfever symptoms all spring, summer and fall. Frequently I found myself in the pediatrician's office. I caught colds, strep throat, and bronchitis repeatedly. I wheezed, I coughed, I sneezed. At a very early age, I learned the art of swallowing pills over taking liquids. I've always had a tissue in hand. When I was three and a half years old, I was hospitalized for bronchitis and pneumonia. My pediatrician suggested that I hold off on having allergy shots; he was hoping I would outgrow my allergies. In general, I was a weak, low energy little girl. Like clockwork, every spring when my ballet school had it's annual performance, I danced with laboured breathing--I was in the throes of the annual spring allergy attack.

I seemed to become progressively worse. I was very allergic to animals--especially cats and horses which brought on wheezing and all of its allergic sidekicks such as sneezing, etc. Feather pillows threw me for a loop. I frequently had headaches. In fourth grade, my mother took me to the opthamologist. She hoped that glasses would relieve me. They didn't. In seventh grade I had a severe case of mononucleosis that left me tired and weak for a year. In eighth grade, my headaches became more frequent and severe. My energy level became even lower and lower.

It was about that time that a major depression set in. It became progressively worse over my high school years as I became sicker and sicker. During tenth grade I was seeing my doctor on a regular basis. I kept coming down repeatedly with sore throats and headaches. As soon as I felt better, I had another bout with something else. He was very concerned and suggested that I have some sinus x-rays taken because I had a sinus infection. When he saw my x-rays, he immediately sent me to see an allergist without delay. I had a large mass in my sinuses and he wanted a specialist to look at it.

The allergist found that my nose was filled with polyps and that several of my sinus cavities had large masses in them. He said if this condition didn't respond to medication that it would require major surgery and that he would remove my tonsils and adenoids as well. I had x-ray after x-ray taken. I began taking heavy doses of nasal sprays, decongestants, antibiotics and a steroid spray. This allergist also took some blood, tested it, then put me on allergy shots. He said he had never seen anyone as allergic as I was. He thought that the shots would prevent me from becoming sick again.

After seven very anxiety-filled months for my parents and me, we were told that my sinuses had cleared up. I was very relieved but I still had headaches and the doctor could offer neither a reason why I had them nor any relief for me. He said I should be fine because my sinuses were cleared up. My mother had heard something about food allergy and headaches, but he told us flat out that I did not have any food allergies.

Meanwhile, I was becoming more and more depressed. My parents were extremely concerned about me so in the spring, they took me to see a psychologist. He is an extremely kind and compassionate man whom I love dearly. He had faith in me when I didn't and helped me through my deep depressions. He saved my life by giving me hope. I am deeply grateful to him for his gentle patience, humor and wisdom in pointing me in the right direction.

Having allergies himself, he recognized the role that they can play. He sent me to see a psychiatrist so that I could give antidepressants a trial run and hopefully find some quick relief for a black mood. We tried two drugs and I had so many side effects from the smallest possible dose and no results, that they were stopped immediately. The doctor said that he couldn't help me on an outpatient basis. I was so sensitive that I would need to go to a large medical center------he recommended the Mayo Clinic.

I continued to see the psychologist. He gave me a book on environmental allergy to read. I found it very interesting and could see parallels in it to my allergies. But, at that point I was skeptical that my allergies could play such a large role in my unhappiness. I knew I was depressed but I didn't realize how sick I was. I had never felt well, so how could I know any differently? I thought I was going crazy or that there was something terribly wrong with me. I didn't want anyone to know, except him, how miserable I really was. I was suicidal; I didn't think I would act on that feeling, but I felt so helpless and hopeless.

Ballet, the big love of my life, only exhausted me and depressed me more. This upset me terribly--the one thing I had always loved to do I dreaded and could no longer find any pleasure in. My psychologist and I talked and I decided I wanted to go away for my senior year to a boarding school. We hoped that the different atmosphere and the more challenging academics would busy my head enough so that I might feel better.

We were wrong. My health only worsened. I woke up in the morning with very red, dry eyes. My headaches became very severe again. I kept getting sinus infections which concerned everyone--I didn't want another problem like the one I had just gotten over. I was extremely fatigued. Moving felt like a terrible strain. I couldn't concentrate through my pounding, throbbing headaches.

In the spring, I became very depressed. I wanted something to be resolved; I hated being at school when I felt so horrible, I wanted some relief. I came home to start taking lithium. I felt like a horrible failure that I couldn't just stick it out but my misery superseded that. An antidepressant was added along with the lithium when I wasn't feeling any relief. The psychiatrist I saw who administered the medication said I didn't look depressed at all to him. I thought this was a wonderful victory. I was very uncomfortable with anyone knowing how depressed and sick I really felt.

Soon the side effects from the medication were so severe that I had to discontinue them. Once again I had been disappointed. I had placed so much hope in those drugs and again I was left with what felt like fewer and fewer options. I returned to school, made up my work like a whirlwind and graduated with high honors.

I had been accepted at Sarah Lawrence College for the fall. I didn't know what to do. I had fallen in love with the college, yet I knew that there was no way I could possibly get anything out of it when I felt so horrible. I decided to take the year off and straighten out my allergies once and for all. I remembered the psychologist's words that he thought that if I could have my allergies helped in some way that I would be fine. I reread the book on environmental allergies and I became hopeful.

I began seeing a doctor who specializes in environmental medicine on the psychologist's recommendation. He took an extensive medical history and tested me for sublingual allergy drops. I was pleasantly surprised when I saw that these drops actually did help me a bit. The shots that I had been taking might have actually worsened my allergies—they certainly didn't help. He had me eliminate common allergens from my diet. I was surprised and immensely relieved to discover that I did have multiple food sensitivities. Many foods provoked headaches, depression and fatigue.

He also taught me about environmental controls. I ripped the carpeting out of my room and bought an air purifier. I began to switch everything over to cottons. I started the rotary diversified diet which I found nearly impossible to stick to for very long. My severe cravings soon lead me to eat something forbidden. I found this lack of control very frustrating. I was still very depressed. I had learned an immense amount about allergies, but unfortunately I wasn't finding much physical relief.

I was very glad to know what I had was a vast amount of allergies and that I wasn't crazy. These were things that were out of my control. It wasn't because I was a weak person that just couldn't overcome these problems. I seemed to be allergic to everything and it was wreaking havoc on my entire body. I am very appreciative of all that he taught me. He showed me how to look at my depression in a different light.

By spring I was deeply depressed again. I discussed with my doctors, and I decided to try another round of chemically different antidepressants. We wanted to find some quick relief for me while I worked on my allergies. Again I was full of hope, but I had nothing but side effects from the drugs. I continued with my allergy shots and drops and the modified diet. I was beginning to find it difficult to find foods to eat that didn't bother me. I was very concerned about going to college in the fall when I didn't feel much better. I had the tools of environmental knowledge but I couldn't find much relief.

In the summer I went to see a doctor that my parents heard had amazing success with depressed patients. I was in the throes of "which is worse, the allergies or the depression?" I decided that if I weren't so depressed I could possibly deal with my allergies better. So I went to see this man.

He talked to me and told me that he thought I was having

panic attacks. When I told him about my allergies he told me that I didn't have any food allergies at all because I didn't have hives. I was enraged by this after all that I had learned from the ecologist, but I bit my tongue. I had really hoped this doctor could help me. He told me he thought I was having separation anxiety from my mother about going to college. This upset me terribly.

Again, I felt like there was something wrong with me and that I had brought all this upon myself. He prescribed an anti-anxiety drug for me. I would have tried anything so I took it, but again I was so sensitive to the medication, that all I had were side effects that made me very ill. I think he thought that they were fabrications of my mind. He told me that I would have to learn to live with being sick--I should take naps and push myself in order to overcome this. I discontinued seeing him. I felt like I was a very weak person.

Reluctantly, I went to Sarah Lawrence College in the fall. I didn't know if I could study under these conditions. I had a fever and bronchitis from fall allergies. I packed my oxygen, air purifier and humidifier and off I went determined to make it work out some-how. I was very lucky to have a dear roommate that did not smoke and who was very concerned about my health and well-being. Without her, my freshman year would have been impossible.

I became progressively worse: my chemical sensitivities plagued me, everyone smoked all over campus, non-smoking areas seemed non-existent, my headaches worsened, every time I ate. I felt nauseous, bloated and headachy, my eyes were red and swollen, my ears itched, my throat itched and broke out in little bumps whenever I ate, I had severe sweet cravings.

I could only work by the energy created by the grace of sugar highs which always ended up giving me pounding headaches. The dust and mold from library books put me to sleep and the print from new books started my head throbbing. I couldn't concentrate on work that truly interested and excited me. I felt stupid, freakish and inhuman. It was very difficult being around people of my own age when I felt like I was old and sick before I was even twenty. I didn't know why anyone would want to bother with me. I felt terribly alone and cheated. I had to start taking a small air purifier to class which only made me feel more of a freak.

Everything was out of control--the slightest thing could make me sick--perfume, a cigarette, a moldy classroom, a cleanser. My nose had become so acute that I could smell things no one else could. I tried to hide all of this. Who could possibly believe the extent of this all and still think that I was a sane human being?

I had stopped taking the allergy shots because my sensitivities had changed and the dosages needed to be adjusted which couldn't be done while I was at school. In the spring, I became severely depressed again. I didn't know what to do. I began contemplating finding a doctor to prescribe MAO inhibitors for me (a dangerous antidepressant), as I hadn't tried those yet. I went to the library and read the Physician's Desk Reference on these drugs and then I realized how ridiculous it all was. I read about the food interactions and it scared me--these drugs had serious side effects and I would probably experience them if past experiences were any guide. I called the doctor's office for a referral to an allergist in New York City, all the time remembering the psychologist's words that if my allergies were better, I would be fine.

I started to see another, my second ecologist. He too was amazed by the extent of my allergies and started me on shots after testing. I began to notice that my allergic reactions felt like they were effecting my throat. We ruled out a possible thyroid problem and crossed our fingers hoping that dietary adjustments, medication and allergy shots would kick in soon. He was extremely kind and compassionate. He knew how frustrated I was at this point and he really wanted to help me.

In the fall, I returned to Sarah Lawrence for my sophomore year. I was afraid that I wouldn't be able to make it through the year--I was becoming sicker and sicker. Soon my depression became nothing compared to the severity of my allergies. I was very dizzy all fall and my ears felt plugged. Sitting in class, I would feel like I was free falling in an airplane. My headaches were incapacitating and I slept constantly.

One Friday afternoon, my throat started to close. I spent the entire weekend in my room with my air purifier and oxygen, fasting. I called my ecologist and he told me that the mold count was high that day. He was reluctant to prescribe any new medication for me for fear that I would react to it. I felt better on Tuesday and was able to return to class. Right after Thanksgiving break, the anaphalaxis happened again. This time I was sitting in class when it happened. I left immediately and went to my room and turned on the air purifier and took an antihistamine. I called him again and he prescribed a steroid spray for me.

I was unable to leave my room for <u>ten</u> days. I was afraid to go to the emergency room because I knew the disinfectants and outside air would only make me worse and that they would not understand the complexities of my allergies. I had adrenalin in case I needed it, but I was reluctant to use it. I didn't know how I'd react to anything. I could barely breathe and I honestly thought I might die.

I had never felt so scared and alone in my entire life. The injustice of it all saddened me. The only thing I could do was wait it out. I didn't eat for days because I was still experiencing the anaphalaxis and eating only made it worse. I telephoned him daily. He was extremely concerned. My entire world was collapsing. I thought I was ready for living in a bubble--I was only twenty years old. I had planned on studying in Paris my junior year for a long time, a plan that had become completely ridiculous. I had wanted to go to graduate school to become a psychologist, I had wanted to take ballet class--but now I just wanted to be able to go outside and be able to breathe. Everything had become impossible as I lay there on my bed for days.

My ecologist and I couldn't figure out what had brought this on. The day this began he told me he had several emergency calls with asthmatics being sent to emergency rooms. Mold counts were extremely high. We were both waiting for cold weather to set in. I hated the fact that I was at the mercy of the mold count. I was angry and sad about the ridiculousness of the whole situation. It was ludicrous that my body would not let me go outside until there had been a hard frost with consistently cold weather.

My throat gradually started to open up during the next few days. I started on foods that I rarely ate and that seemed to be harmless. I ate sweet potatoes, cashews, black olives and Gerber peaches--fresh peaches were out of season. It was a very depressing time for me. I was twenty years old and reduced to baby food. I couldn't leave my room. I had no idea how this attack was caused or how it could be prevented. I had to show my housemates how to use my adrenalin pen in case I was so sick I couldn't do it myself and I needed someone to help me to the bathroom because I was so dizzy.

If I laughed too much I couldn't breathe. My room was incredibly hot and humid from my vaporizer. The antihistamines I needed to take dried out my lungs incredibly, but without that medication my throat closed. It was December yet I was wearing my bathing suit. My friends would come in to check on me and start peeling their winter layers off--it was like a Florida summer!

My doctor, very concerned about my condition, told me he normally didn't turn patients away but he no longer knew what to do for me. This was a true act of kindness on his part. He didn't keep me as a patient and try to fix me for his ego's sake. Instead he referred me to another ecologist. He told me that she was one of the top environmental allergists in the area and he hoped that she could help me. I am very grateful for his kind recommendation. It has changed my life.

I called the office and set up an appointment. I made all the arrangements to leave school early for the month long semester break. Then I waited for my throat to stop swelling closed so I could travel home. On the way home in the car, I had to use a mask because the exhaust on the highway plus the cold winter air irritated me. I was scared for a long time. I didn't know what would set my allergies off--nearly anything could--and there really wasn't any way to remedy the situation except for waiting it out in a clean atmosphere.

When I went to see the doctor for the first time, I was desperate. There wasn't anything I wouldn't do to get better. I would have tried the most unorthodox approach if it had worked for one other person. I had talked to several people from home who had gone to see her and were feeling better. They also told me how sick she had been with her allergies which really gave me hope that she would be the one who would understand and be able to help me.

My mother and I were sitting in an examining room when the doctor walked in. I was immediately struck by how lively and healthy she was. She had a very positive and upbeat attitude, yet no nonsense approach that really appealed to me. She took my history then started to tell me animatedly about the macrobiotic diet. I really was quite clueless as to what that diet was; I had heard about it but was lacking in specifics.

She assigned me two books to read, one on allergies which I was basically familiar with from the information from my former ecologists, and one on macrobiotics for allergies which really fascinated me. I liked her approach. I was going to be in charge of taking care of my health. I could tell she would be very helpful, but that she wouldn't baby me and hold my hand. She is a very busy doctor and doesn't have time for that. She only works with those patients who are health-oriented and I was going to be one of those patients. This was my last resort--I didn't know what else was left to try. I was going to give it everything I had because I was sick and tired of being sick and tired.

The doctor took blood to check vitamin levels and began testing me for shots. I was allergic to the preservatives in the shots so it was a longer, more complicated project than it is for most. Before I left, the doctor told me I would be feeling better within a year in response to my mother saying that I had decided not to study abroad the next year because of my allergies. I nearly started to cry when I heard this. So many times I heard that from so many doctors only to find myself deeply disappointed and still sick. I really wanted to believe her, yet past experience had embittered me. Nevertheless I was going to give macrobiotics a try.

It was a very difficult time of year to try to start on macrobiotics. There were scads of Christmas foods around the house plus lots of get-togethers with even more food. I started on a very basic macro diet but found myself supplementing it with desserts. But, what amazed me was that I found I didn't feel nearly as sick as I would have had I not had the macro meals before the slip-ups.

On December 28, 1989 I decided to go macro cold turkey. Most of the offending treats were out of the house at that point, thanks to my cravings. The first week I felt horrendous. My body was going through withdrawal from all of the foods I normally ate because I craved them. My head pounded, my joints ached, I had diarrhea for weeks, I could barely stay awake, I was incredibly nauseous, irritable and very depressed. I craved everything I couldn't eat and saw everyone else eating. Mostly I ate brown rice that week. I was too nauseous to handle vegetables. As the days passed, these symptoms lessened. The very first thing I noticed was that I didn't have as many headaches. I began taking vitamins for the multiple deficiencies that the doctor had uncovered.

On New Year's Eve we had an open house for some dear friends who had moved to Alaska and were visiting during the holidays. One lady from Alaska had gone macro on the same doctor's advice because of difficult allergies, and had improved. She gave me cooking hints and encouraged me. She assured me that I would see re sults despite the long, hard road if I was patient. Her sweet encouragement helped me as well as the sight of her eating carrot sticks during the party!

At the end of January, I returned to school. I was more hopeful than I had ever been. I hadn't been macro very long, but I had a tool with which to become healthy. I had made some important decisions and decided to change my life in certain ways. I was putting my health first and I wasn't going to ignore it anymore and pretend I was okay when I wasn't. I was sick and the only way I could change that was by taking control of the situation. So I packed up a kitchen plus macro staples and headed for school.

The second thing I noticed from the diet was that I lost what was a lot of weight for me; about fifteen pounds. Gradually I gained almost ten pounds back. I no longer felt bloated. I was able to start taking ballet class again. The little improvements encouraged me along a difficult and sometimes lonely path. Sometimes I felt ridiculous explaining to people what the odd odors and foods that emerged from my kitchen were. But mostly I didn't care; I was doing what I had to do.

When spring arrived, I did not suffer nearly as much as I had in the past. I had the annual spring depression but this time it was so obvious to me that allergies were the cause of it that I felt relieved. My parents picked me up for spring break. My mother had put a box of tissues in the car because in the past I had to constantly blow my nose. She was amazed that I didn't blow my nose once in the four hour trip home. I no longer suffered from sinus pain and headaches. Throughout the spring I was very pleased at the vast improvement of my spring allergies.

In the spring I also started seeing an excellent chiropractor. I had been experiencing some neck and back pain. I found the chiropractic adjustments helped those conditions and could completely get rid of some of my headaches. I also just felt generally better and more comfortable after an adjustment. I could feel my alignment changing and my muscles becoming stronger in ballet class. Finally I was starting to feel like my body wasn't my enemy.

Over the summer, I noticed an increase in my energy level. I didn't need several naps a day anymore. I could concentrate better; something that was impossible before. I took ballet class and worked in a ballet studio, a physically rigorous trial for the macro diet that it passed beautifully. I think that macro would have wonderful applications for dancers. It makes one feel incredibly healthy and energetic plus it is very easy to stay thin on the diet. I not longer felt bloated, heavy and tired after eating.

My chemical sensitivities are starting to improve also. Perfume is less of an irritant as well as exhaust. When I have a headache now, I can identify the cause. I haven't taken a Tylenol in nearly a year. My periods, which have always been painful and irregular, are regulating themselves. I no longer have PMS.

I returned to Sarah Lawrence for my junior year with hope and excitement, something I had never experienced previously. I felt apprehensive about what would happen to me in the fall, but I knew that I was so much healthier now than a year ago that whatever happens couldn't be as severe.

As of this writing, I have been macro for nine and a half months. It has completely changed my life. There is no way that I would go back to eating as before; it is not worth it. I am starting to feel healthy and happy and that makes all the effort worthwhile. Admittedly it can feel isolating at times; I don't have people around me that are macro, I'm doing this by myself. When I feel discouraged, I just look at the big picture and see how far I've come.

It is a slow process, not a quick cure. I've been sick nearly my whole life, so it will take some time to heal. Sometimes I still wish that I didn't have to be so strict with my diet. I live among pizza, Chinese food and chocolate at college. But then I have to remember that at least I have something that I can eat; for a while I didn't know what to eat at all without reactions! I do spend a lot of time cooking. I really can't have a quick dinner very easily.

If I know I'll need to eat, I fill my thermos and bring it with me. I've had to put aside any uncomfortable feelings, let the comments and second glances roll off me. This is just the way it is for now. Someday I will be able to have the occasional treat, but not now. I've come too far to backslide now. I really don't have much of a choice. My body can't take abuse; it is still trying to heal.

Macrobiotics is nothing short of a miracle to me. Every morning when I wake up I thank God that I'm alive and that I feel better. There was a time when I was not happy to be alive and I don't want to forget that. I don't deny that there is still a lot of room for improvement. I still don't feel well; I have good days and bad days, but I know that the longer I am macro, the better I feel. I can only continue to improve. I really enjoy taking ballet class now. I watch myself become stronger. The addition of my greatest love, ballet, back into my life is a gift for which I am deeply appreciative. A weak body and a love of dance is a painful combination.

At 21, I am happy for the first time in my life. I know I risk sounding corny if I haven't already. I am just so thankful that I was lucky enough to find macrobiotics. I don't know where I would be without macro today. I don't believe anything else could have done all this for me.

-Contributed by Amy

A WORD FROM AMY'S DOCTOR

Pediatricians seem particularly resistant to the idea of allergies as Amy's case demonstrates. Early recognition and treatment could have helped her avoid ever becoming so severe. But Peds usually insist the kid will outgrow their allergies. All I ever see is they have outgrown the pediatricians.

Also now you can understand that the brain is also a target organ for people with multiple allergies and target organs (universal reactors). However, when researchers who are pro-pollution/anti-ecology examine these people, they conclude that they have "personality disorders" as their primary problem. Of course, most of these researchers' studies were funded by workman's compensation, too (Black, et al, JAMA, 1990: 264, 24; 3166 and Terr, et al, Arch. Intern. Med., 1986: 146; 145).

Amy demonstrates again how the ego of medicine gives the unspoken message "If I don't know what's wrong with you, then no one does. Furthermore, if you don't get better on my medications, then you must be fabricating your symptoms." Rule: When you feel your *sense of self worth deteriorate* with a doctor, leave. He's trying to cover up for his inability to help you.

Also it points out another rule: usually when all medication makes you worse, it's because you are missing some important nutrients that are needed in order to metabolize medications.

This was a wonderful learning experience for me to read Amy's story, because it taught me so much more about her suffering and perseverance to get well than I knew from taking her history in the office. Also I had no idea what a terrific writer she was. Because she is a strikingly tall, svelte and beautiful ballerina with a gorgeously long mane of blond hair, I figured she had to have a limit somewhere on her gifts. I was wrong. I asked for her story because I thought it would be easier for young people to identify with the trials and tribulations of a fellow college student with E.I. rather than hearing about it from a middle aged doctor who had to sleep in the bathtub of a hotel or climb into a plastic bag as flight attendants sprayed an airplane with pesticide. This young lady is incredibly special, as I think you have seen for yourself. She is indeed a very special and gifted young lady and I have a feeling we'll be seeing more of her either on the dance stage or in her chosen profession as an outstanding psychotherapist.

MULTIPLE SCLEROSIS

W.D., a 22 year old airline reservationist, was helped into the office wearing an eye patch for diplopia (double vision due to weakness of eye muscles), and had oozing pustular acne on both cheeks. She was too weak and unsteady to navigate the corridor unaided. She had been in bed much of the last 5 months after a hospital evaluation for the diagnosis of multiple sclerosis. She had positive evoked potential responses and optic neuritis. While hospitalized, she developed hepatitis from the multiple drugs she was given. She had consulted two neurologists who agreed there was nothing more that could be done for her. The nuclear magnetic resonance imaging scan showed demyelinating lesions in the cerebrum, cerebellum and brain stem. There was no question she had severe multiple sclerosis and could look forward to permanent wheelchair status any day.

She was started on the program of simultaneous nutrient assessment, inhalant testing, nystatin powder (152 colonies of Candida grew from vaginal culture), and the modified macrobiotic diet (no ferments for yeast sensitive individuals until they are able to tolerate them). In 5 months, she was radiant, walking normally, no longer needed the eye patch, and was back to work. Her face cleared and she turned out to be a strikingly beautiful Latin woman. She described herself as having more energy than she ever had. She did, however, have recurrence of weakness when exposed to the jet exhaust fumes and remained well if the ventilation was improved and continued to work adjacent to the airplane hangar.

One day her mother noticed her limp. She quickly searched her refrigerator and found she had stopped the whole program. She had acquired a boyfriend (I told you she was beautiful) and thought the program too much an interference in her social life.

You would think that with her mother and I urging her and most of all with the fantastic recovery she had made that she would go right back on the diet. Not true. She had abandoned the diet and

-255-

stayed off, and ended up in the hospital on high doses of steroids by intravenous and continued to deteriorate. Not every story has a happy ending. Her doctors called her improvement a spontaneous remission.

MY BATTLE WITH RHEUMATOID ARTHRITIS

It has been 23 years since I was diagnosed with Rheumatoid Arthritis, which affected most joints in my body, particularly my hands, feet and right wrist. For many years I had the usual drugs and treatments offered for arthritis. Many of the drugs gave me disturbing side effects. It also became necessary for me to have surgery involving both hands, feet and wrists including a left wrist replacement. The various drugs helped control pain and stiffness, but did tremendous damage to my immune system.

In 1983, thanks to a health magazine article, I met an allergist specializing in environmental medicine. She had achieved good success working with some arthritics and agreed to take me as a new patient. Testing revealed allergies to yeasts, molds, pollen and dust. Food testing indicated many food allergies, especially milk, corn, wheat, beef, eggs and chocolate. Blood tests showed a high level of rheumatoid arthritis factor in my blood and severe Vitamin B-6 deficiency, which I tracked back approximately 20 years.

With the doctor's suggestion I tried the rare food diet, food injections and using a 4 day rotation diet. By eliminating certain foods and using the food injections, I was able to eliminate all medications and control the pain and stiffness. This worked well, but did not improve my immune system. I healed very slowly, often developing infections and flu. My new knowledge made me realize that using antibiotics frequently is unwise.

In 1988 the doctor introduced me to macrobiotics. I read the book, "You Are What You Ate" which explained the diet, how to begin, suggested reading material and answers to questions one might ask.

The macrobiotic diet does require a great deal of reading as an ongoing process of learning. One must make a real commitment and be willing to make changes in their lifestyle. I found it difficult to decide if I could make such changes, but I did so desperately want to be able to improve and control my arthritis without the drugs the rheumatologists offer as the only treatment.

I started the diet in October, 1988. It is a bit confusing until one becomes familiar with the various foreign sounding names of Japanese radish, seaweeds or beans one may have never used. The counselor I went to is a young woman who developed rheumatoid arthritis, switched from her vegetarian diet to macrobiotic diet and halted the progress of her arthritis with very little joint damage.

She instructed me on what to eat, what percentage of grains, greens, beans, seaweeds, miso soups, root and other vegetables to use, etc. Also she told me what to avoid and why. She cautioned me of discharge also known as healing crisis. She said it would bring on severe symptoms for a week or more. Afterward one feels better. The more discharges one has, the more toxins will be removed from the body and one will feel much better.

Luckily, the local macrobiotics group met weekly in a nearby city. They were having macrobiotic cooking class just at the right time for my desire to learn more. I went there for two cooking classes and dinner. It helped to see so many there and know one is not so isolated as they might feel with such immense changes in diet.

Even with all this help, I found the diet difficult, disliking some of the foods. I felt like I didn't want to continue, but I so desperately wanted to be well without all those dangerous drugs, that I realized I need a firmer commitment. I read "Recalled By Life" by Dr. Anthony Satillaro, who cured his cancer on the macrobiotic diet. His book helped me realize if this diet could save someone so close to death, I should see how much it might help me.

In December 1988 I had my first discharge. It was 10 days of terror. I was so stiff, had severe pain, swelling, diarrhea, vaginal discharge and body odor. Each day was worse. I could barely handle dressing or walking. After the discharge ended, I felt much better. As the weather permitted, I began walking, first 1/2 mile, later building up to the present 2 mile level.

Things were improving. Day after day, I wrote in my journal "Feeling O.K." I was losing weight, as is to be expected; getting more organized, meals improving and learning to like foods I had disliked.

As time went on, I had 3 or 4 small discharges, consisting mostly of pain and stiffness. After each discharge, I felt better.

Now, after over 2 years on the diet I can say I truly feel much improved; I have more flexibility, energy and strength. I am amazed to know how powerful this diet is and so happy I didn't allow my first thoughts destroy my opportunity to succeed.

My most recent discharge was in December, 1990 and was a rough 7 days, similar to my first discharge. Being fearful of further deformity, I worried about hand swelling. I used buckwheat flour in a paste form spread over the swollen areas and it does reduce swelling. I also worked to keep my fingers flexible. I heated water with ginger root and soaked my hands in it. It felt so soothing.

I notice I feel so much more clear headed now than when I took 12 or 14 aspirin a day. Since I began the diet my right wrist is much stronger. I broke it many years ago and it would be very weak quite often.

The doctor recently told me each time she tests my blood for rheumatoid arthritis factor, the results are a weaker reading. She truly believes if I continue to practice macrobiotics for perhaps 2 more years, the rheumatoid arthritis may be completely out of my blood. This news really surprised and thrilled me. I thought I had achieved as much as possible.

Many have asked me about macrobiotics, some requesting me to write out instructions for them; others don't believe diet can do anything except control weight. I tell them all how wonderfully the diet works.

It is my personal opinion that anyone who is suffering and wouldn't try this diet doesn't have a genuine desire to recover. It is quite a sacrifice, but I feel it is well worth any inconvenience.

It is thrilling to know I can take the responsibility for improving my health and future. Now I feel I have a future I can look forward to, instead of worrying how much worse I might feel.

I thank God for directing me to a doctor who is so helpful and knowledgeable and for giving me the courage to make the right choice.

It is my hope that in the near future, people can easily find many restaurants that are more health conscious and serve wholesome natural foods.

-Submitted by Anne

A WORD FROM ANNE'S DOCTOR

When I first met Anne, she shuffled into the room with the gait so classic of rheumatoid, with swollen deformed hands held at chest level. She had had multiple surgeries and was accustomed to a life of pain. To my amazement, this was a young lady who worked every day as a secretary, looked after her aging parents and always brought a ray of sunshine with her wherever she went.

After years of heavy duty arthritis drugs, Anne developed a leukopenia, which she had for well over 10 years. This means the arthritis drugs poisoned the ability of the body to make as many white blood cells as a normal person does. That's why she had so many infections. Nothing any of her doctors (including me), could think of, ever restored the white count to normal. But since she has gone on the macrobiotic diet and had her discharges, the white count has finally improved for the first time in the many years that we have on record.

Sure, the diet was difficult, especially the social aspects that are so very much needed. But for Anne, nothing seems impossible, she just works a "little" harder. I admire her in more ways than I've ever told her.

MACROBIOTICS BRINGS LIGHT
THROUGH A TUNNEL OF LIFELONG E.I.

As I sit here writing, my heart is filled with praise to my precious Lord for his bountiful blessings. I have everything I need and more! I have eyes to see God's beauty all around me. I have legs to walk so I can be outside and really enjoy God's handiwork. I have ears to hear the birds. It is cold today at zero degrees Fahrenheit, with a chill factor of 15 degrees below zero. I just returned from a walk. If I had been told, even six to eight months ago that I would or could walk over five miles on a cold winter's day like this (or any day for that matter), I certainly would have said "No way!" Never before have I really enjoyed walking any distance without experiencing undue fatigue.

Since I am 57 years old, (and perhaps one of my doctor's chronologically older patients) I may find it more difficult than others to recall specifics healthwise of my early childhood. I do recall playing alone a great deal as I could not "keep up" with my friends. I was content to stay near home and help care for my six younger siblings. I was the eldest daughter so everyone felt I was a "good girl" because I helped my "tired" mother a great deal.

I do recall having a great many painful ear infections (then called "gatherings" of the ears), a chronic sore throat, many chest colds, headaches, periods of undue fatigue, lethargy, vertigo, etc. All of us had styes on the upper and lower lids every winter and spring which were treated daily with Brewer's yeast tablets. Certain foods caused generalized hives and headaches, such as strawberries, wheat, and chocolate. There were no foods I didn't like, but I would leave the "reaction" foods alone for even up to a year and then find I could return to them.

No one even thought about allergies per se. I often had extended periods of nausea and vomiting, generalized aching of joints and muscles and, what I then termed as an "all gone" feeling. I missed a great deal of school and was referred to as a "nervous child." I also had chronic lower back pain.

My mother felt I would feel better once I started my menses. This only increased the lower back pain. My periods were always sporadic; sometimes only two to three per year even through college and years of nurses' training. During these years I was diagnosed with hypothyroidism (per basal metabolism testing) and started on supplementary thyroid drugs. I lost a great deal of weight and felt even more anxious. After a year I discontinued the thyroid prescription on my own.

I can never recall feeling really great. The headaches increased with the years, along with the chronic intestinal problems. I often broke out in a cold sweat during the day, having to change my clothing. I had daily night sweats and severe generalized itching, especially at night. From childhood I always had cold, sweaty hands, to the point of perspiration literally dripping from my hands. I always carried three to four cloth hankies with me to dry my hands.

I loved bedside nursing, but during my nursing career generally found myself in a position of authority. I consoled myself with the realization that this position allowed me to make sure all staff working with me gave the patients the kind of care they needed. In 1965 (age 32), an upper G.I. series of x-rays showed a large duodenal ulcer and I was subsequently placed on a bland diet with "plenty of milk and milk products." My physician could not understand why I did not tolerate this diet well. Nausea and vomiting increased and I often was forced to "rest and relax" for two to three week periods. This became increasingly frustrating as I loved my work. Seven years later I had a subtotal gastrectomy for a bleeding ulcer with 3/4 of the stomach removed. I had asked to have a pyloroplasty done, but my doctor felt a subtotal gastrectomy would be best. I didn't understand, but I trusted his judgment. At that time I was coordinator in the "newly built" skilled nursing facility. Little did I realize I was reacting to "all things new" including paints, chemicals, carpeting, equipment, etc. I tired very quickly, having to lie down to rest during midday at work.

Over the years I had numerous bladder and kidney infections. I was treated with sulfa drugs and long-term antibiotics. I had a chronic vaginal discharge for which I sought help. The doctor laughed at me and had no suggestions. I had to change sanitary pads six to eight times per day. I did have several urethral dilatations as I found it impossible to void without pushing. In the 1980s, I had work-ups for "kidney problems." I was told I had only 25% total kidney functions and was urged to force fluids day and night and was placed on a low salt, low protein diet.

I was at this time already on a low carbohydrate hypoglycemic bland and low fat/diabetic diet. I couldn't find much to eat and lost weight to 78 pounds. By this time I often had three to four plus pitting edema of legs and feet plus edema (swelling) of abdomen and hands. I went from a size six shoe to an 8 1/2 to 9, and was placed on a diuretic. This was a great "game" trying to maintain a normal potassium level. I took potassium supplements but was often hospitalized with electrolyte imbalance, or simply fatigue, confusion, anxiety and tremors. I would receive I.V. fluids and rested but never slept when in the hospital. As far back as I can recall, I have frequently slumped to the floor at home or in stores. I would be taken to the emergency room where routine blood work would be done and I was subsequently told all was "normal". During these times, I was often told "you let your emotions rule you" and the inference was that I would profit from proper counseling or psychiatric help.

Through all this I was sent from specialist to specialist and acquired several diagnoses for my numerous "symptoms and problems." Among these diagnoses were post-gastrectomy syndrome (with dumping, excessive vomiting, fatigue, and vertigo), Hashimoto's disease of thyroid, Barlow's syndrome (with frequent "cluster periods" of chest pain and ensuing weakness), chronic pancreatitis, diabetes (and was frequently treated for hypoglycemia) and arthritis of the cervical spine and hands. Along with the other symptoms, I experienced tremors of my entire body, palpitations, tachycardia and constant nausea with frequent vomiting. I was having strong feelings of anxiety, inadequacy and dependency, fleeting aches and pains in different areas of my body as I went from room to room in my home. I was becoming very clumsy with codeine every four hours around the clock. I'd waken during the night and feel as though my head was about to explode. Tremors and anxiety were worse. I cried a great deal, awakened with clogged sinuses and constantly relied on nasal spray. I slept with a mist humidifier.

I visited an ENT specialist and was ultimately tested for about ten foods. I was given sublingual food drops and was told to rotate these foods. Rotate? I didn't dare eat anything else. I told the nurses I was afraid to eat and was simply told "don't be." The symptoms subsided somewhat, but if I tried any different foods than the ones covered by the sublingual extracts, they returned full force.

In December 1988 I had another stomach/intestine surgery (Bilroth II) with rerouting of bile flow. This helped somewhat. At least the constant nausea subsided. However, as I added more foods to my diet, in due time my other presurgical symptoms became markedly worse. I returned to the ENT doctor to be tested for added foods and was told I couldn't be tested further. By then I had developed a chronic cough, severe nasal congestion, had no sense of taste, extremely dry mouth, had difficulty swallowing, extreme fatigue and massive headaches. I was experiencing more muscular and joint pain, nausea and vomiting daily, numbness of face, hands, and arms, along with stiffness and pain in hands and arms. I found it difficult to use my finer motor skills.

Everything was an effort; even brushing my teeth. I was treated for myasthenia gravis for three months and then was admitted to the hospital neurology department where myasthenia gravis was ruled out. I was again told by the chief of staff that I needed psychotherapy. As a last ditch effort I did go to a psychologist for several sessions. She kept telling me I was getting better. I tried to believe this, but in truth was feeling worse day by day and the symptoms persisted. My faith in God plus my God-given husband's faith in me sustained me, however. Francis believed in me until I was again able to believe in myself.

In October 1989, I consulted an ecologist. I read the book, The E.I. Syndrome and thought it had been written with me in mind. Most of all, the author understood (from personal experience) my every symptom. I have frustrated many doctors, many of whom had treated me symptomatically. I was at one point on 17 different prescription drugs plus vitamins and minerals by the score. Talk about "junkies."

I did, however, go to the ecologist simply to get my food allergies under control. Little did I know that not only was I allergic to all 67 foods I was tested for but also sensitive to a variety of trees, grasses, weeds, house dust, house dust mites, and several genera of fungi. I also react to plastic, aluminum, chemicals of many kinds, many fragrances, odor of some foods while they're cooking, man made fibers and on goes the list. I have known for years that I would become irritable, tense, anxious, weak, spacey, and would physically hurt when ironing, cooking, doing laundry or working around any electrical appliances. I didn't dare tell anyone this because I was sure this would absolutely clinch the supposition by many people (especially physicians) that I needed psychiatric help. I also realized that while outside walking I was more "comfortable" walking around in our fruit orchards or open fields, with my charcoal mask, than down the road near the electrical wires. Now I understand that I am electromagnetically sensitive.

Besides all of this, the doctor found my magnesium level was extremely low (as shown by the magnesium loading test) which can cause symptoms such as weakness, depression, palpitations, uncorrectable low potassium, fatigue, etc. She helped me realized that I was indeed at high risk for a fatal cardiac arrhythmia. Since I couldn't tolerate prolonged magnesium by mouth, she had my husband give me magnesium sulfate injections at home. (After correcting this deficiency, I felt stronger, palpitations were less common and I could think more clearly.)

When I first read about the macrobiotic diet, I thought "No way would I consider this." I dislike cooking for myself. Then, I came to the realization that with the enormity of my problems, I had no choice but to go macro. I am a slow learner so I struggled to accept the drastic changes we had to make in our home and indeed in our whole lifestyle. I would often cheat on the diet. These periods of "cheating" are becoming less and less frequent and I find myself feeling so much better. At this point, I realize what *real health* can feel like and there is "no turning back."

This past summer I came to the realization anew of the magnitude of God's blessings in my life, not the least of all being my warm, sensitive, caring, precious husband Francis. For the 25 years of our marriage, he has not only taken me to doctor after doctor, nursed me back to my optimum health, believed in and loved me, but has lovingly planted a vegetable garden. This year for the first time in all these years, I watched him plant it and watched it grow with an excitement I had not experienced before. It was great to get up every morning, go out and pick fresh vegetables to cook for our soup for the day along with my delicious seaweeds. Oh, the new taste sensations I experienced! Fresh beets and beet greens, fresh carrots, chard, onions, string beans, squash; as God intended them to taste. I feel certain the dietary changes with God's help, have been the biggest asset as far as my quest for total physical wholeness is concerned.

I presently take injections for dust and mold. I have stopped the biweekly pollen injections. Along with these I take daily injections for the 67 foods for which I was tested along with biweekly injections for yeast. The palpitations are a rarity now and so is the tachycardia. I have taken nothing for headaches in well over a year. I am decidedly stronger and have been able to increase my daily walks from 1/10 of a mile to nearly five miles daily. I have never in my entire life been able to walk even nearly this distance without severe undue fatigue. After my walk I run from five to ten minutes with our dog. This is another first. I have had no chest pain in nearly one year. I have only occasional periods of nausea/vomiting, weakness, irritability, forgetfulness, and depression. These generally occur when my "total load" is high, i.e., working around electric appliances as indicated before. Watching TV and talking on the phone cause palpitations, anxiety, fatigue, and a spaced out feeling. At least I understand this now and I am trying hard to limit my time periods in the areas where these symptoms occur.

My hands no longer drip with perspiration and the severe constant pain in my hands only occurs when I handle plastic, aluminum (foil, etc.), vinyl, newspapers, new books and magazines. No longer is there a need to force fluids. I drink water only when I am thirsty. My soups three times daily and other foods provide the liquid I need to urinate freely in large amounts. I have had no lomotil for diarrhea, nor do I suffer constipation. The dumping has ceased and hypoglycemia is not a problem now. I occasionally find I need carrot or squash juice to give me a physical boost. The night sweats of nearly twenty years have ceased. Chronic pancreatitis is no longer a problem. The plastic lenses in my glasses have been recently exchanged for glass lenses. (I used to become anxious and unable to concentrate while reading.) An auto air purifier has decidedly helped in reducing my reaction to exhaust fumes. As we live in an old farm house, we are continuing to make changes so I will be more comfortable inside. There is yet much to be done in this area. The bedroom is sparsely furnished with a bed (with all cotton linens), and a stand with an air purifier. I have recently removed my bedside lamp and exchanged the electric clock for one which is battery run. We are "chipping away" in other areas of the house which cause untoward symptoms.

Stress and how it is dealt with play important roles in allowing total wellness to occur. I find myself frequently drawing on my faith in God and praising him for providing my greatest earthly blessing; my precious husband. Both are a source of great strength for me. I try to avoid fragrances and chemical containing products and find I am able to do my own housework now. I do have to wear a charcoal mask if I need to work in certain areas of our home. The macro diet gives me the strength needed for my daily activities, and I am no longer completely exhausted and racked with pain upon retiring. Six to seven hours of sleep is all I require now and I waken a bit stiff, but refreshed. (I found myself retiring at 5:30 to 6:00 p.m. daily for years; waking as tired as I was when retiring.)

I feel I have been given a new lease on life. I am so grateful for the doctor's willingness to be used of God to help others with their E.I. problems. She is indeed an inspiration to her patients. I am gradually seeing the light at the end of the tunnel of total emotional, physical, and spiritual wellness. Listening to my body, finding food is my friend instead of my enemy, and daily turning my entire self over to God is the secret to this wellness. There will still be mountains to climb and valleys to go through, but each day is a new adventure.

-Submitted by Jacqualyn

A WORD FROM JACKIE'S DOCTOR

People like Jacqualyn always fill me with amazement. How on earth do they survive? The era of molecular medicine cannot come too quickly. The current evolution in medicine will leave in it's wake many such people who have been repeatedly medicated and surgerized because we were not smart enough to look for the environmental trigger, correct the biochemistry and nutrient deficiencies and put people in charge of their diet and lifestyle changes necessary to bring about wellness.

There are many examples in the scientific literature of arthritis, gall bladder attacks, hyperactivity, migraine, ulcers, colitis, asthma, and much more being caused by hidden food allergies in certain people. But medicine still ignores it. Since insurance companies reward doctors for quick office visits and prescribing drugs, and penalize them for lengthy visits to instruct and teach patients in allergy diets, there will not be a rapid change.

It is obvious that when prescription drugs and surgery fail, however, and doctors insist on falling back on the psychiatric diagnosis to salve a wounded ego, it is time to bail out. Reading and self-education is what has helped most people to get on the track of wellness.

Jacqualyn had just about every magnesium deficiency symptom there is, but no one ever checked it, in spite of years of diuretics and 3/4 of her stomach removed.

I'll tell you something else. I had no idea what I was getting into when I haphazardly mentioned to a few people who had turned their lives around with macro that they were welcomed to write their stories a book. I knew they had things to teach and would be better at it than I. But, wow! I never knew how really sick they were. It has been a monstrously humbling experience to learn how these people endured against all odds. I'm overwhelmed with admiration and respect for their abilities to not only withstand all they did, but persevere in order to reach their goals.

As for Francis, Jackie's husband, you need only see the twinkle in his eyes once to realize there isn't anything he wouldn't do for her.

ACUTE MYELOGENOUS LEUKEMIA
Clear Cancer With A Diet?
Let This Attorney Help You Judge For Yourself

It was just over twenty-six months ago that I was diagnosed as having acute myelogenous leukemia: Friday, the 13th day of January, 1989. I had been very sick for about two months with various symptoms. I had a cough for 32 days straight. In November, I had a big, black bruise on the back of my right leg. My mother had noticed it and told me to go to the doctor. I, of course, had ignored it as nothing.

I had gone to the ear, nose and throat doctor for my sinuses. They had been plugged for months. He said my throat was red, but he could see nothing wrong. I remember discussing his son going to law school and the lady in the waiting room. She had cancer of the throat and wasn't expected to make it. I never suspected that I, too, had cancer and neither had this doctor.

I then went to my family doctor who treated me for a hiatal hernia with a popular capsule to suppress acid secretion, and a sinus infection with antibiotics. Neither doctor drew any blood. I went to the dentist because I was grinding my teeth. I actually bit my tongue on each side removing a chunk. The area around the sore turned black and took about a month to heal. The dentist x-rayed me and found no cavities. He was going to make me a mouth guard to protect my teeth. I was hospitalized before my next appointment.

Six months prior, I had complained to my gynecologist of hard stools, dark urine and a falling asleep or dead feeling in my limbs. He said I was under stress with two small children and my law practice. He offered no treatment. I also went to a cardiologist as my heart was jumping, but on the treadmill machine I checked out O.K. No treatment was offered and no blood was drawn. A blood test may have shown the leukemia.

Leukemia is a cancer of the white blood cells that are crucial for fighting off infections. It is really a cancer of the precursor cells (stem cells) which form white blood cells. Acute Myelogenous Leukemia is a malignant disorder involving the production of abnormal, immature white cells in the bone marrow. In advanced leukemia, the uncontrolled multiplication of these abnormal cells results in the crowding out of the production of normal white cells needed to fight infection, of platelets to control hemorrhaging, and of red blood cells to carry oxygen to tissues. As these overpopulated abnormal blood cells circulate throughout the body, they infiltrate and choke out the vital organs and glands causing them to enlarge, malfunction and eventually die.

One does not usually die of leukemia itself, but of internal bleeding or the spread of infection which the immune system can no longer control. Since white blood cells defend the body against disease producing bacteria, viruses and fungi, when there are too few white blood cells, the immune system cannot function. A third common cause of death is the chemotherapy itself, as you will learn. For that can kill off so many of the healthy cells that you have insufficient white cells left with which to defend the body. Hence, you can die from a simple cold.

Excessive exposure to radiation and to certain chemicals, such as benzene, have been linked to the development of leukemia. For example, a common source of radiation could be the radon (radioactive gas from the soil that leaks into basements) that is endemic to some areas of the United States. A common source of benzene is from cigarette smoke or pumping your own gasoline at the filling station. In my case, my natural father was in the war in Hiroshima. He, at the age of 65, has a chronic form of leukemia.

I also worked at an automobile plant summers while attending college and the year after I graduated from college. During the summers, I operated a machine. After the completion of the production of my cast iron automobile part, I would dip the part into a liquid solvent to rinse it off before measuring it for proper size. The solvent I dipped my bare hands into was gasoline, which contains much benzene. As a machine operator, I would dip my hands into this gasoline many times a day over a period of several summers. The automotive part was cast iron. I would be covered with black iron which would go into my pores. I would shower and even on my days off, black would wash out of my pores. This iron may have offset my other minerals and weakened my system, increasing my chance for leukemia.

On January 11, 1989, I had been to my gynecologist for an exam. I appeared to be pregnant or having a miscarriage. I had in the last few years miscarried a child in my fourth month in December of 1984, and then delivered my son on December 23, 1985 and my daughter on February 2, 1987. The last thing I thought I needed was to be pregnant again. If only I knew then what would be discovered in the next few days, another pregnancy would have been a blessing. I was examined. Something was obviously wrong. I had a sonogram in the doctor's office (the tenth sonogram in three years) and a pregnancy test. I was not pregnant, but there was tissue in my uterus. I was sent to the hospital to make arrangements for a D & C. They drew my blood at the hospital; I then went home.

Later that afternoon, I got a telephone call. My doctor told me that I had abnormal blood cells and that I should call an internist. Thank God I was sitting down and no one was around because that was more than I could take. It was my worst nightmare come true. The man had just told me that I have cancer. What else could abnormal blood cells mean? I got off the telephone and cried. Boy, did I cry! After a while, I called my friend and said, "I have something to tell you." She asked, "Is it bad?" and I said, "Yes, I have abnormal blood cells." She told me not to worry until I saw the doctor the next afternoon. I agreed and hung up. I called my husband and told him that I had to go to the doctor the next day. He said, "O.K.," but I didn't tell him about the abnormal cells.

I didn't sleep that night. When I got up, I went to work to await my appointment. I felt like I was bleeding to death so I called the internist and asked if I could go in early. He said to go right in and to make sure someone drove me. In the office my blood was drawn and I was given the first of what was to be many bone marrow biopsies. I was laid on my side. My upper hip region was injected to numb one area. A large corkscrew was screwed into my hip and a piece of bone was removed along with some bone marrow. It was a very painful procedure. It made having a baby seem like a piece of cake. The samples were then examined for abnormalities and sent off to a lab for more detailed examination.

I told the doctor to be honest with me. Quite frankly, this was still a bad dream. He told me that he thought I had leukemia. I must have known something, he said. I was new to the medical world and brainwashed that they could cure anything. Also, as I was later to learn, there are other types of leukemia that have a pretty fair chance of recovery. Mine, however, was one of the more aggressive ones with a very poor track record. I did not yet know that at age 33 I had just been given my death sentence, and was not expected to see the new year.

I was wheeled to the hospital for further testing. At that point, I had never dreamed that I would not be leaving for another twelve days and that during these twelve days, my body, mind and soul would go through a fight for my life beyond my wildest nightmare.

I went through the routine check-in procedure, and was wheeled to my room. I remember when I finally got the heart to tell my husband Andy. Oh, how we cried! How could this happen to us? We had two small children. I was an attorney, he was an attorney. My career was really taking off. I was considered one of the best matrimonial attorneys in the city. I made a six figure income. We had a house, owned our office building, I drove a BMW. I had two law degrees. We had all that money could buy and me, I had leukemia. There must be a mistake. This was not happening to me. And yet it was.

So for the next several days, I was given blood transfusions. Normally, one no longer gets whole blood, but blood products instead. That is, when you need platelets or red blood cells, you get them only and not the whole blood product. It is more economical. You can also get just white blood cells, but this is rarely done. And when the white blood cells are dangerously low, they give broad spectrum antibiotics intravenously to fight the infection. The goal was to strengthen my body so that the chemotherapy would not kill me.

I was presented with a contract. This contract stated the various chemotherapy drugs that would be used and their numerous side effects. I was to read it over for a few days and decide if I would be treated in Syracuse or go to New York City. My brother-in-law is an oncologist (cancer doctor) in New York. He told me that it did not matter where I got my treatment, as the protocols are the same throughout the country. He also told me to get my affairs in order. I was going to die.

I cannot begin to tell you the impact that this statement had on me. You figure that if your brother-in-law, a cancer specialist, tells you to get your affairs in order, then there is no hope. My personal oncologist said that I had a 5% chance of surviving the year. Later, in my research at the medical school, I learned that the best statistics with optimal triple session chemotherapy and a $100,000 bone marrow transplant report a 10-50% chance of living five years. As you will see later, I did not have optimal chemotherapy.

My first chemotherapy consisted of two different drugs in combination to put me in remission (to poison and stop the production of the abnormal stem cells that were trying to take over my body) and then a second treatment of two different drugs in combination called consolidation treatment. I had been scheduled for three treatments, but I refused the third.

When you think of medical drugs, you think of something that heals the body. But chemotherapy drugs are very powerful chemicals: their purpose is to kill cancer cells. In the process they also kill a majority of the remaining healthy blood and bone marrow (where blood cells are made) cells. The theory is that cancer cells are faster growing than healthy cells so the chemicals will kill them first. The problem is, because they function on a logarithmic basis, the can never kill every blood cancer cell. There are always some cancer cells left. So it's only a matter of time before they regrow in sufficient numbers to cause recognizable disease again. Chemotherapy drugs also directly attack the genetic material of the cell and can be stored in organs of the body; as well, they have a side effect of causing (a new) cancer several years later.

I received Daunomycin for three days intravenously (in a vein) and then Cytosine Arbinoside for seven days. For twenty-four hours a day for ten days I had these chemical poisons running through my veins. They were attempting to kill the cancer cells without killing me. I had transfusions of blood almost daily as my system was no longer producing enough blood. I was living on other people's blood, risking AIDS and hepatitis; if I lived that long. I threw up almost round the clock for the entire ten days. I was given steroids to reduce the vomiting. It helped some.

The side effect was I had a fat "moon" face for months afterwards. I lost about ten pounds. My beautiful long blonde hair that was below my butt fell out in bunches. I was bald. My head looked like a newborn baby's. My mouth was full of sores as I had no white blood cells to fight the normal bugs in the mouth. My hemorrhoids grew to a size that I never thought possible. My bones ached. I was always cold. I would shiver and need more blankets. I could not eat; my mouth was too sore and the hospital food was disgusting. I spent a lot of time praying, spacing out with the TV set, and talking to friends on the telephone (more than once I had to hang up to vomit). I had constant diarrhea and red colored urine. I had to urinate constantly due to the large volume of chemotherapy fluid taken intravenously.

If you want a taste of hell, then do chemotherapy. I honestly do not believe there could be a closer experience here on earth. The good part is that I went into remission. That means that when I had another bone marrow biopsy, the bone marrow no longer showed cancer cells. Throughout the ten days, I had several tubes of my blood drawn on one or more occasions per day. Between the blood work, the transfusions and the I.V., my arms were pin cushions. They ran out of places to prick me. My veins were bruised and swollen. I had edema (swelling) in several places that would take months to heal.

They discussed placing an I.V. Hickman catheter in my chest. This is a metal plastic combination that puts a porthole in your chest into a main artery so that they can plug you into the I.V.s and give or take blood without sticking you. I had read, however, of the infections that could be caused, the scarring that was left and the danger of a piece of the catheter breaking off and entering the blood system and lodging in the heart.

I had cancer alright, but I never planned to die from it or any of it's complications, to include errors of the medical staff or their equipment. I watched each and every person who touched my body, let it be day or night. I asked questions, read labels and overall policed the entire situation to ensure that I would be one of those who walked out of that hell hole.

After the first course of chemotherapy and my remission, I begged to go home. You usually stay in the hospital for the first month. After the treatment, you are not yet producing blood normally. There is still a need for transfusions. You also do not have any white blood cells to fight infection. Even the slightest infection can be deadly, for example, anyone's cold germs could kill you. Therefore, it is advisable to stay in the hospital to have reverse isolation with visitors gowned and gloved and to have your temperature checked regularly. At the first sign of fever, I.V. antibiotics are necessary.

I had a theory, however, that it was more dangerous to be in the hospital than at home. Where but in a hospital would the most deadly germs be? After all, that is where all the sick people go. I begged to go home. I remember the doctor coming to my room with his nurse to talk me out of it. They tried, but I said that I could either go with their blessings or without. He gave me a big hug, and made me promise to call him and get to the emergency room as soon as I had a fever. I had to check my temperature every four hours or if I felt warm or sick. They noted in my chart that I requested to go home (against medical advice) and checked me out.

I went home. It felt good to be with my husband and my children. It was nice to be in my own bed with my husband instead of alone in that cold hospital room. No one came into my room in the middle of the night to check my vital signs. I could sleep through the night. I had to wear either a scarf or my wig as I had no hair. I had to soak in the bathtub three times a day as my hemorrhoids were swollen. I ate more than I did in the hospital. I wore a gauze mask for germ protection if anyone came to visit. I started to read about holistic medicine and became very interested.

Throughout my stay in the hospital, I was in what they called reverse isolation. That means that I had my own hospital room and bathroom. I was allowed no flowers or living items that might carry germs or infection. No one could enter my room without washing their hands and putting on hospital clothes to include shoe covers and a mask. No one with any sign of a cold was allowed in. This all set the scene for a lonely stay. I had many visitors, but they usually came at night or on the weekend, since during the day most people worked.

Well, it was only a couple of days before my hemorrhoids got the best of me and I got a fever. I had to return to the hospital. I called the emergency room and I went in. Of course, there was a bed shortage so I spent about half of the night in emergency. Talk about germs! You should see what goes through emergency. Then more x-rays, blood work and another complete physical. I would soon have this routine down pat. Then off to my room for my I.V. antibiotics.

One of their wonderful rules was to put the I.V. into the arm with only saline solution in emergency to save the nurses time up-stairs. That meant you had to have this needle in your arm for no useful purpose for hours before it was ever used. I refused to allow this after the first time. Sometimes I felt they forgot that I was still a person. Sure I was supposed to die of this dreaded disease, but be-tween then and now I would like to endure as little pain as possible, and with as much dignity.

During the period after my first chemotherapy when I was waiting for my blood and bone marrow to grow back, I began to do a lot of thinking and reading. I read "Love Medicine and Miracles" by surgeon, Dr. Bernie Segal. I started to take vitamins and to question my diet. As I got stronger, I began to run three miles per day with a friend. I went to the medical school to research my illness and I read a great many holistic health books on diet, nutrition, and lifestyle.

I had thought deeply about refusing all further chemothera-py. I figured I was in remission, so if it wasn't broken you didn't need to fix it. But fear got the best of me and I took a second set of chemotherapy. This was VP-16 given over thirty-eight hours fol-lowed by cytoxan over two hours for three days. I was continuously on intravenous.

When I was diagnosed, my white blood cell count was a few hundred cells (normal 4,500 to 10,000) with most of them cancerous forms. After my first chemotherapy treatment, when the healthy stem cells multiplied and replaced the diseased or cancerous ones which the chemotherapy had killed, my blood counts were checked and they were normal at about 8,000. But after this second treatment, I was not so lucky. My counts for the next months never reached 3,000. Too many healthy stem cells were killed by the second chemo-therapy.

During this second treatment I thought I was going to die. One night my body just started to bloat up; I had retained water and was unable to excrete it. I got very nervous. I demanded to see the nurse and when she could not help, the doctor. No one wanted to help me. After all, these drugs were prescribed for a certain dosage and that dosage was not to be changed. There was no such thing as an individualized dosage. If you had a problem, no one knew what to do. Thinking was off limits. We had a protocol to follow!

As I mentioned before, I was not going to be a victim of this disease or the medical staff or their treatments. I therefore demanded to see my doctor and said that my dosage was either to be lessened or I would unplug the I.V. myself. My "medicine" was lessened and the swelling began to subside. I began to excrete normally. That night I almost died. The drugs were poisoning my kidneys that I needed in order to live. And I not only had to make the diagnosis, but to fight the staff in order to carry out the life saving step of reducing the drugs.

Then there was another scene where I was begging to get out of the hospital as soon as I was unplugged from the I.V. But after several days at home, I had to return. This time I had burned my finger on a hot cup. As I had no white blood cells necessary for normal healing, it was a miracle that I didn't need a skin graft. Amazing that just a small burn from a lightly hot cup could land me back in the hospital for another transfusion.

After I was released, I was to wait for my blood counts to return to normal and then I was supposed to have a third course of chemotherapy. My counts started to go up, but then they went down again. I either had leukemia again (which was very possible), or I could have been exposed to a virus or germ. Or if I was really unfortunate, I could have something like organ damage. Well guess what? I had hepatitis. Can you believe it? Not only did I get leukemia, but I was one of the select few who either caught hepatitis in a blood transfusion (thank God, not AIDS) or it was chemically induced by the chemotherapy. Whichever, hepatitis can be fatal, as it destroys the liver. If I thought I was a goner with leukemia, you can just imagine the statistics with hepatitis to boot.

And the irony is I had done my homework and gotten blood from friends and family reserved for me. But my doctor said it was unnecessary and so I was given stock blood from anonymous donors for my transfusions.

And now my blood count. The few long term survivors that there are have blood counts well over 3,000. My counts after the first treatment were 8,000. They had destroyed many of the cancer cells without killing too many of the stem cells that produce normal white blood cells. But during my second chemotherapy treatment, many more healthy stem cells were killed and my body was able to produce less than half of the white blood cells than it had produced before. My counts were now always below 3,000. A normal person has a white blood cell count between 4,500 to 10,000. I had reached a point where I questioned whether the chemotherapy would kill too many healthy stem cells to sustain my life compared with the number of remaining cancer cells. There is a delicate balance. I knew that the chemotherapy in theory (because of its logarithmic destruction of cancer cells) could not ever remove every cancer cell.

So I stopped further treatment, as I felt I had two bad signs since my second treatment: hepatitis and a dangerously low white count of 2,200. Also, my platelets were far less than the minimum allowable. I had several fears at this point. Could my liver take any more chemotherapy or would it fail to function and I would die of hepatitis? Would I have further kidney trouble and die of renal failure? Would I hemorrhage to death from low platelets. Would I be exposed to someone's cold and die from that? Would I get another cancer in years to come from too many chemical exposures from my chemotherapy (which is known to cause cancer years down the road)? Would my blood count be reduced to half or less of it's present level, leaving me statistically to die even after another treatment? Or would I die because I had not received optimal treatment (namely three courses of chemotherapy)?

Somehow, I still thought I was going to live. It seems that I was the only one who thought so based on the medical information I had received up to this point.

My oncologist was pushing strong: I had to take this next treatment or I would not have a chance. But from everything he said, I didn't have a chance anyway, so why bother? I didn't. Prior to making that decision, however, I ran a lot of miles, read a lot of books, got the opinion of two other oncologists, saw a social worker who deals with cancer patients, a macrobiotic counselor, and a new doctor.

I went to Roswell Park to see an oncologist who specializes in AML leukemia. She requested my former bone marrow and blood work studies. I explained to her my concern of my blood counts and

and my hepatitis. She was very understanding. She did contact my first oncologist. He explained to her how I had been taken off my protocol with noncompliance. In a nutshell, I refused many tests so I was no longer a good case study. I was more concerned with my own health than with performing his research. In fact, had I elected to do a third chemotherapy I would have been precluded from using one of the drugs originally assigned to me anyway, because AZQ, as it is called, was experimental and given only to patients in the strict protocol.

The funny thing is that before I was given any treatment, I remember saying that I wanted the drugs that my doctor had the best results with. I was told I must go on a protocol and that the drugs that would be used were NOT experimental as they had been used many times before. Why then couldn't I get AZQ? As I was later to find out, my protocol was only used at two hospitals and the statistics were not yet in on it's success rate. The oncologists at both Roswell Park and later at Strong Memorial Hospital in Rochester were not optimistic about these drugs.

The bottom line, as per my doctor's clinical chart note dated May 22, 1989, was that "It is impossible to know with certainty whether she would benefit from a second course of consolidation therapy, however, there is clear cut benefit from intensive consolidation therapy and it is usual to give at least two courses. Therefore, I recommend as her home physician, that she receive a second course of consolidation chemotherapy. My choice would be high doses of ARA-C for 12 hours, four to six days with three days of Daunorubcin infusion or mitrosantrone. She does not have an HLA matched sibling and, therefore, it seems imperative that she have her bone marrow harvested immediately following completing and recovering from her consolidation or if she chooses not to have further consolidation therapy, she should have her bone marrow stored now." Further, my liver function tests were assessed, and although they confirmed the hepatitis, they determined that it would not interfere with my chemotherapy. How they could make that determination, I am not sure. Obviously, the liver was damaged; why damage it more? I guess they figured the cancer would get me before the liver damage would.

I began counseling. I was taught imagery: the Dr. Bernie

Segal way of going into a meditative state, entering your body and either becoming a body part or some other image that is going to remove your cancer. I would visualize myself going into my blood stream as a healthy, large white blood cell that moved all throughout the blood and bone marrow system removing any bad or malfunctioning white blood cells. I would engulf these malfunctioning cells and they would be excreted from my body. I would do this three times a day. I felt good about this meditation state. As I was becoming more and more aware of the mind, body and spirit connection, I was also aware that when I finally believed that I no longer had leukemia, I would no longer have it.

I discussed various personal problems that may have had a bearing on my illness. I had never met my natural father. I had been adopted by my father as a child and had never given myself the opportunity to meet my natural father. It was something my counselor highly recommended. I intended to, but was not then ready. We discussed my marriage and my husband's behavior that I felt was deteriorating. We discussed the embarrassment that I would feel as a person, mother, wife and fellow attorney when he did certain things. My counselor made me understand that his poor behavior was not my fault, but his own. I began to realize that maybe this person that I was devoting my life to was taking more than he gave, and that I might even be killing myself over it.

Life has a funny way of presenting us with the same problems over and over again until we learn the lesson it was meant to teach. I eventually met my father, but have not yet resolved all of these issues. I divorced my husband. I am beginning to understand that we all need our freedom and we all cannot sit down and discuss personal problems or emotions. You must accept people as they are. There is a reason for everything that happens. It was with my counselor that I learned to listen to my inner self or spiritual self: a part of me that I did not even know existed. I knew what religion was and the Holy Spirit, but not my own unique spirit with it's own thoughts, intuition and direction.

So I told my counselor that I didn't think chemotherapy was a good idea for me. We would meditate and I would go inside and ask myself if I wanted or needed any more chemotherapy. The answer was always the same, "you don't have leukemia anymore, so why take a drug that might kill you?" My mind, body and spirit did not want chemotherapy. I knew then that I would have no further traditional treatments. I would continue to investigate what modern medicine had to offer, but inside I knew that I would never seek traditional oncological treatments again.

When you have AML leukemia, after you complete the chemotherapy treatment, you have a bone marrow transplant. I remember when my doctor told me I should have a bone marrow transplant to give myself a second year to live. (But, also that I had a one in three chance of dying from complications of the bone marrow transplant within the first month.) My doctor referred me to another doctor at Strong Memorial Hospital to have my bone marrow stored. As I was adopted, my bone marrow did not match any members of my family. My four half-sisters and my mother all had their blood typed, but no one matched. That meant that I would have to have an autologous bone marrow transplant: my own bone marrow would either be removed and immediately transplanted or it could be frozen (for up to seven years) to be transplanted if I ever came out of remission.

The better form of bone marrow transplant is the allogeneic transplant. That is when one of your family members or a matching donor donates bone marrow to you for transplantation. The difficulty with an autologous transplant is in receiving bone marrow from your body which may contain leukemic cells versus from a donor who is cancer free. The plus side is that you will not get graft-host disease or reject the donor's bone marrow and die from that.

So I went to Rochester to discuss storage of my own bone marrow. The doctor was very interested in having me do a transplant at that time. He was not very optimistic with my rate of cure or survival based on my having only taken two of the three recommended chemotherapy treatments, nor with the specific drugs taken and my not having any matching donors. He explained all of these procedures to me and sent me home to think about things. He actually called me at home at 7:00 in the morning to give me the gruesome statistics. He basically told me that without the bone marrow transplant immediately, I should know what the end result would be. *I would die.* He told me that if his own sister had leukemia, he would tell her to get a transplant.

Well, I knew I was not going to take the immediate bone marrow transplant. I had read in the medical school library that one in three patients die in the transplant itself from complications. I was alive and "well" and I had no immediate death wish. I also knew that the hospital would receive $100,000 from my insurance company if they completed this procedure on me. I felt that maybe they had more to gain than I did. My two chemotherapy treatments had each cost $20,000 for a total of $40,000, but somehow $100,000 had a ring of profit in it that may have clouded the vision of even the most honest of men. Whatever their reasons, I was not ready to die.

I did check in to have my bone marrow stored. The procedure seemed simple enough and I felt that this would be my backup security. However, during the first night with the procedure scheduled for the next morning, I walked out of my room and left. My mother was with me and she had planned to spend the night. We had discussed the procedure with the doctors, nurses and anesthesiologist. The stories just didn't seem to jive. My inner self said to leave and I did. I would go back for blood work on three other occasions at Roswell Park over the next year, but by May of 1990, I had decided to give up my oncologists. I had abnormally elevated liver enzymes from the hepatitis and my counts, although far from normal, were improving. At first they thought I was crazy when I told them of my vitamins, minerals, amino acids, diet and lifestyle. On the last visit I recall the nurse saying, "You know, Karen, some of you do make it." This was the first sign from the oncology community that they actually believed that I was going to live. If only they could believe that their patients could survive. They send such hopelessness with each statistical determination and each look of fear.

On April 13, 1989, I went to see a nutritionist. She checked me for various food allergies. I eliminated many foods from my diet as I had a sensitivity to them as confirmed by applied kinesiology (muscle testing). By eliminating these foods which included among them wheat, vinegar, mushrooms, yeast, the gourd family, the grape family, laurel family, peas, coffee, maple, mint family, olive family, palm family, poppy seeds, cocoa, chocolate, honey, dried fruits, synthetic sweeteners and all ferments, I had a great deal more energy. Instead of my body fighting to remove food items that I was sensitive to, it could begin to heal. The nutritionist also tested my vitamin and minerals, nutrients and digestants via muscle testing. I had various deficiencies. I did what the nutritionist said and follow her advice to this day. I must still avoid some of these foods, but others I am now able to tolerate. I began taking supplements. I was not aware of my next doctor at this time and the fact that she could test the levels for each of these things in the blood and urine.

I next went to see a macrobiotic counselor. She and I now laugh at the first time she saw me. I asked her if she had thought I would make it when she first saw me and she admitted that she was surprised that I had. Anyway, without her help and the help of many others, I am sure that I would not have survived. You see when you look to heal and no longer to cure, you realize that we are all one, and only with the help of each other can any one of us survive. The counselor taught me about macrobiotics. She adjusted my diet and told me what to eat and what not to eat. Her advice complimented that of the nutritionist in the elimination of various foods, but it went further and eliminated more foods and required a special type of preparation. I saw her in mid-May. I was told to eat 40-60% whole grains and grain products, 25-35% vegetables, and 10-15% beans and seaweeds. I was to drink bancha tea and dandelion tea.

On June 4, 1989, I saw an ecologist for the first time. I remember that day clearly. I was excited, for I knew then that I was going to get well. I liked the ecological style of the office: wood floors in some areas and quarry stone tiles in others, a sign asking people to refrain from wearing perfume, cologne, aftershave and disallowance of smoking. I also liked the fact that the doctor looked younger and healthier than the age suggested by the wall diplomas. The doctor later told me she thought I was one of those "punk" kids. You see I had very little hair at this point, no more than a quarter inch or so. I had tired of my wigs a few days before and decided that it was warm enough to leave them home.

On my application to the office I listed my symptoms as leukemia, sinusitis, tiredness, gas, bloated stomach and yawning. Inside the form, I also mentioned hepatitis, lack of taste, lack of smell, constipation, arthritis, leg aches, back aches, weakness, tingling, racing heart, undue fatigue and sweating spells. Besides the exhaustion, I no longer had a period. I complained of vaginitis, hyperactivity, compulsive eating or binges, inability to think clearly, insomnia, frequent urination, inappropriate behavior, mood swings and even more.

I wrote that I didn't expect miracles, but with her aid, I felt my chances were going to be greatly increased to stay in remission. I had improved my situation greatly, but I knew her knowledge would be beneficial. So when all of the other doctors had left me to die, and no one but me felt I had a chance to survive, this doctor agreed to try to help me get healthy enough to heal my body and recover. I've read in the Sunday paper column "Your Best Friend" where all of these different people write in about their best friends. I have thought of telling my story, but I have a feeling she would be too embarrassed. Instead, I offered to write this article.

My blood work at the office showed a 2,700 white count, abnormally high liver enzymes (my hepatitis), a magnesium deficiency, very high iron, low platelets, enlarged red cells, no chromium, and low zinc. I was tested for various allergies to include dust, mold, and Candida albicans. I also exposed petri dishes (mold plates) to measure the fungal load of my environment. The doctor prescribed vitamin, mineral and amino acid supplements to correct my documented deficiencies as well as prime my detoxification system, and prescribed nystatin. She also encourage me to continue the macrobiotic diet.

I cleaned my home and office environment according to The E.I. Syndrome. I drank spring water, ran air purifiers, put gutters on the office, and cleaned the mold and mildew.

She also suggested that I take a few extra days a week off just to relax and have fun. I have worked a regular court schedule since being released from the hospital. I still try not to schedule court or appointments for Wednesday and Friday. I have learned to do and enjoy things that I never took the time to enjoy before. I ride horses, play tennis, swim, sail, jog, attempt to play the piano, write articles and am very active in several organizations. And I planted an organic vegetable garden and a perennial flower garden this year.

In January of 1990, the doctor went with me to consult with Mr. Michio Kushi. Mr. Kushi adjusted my diet and told me leukemia was not my problem. I had been macrobiotic for seven months at that point, but after spending the weekend in Boston, I became more knowledgeable and more dedicated than before. I also began to grow spiritually.

My mind became very clear and I felt energy that I had never felt before. My blood work continues to improve. I no longer have hepatitis. All of my various complaints on my original worksheet for admission are gone with the exception of my facial acne which I have had for over fifteen years. Up until the time of my illness, I took antibiotics on a regular basis in an attempt to control my acne. I am now taking homeopathically prepared sulfa and silicea salts and my acne has almost cleared. I wash my whole body with a rough wash cloth at least two times a day. Many dermatologists say to wash your face three times a day. I have a theory that if you scrub your whole body, the body can discharge over a larger area and not just the face leaving less discharge for the face. I have more energy than I ever remember having before.

At one point, I obtained a second opinion from Roswell, a cancer specialty institution. I think I'm the only one from my group of newly diagnosed people with AML who did not follow the chemotherapy and/or transplant protocol. Also, I'm one of the only ones left who is still living. I am more alive now than I've ever been in my life.

Most importantly, however, is that I *am* still alive. I have been in remission for over 33 months with no sign of illness, and am healthier than ever before. As strange as it may seem, I am actually happy that I had my illness. It has been a great learning experience for me. I have learned a great deal about our medical system and unfortunately much of it dismays me.

We are spending millions of dollars annually for cures for cancer, heart disease and other illness. We continue to look in the area of chemotherapy and drug methods that can be easily patented by the large pharmaceutical companies. We refuse to look at the alternative treatments that are as simple as diet and nutrition (macrobiotics and nutritional biochemistry), because, these things cannot be patented. And health freedom is eroding in the U.S.

The scientific and medical communities are just barely beginning to recognize that diet and nutrition not only prevent cancer, heart disease, multiple sclerosis, allergies, environmental illness and other diseases, but they also heal or cure them. Are they so selfish or possessive of their patients that they can't see the need for a simultaneous referral to a specialist in environmental medicine and nutritional biochemistry where their blood nutrient levels, environment and allergies can be assessed and corrected?

Food manufacturers are prolonging the shelf life of products with chemicals which are weakening our immune systems. Who more than the cancer patient should be taught how to avoid adding further insult to an already over-compromised system? Who more than a cancer patient should be encouraged to drink natural spring water to avoid the added chemicals and pollution in drinking water, or to breathe clean air even if it means running an air purifier, as air is the basis upon which all human life is sustained. Polluted air full of chemicals can further weaken an immune system already damaged by benzene. It is only logical that regardless of the route you chose for yourself, you have a much better chance of recovery if you unload the system of it's environmental insults and correct it's biochemical glitches. And, more importantly, each person must learn to be ultimately responsible for his own health and healing.

I am not proposing that we forego our present medical system for alternative remedies, but that they compliment each other. What harm would be done if patients were taught to heal themselves? Strong drugs are used for chemotherapy, for high blood pressure, pain, headaches, etc. How many vitamins, minerals and nutrients are destroyed by taking these drugs? Doesn't it make sense to correct these deficiencies immediately to give the patient a fighting chance to live? Instead, we send him home and tell him that there is nothing more to be done. When he gets sick again, he should come back and be treated again.

The medical school library is full of articles on nutrition. We have normal values for the various nutrient levels and yet patients are not tested to see what their deficiencies are. Diet, exercise and a positive mental attitude are also ignored. Allergies have also been extensively studied and yet are ignored. Candida albicans is well-documented as an immune system modifier and ignored. Chemicals have been proven to be very detrimental to the immune system and yet are ignored. Why do we ignore the obvious and let so many people die or live unhealthy lives? Is it out of ignorance or greed? Or is it that the answer is just too simple and doesn't glorify the doctor like high technology medicine does?

When I was in the hospital, my sister was one of the nutritionists. She would regularly bring me sodas, candy and ice cream. The diet in the hospital was very bad even by American standards. The meat was overcooked as were the vegetables. They served Jello, pudding, and always a sugary dessert. The American diet is not healthy and the American hospital diet is even worse.

The macrobiotic diet is the most perfect diet that I have seen. It is not a vegetarian diet, as it employs a small amount of fish and shuns all the baked goods and dairy that vegetarians eat. The theory is that if the human mouth consists of teeth, the majority of which are for grinding grains and vegetables, then God must have been trying to tell us to eat grains and vegetables. Macrobiotic cooking is used to make digestion easier, but avoid overcooking which removes the nutrients.

Foods are eaten in their whole, unprocessed state to avoid the destruction of the nutrients. Chemicals and preservatives are avoided by purchasing organic foods. Sugars and other non-nutrients are avoided. Every mouthful counts and excess is not eaten. The body is therefore provided with the nutrients it needs so that it can better heal or move on to higher levels of well being and creativity. For generations, people ate well, and yet in our sophisticated society we don't even know how to prepare a healthful meal. Why is it that we have ignored the basics? We have forgotten the importance of our health, and decided to delegate it to men in white coats with prescription pads.

Another very important part of my healing is and was body work. When I was in Boston to see Mr. Kushi, I had a shiatsu massage. Massage is wonderful in that it gets the energy flowing throughout the body. When I returned home, I started to see a chiropractor. I went every day for the first two months before my spine would even begin to adjust. It made sense that with a bone marrow disease my spine would be out of alignment. I began to feel energy that I had never felt before move throughout my body. As my spine became properly aligned, the body energy began to heal my body. The shiatsu massage balanced my meridians and the energy flowed. I continued to have the shiatsu massage and to see the chiro-practor. Together these two body work arts also helped me to heal.

Hugs and human contact in the form of love were also very healing. Prior to my illness I almost never hugged my friends. Now I make it a matter of course and find that it is very healing to both me and my friends. My children also provide me with very special hugs. There is nothing as innocent and genuine as the love of a child and probably nothing more healing. A spouse or significant other is very important as are close family ties with an extended family.

So avoid getting confined to one niche: the oncologist will clear my cancer, or a macrobiotic diet will clear my cancer. You need an eclectic approach of doing as much good for your body as possible.

In conclusion, I honestly believe that you can heal your body of any illness no matter how severe, if you believe you can and if you have the discipline required to take self control and work at your health each and every day, from as many angles as possible. The quick fix of modern medicine is not going to be the long term solution to any medical problem. We must change our daily habits to heal. After all, whatever we were doing is what got us into the trouble, so it's only logical to change our tack. We have to give our bodies the proper nutrients so that they can function at their full capacities. We have to avoid chemical pollutants in food, water and air.

You cannot let some doctor tell you that you will never get well or that you are going to die. If you believe him, you are as good as dead. You must believe that you can get well (once you decide that you want to), and then take the proper steps to make it happen. Alternative medicine has been a challenge for me. I am enjoying my life like I never did before. I have energy to do things I never thought I would have time for. I have a new attitude about life. I remember before I was sick I would walk around and say I was bored. No longer.

I was given a second chance at life and I intend to use every waking minute working toward the improvement of our society and world. We need some major changes: it is about time that man stopped believing that he could improve upon what God has provided him with, through some chemical or medicine, law or religion. We have been given all that we will ever need, if we will only take the time to look around and see. I wish you all the best in your quest for health.

-Submitted Karen

A WORD FROM KAREN'S DOCTOR

Karen taught us a great deal. First, that many may need an individualized course of chemo to allow them to live long enough for macro to work. But the oncologists seem to take an "all or nothing" approach because their first goal is to fulfill a scientific protocol to the letter. With <u>NO</u> white blood cells, she had to have that first chemo. The problem is, once in the program, your protocol, right down to IV doses, does not get individualized as you read....Even if it's killing you before their eyes in the hospital. Does this remind you of the research on one vitamin earlier? It should. It is the same mono-focus mind set. Karen also reminds us that macro is not just a diet.

Meanwhile, it is difficult to express what an exceptional young woman Karen is. I have steadily admired her organization, thoroughness and perseverance in making herself well. At the same time that she continued her jobs as mother, attorney and more, she also gave of herself in many community endeavors. These included board of directors and newsletter editor for the local H.E.A.L. and macrobiotic groups and more. She even won a city jogging race in her second year of healing!

Now that she is well past her 2 1/2 year mark [having been given a death sentence of just a few months with a 5% (1 in 20!) chance of making one year, regardless of <u>what</u> she did], she has grown to exciting new depths of psychic and spiritual awareness. She seems to have no limits and I consider myself blessed by her loving friendship. She has enriched my life more than I have ever told her.

****

So here you have it: Rheumatoid arthritis, chronic fatigue and weakness, multiple chemical and electrical sensitivities, anaphylaxis, multiple sclerosis and acute myelogenous leukemia in people between the ages of 20 and 57. What more could you want to convince you to evaluate macrobiotics? There isn't a doctor in the world who could cure these people. But they healed themselves. And all had something else in common; multiple nutrient deficiencies, which once corrected, helped provide the energy to do the diet as well as speed the healing. And age has no bearing, since I have seen infants to the aged do the same. But lest you be exceptionally tough to convince, look at these cases.

STAGE IV INOPERABLE LYMPHOMA
An Open and Shut Case

Klarita is a very special lady in many ways, as I suspect you will agree. She was born 44 years ago in Mexico City and had a congenital hemangioma over one side of her face. This was such a severe birth defect that starting from the tender age of eight months to her teens, she endured 35 operations (skin grafts, etc.) in attempt to correct it.

In her young adult life, she had a molar pregnancy which is like a cancer of the placenta, for which she received many months of chemotherapy. Years later she was operated on again for an angioma of the liver where nearly half of the liver was surgically removed.

Then 8 years ago, she began not feeling well. Many diagnostic tests were done but she stumped the doctors. In desperation they did an exploratory operation on her abdomen and found she had lymphoma (cancer of the lymph nodes) spread to many abdominal nodes, the liver, spleen, nodes in the chest and axilla, groin and neck: they did not attempt to remove any of the cancer because the spread was so extensive that she would not be expected to live to 6 months.

That is when this registered nurse decided to go strict macrobiotic, from which she has never veered. That was 5 1/2 years ago.

I was fortunate to meet this gal when she flew from her home near San Diego to check on her nutrient levels in the office. She has a special warmth and loving air about her that words cannot do justice to. She is happy to talk with people who need to communicate with someone who was an open and shut medical case, for whom medicine has nothing to offer but a death sentence. And, of course, even though she keeps up with her check-ups with her doctor, and he has witnessed her miraculous recovery against ALL odds, do you think that in 5 1/2 years he had referred other patients to her program? I guess he is afraid it might ruin his track record as predictor of death.

THE SAGA OF "C. WEED ED"

About 5 1/2 years ago, a funny thing happened to me on the way to the undertaker's to be embalmed, boxed and planted. My "vicious, terminal" cancer went into "remission". Three years before that I had been diagnosed as having multiple myeloma with a gloomy prognosis. I took chemo for 5 months which did not help in this instance. Matter of fact, I steadily deteriorated. I went to Boston to the Kushi Institute to learn about the macrobiotic way of living and dieting. I was introduced to all kinds of strange foods: nori, wakame, hiziki, arame and daikon. I felt that I had been transported by Dr. Spock to outer space. While there, I met several macrobiotic counselors. Each one of them would look at me and comment, "Ed, you have nice long ear lobes. You have a long life before you." So to help things along, I started giving each lobe 3 tugs daily.

The genes I had inherited were a definite plus also. Cousins in Ireland lived to 102. My grandfather, grand uncles and aunts lived past 90. My mother died at 94. Speaking of my mother, she was terrific! I was in the printing business for about 60 years, starting with a mimeograph machine. That was in the years B.C.– before copiers. She ran our mimeograph machine, even after we installed high speed offset presses. One day she came to me and gave me two weeks' notice. She wanted to take early retirement. She was 87!

My wife died of cancer after 3 1/2 years of chemo. That was in February 1983, the same month my malignancy was discovered. Having witnessed my wife's discomfort and lack of success from the chemo, I said one day to her, "I'll never take that stuff," little realizing that soon I would hear that word, that term that sounds like a death sentence, that sends chills up one's spine-- CANCER! So what do you do? Blindly listen to the doctor. And I, who had used that word "never" so positively, was suddenly on chemo. But the cancer kept advancing and I felt terrible. Even my friends commented on how poor I looked. I was getting too weak to walk. After 5 months I heard about macrobiotics and I went to Boston to the Macrobiotic Learning Center to find out just what this was all about. There were eight other cancer "victims" in our cooking class. I used that word "victims" advisedly, because one of the first things our macrobiotic teachers and counselors said or did was to congratulate us for having identified our disease as cancer. "Now you can straighten out your priorities and start really living." We all thought "Are they nuts?"

Invariably, when people learn that I once had an incurable form of cancer in my eighties, they ask me for a copy of my "diet." Well, just what is macrobiotics all about? Macro means "great," biotics means "life." Macrobiotics is a way of life, a philosophy of LIV-ING.

We are all familiar with AA (Alcoholics Anonymous) and the AAA (Automobile Association of America). Macrobiotics is best described as AAAA; namely, AWARENESS, ATTITUDE, ACTIVITY and APPETITE.

AWARENESS that all the time we can be absolutely sure of is NOW, this present moment. One writer put it very well: "The sacrament of the present moment." Be aware of the present moment, relish the present, precious moment.

AWARENESS is the loving, caring presence of a Supreme Being about us, in us, in each other, in nature, the seeds that are sown, nurtured by the sun and rain to grow and eventually, through food, to become a part of us; a complete cycle.

AWARENESS that there is no room in the holistic approach to living for grudges, anxiety, worries, regrets over the past or fears of the future (regrets and fear are twins). To repeat, we can live only one moment at a time!

AWARENESS of that little old word PRIORITIES! Aware of what is really important at the time, in the moment of time which is all we really can be sure of. Believe me, there is nothing like cancer, a heart attack or any life threatening disease to help one get his/her priorities straightened out in a hurry. What good is it to work 10-12 hours a day, 5, 6 or 7 days a week to the detriment of our physical, mental, spiritual and family health?

ATTITUDE- Sometimes we have the attitude that doctors, counselors, dieticians, clergy are responsible for our welfare, our health, our sickness, our spiritual health and we wait for them to tell us what to do. Actually, we are responsible for the welfare of this body that is on loan to us from the Almighty...that we have to do our own research, get acquainted with ourselves, find out what foods help us and what foods drag us down (substitute the word "activities" for food to get a balance). It is our own responsibility to eliminate those facets of our lives that are pressuring us unduly; eliminate any grudges, animosities (real or imagined) and clean them up. This does not mean that we do not listen to our doctors, counselors and clergy, but that we don't shift our responsibilities on to them 100%.

ACTIVITY- Be a participant of life, not a spectator. (I, myself, am involved in more than a dozen community and church activities). Become involved in helping others. Reach out with love, caring and sharing. Help shut-ins with visits, errands, phone calls. Actually this is almost being selfish because you get so much out of it; more than you can possibly put in.

ACTIVITY- Remember that 8 letter word, EXERCISE. No, not in a rocking chair, or behind the wheel of your car, but walking, swimming, aerobics, whatever.

ACTIVITY- Make it a date a certain time each day to call, write, send a card, a word of thanks, encouragement, love, or invite some lonely person to a movie, luncheon, or just talking together. That does not mean just persons you are very fond of, but that person who irritates you to pieces. Maybe you need changing, not that person. Even make it a point to pray for a particular person (or persons) each day.

APPETITE- It does make a difference how you feed and nourish the physical part of us, namely this body. Study, research, observe what foods help you feel better, what really nourishes your immune system. Listen to your counselor (or doctor) and be patient.

It took me 20 months of rigid culinary discipline before I began to feel better and feel that I might still reach 110 years of age, give or take a couple of years.

APPETITE- One very, very important item—in fact <u>THE MOST IMPORTANT</u> item in any given diet—is to CHEW, CHEW, CHEW, CHEW; 50-100 times. Give your digestive system a break. Digestion starts in your mouth with the God-given saliva to pre-digest your food. This cannot be emphasized too much. Please chew. Count each mouthful until eventually you will know when each particular mouthful is ready to be swallowed. Please relax at the table. See what you are eating. Enjoy what you are eating. Take your time and leave business and cares until later. Another very important suggestion when you are serving your macrobiotic meal (or any meal for that matter) is to dress it up, make it appealing not only in aroma but in appearance. Yes, even dine in candlelight. We don't have to wait for special company. Each one of us is very special; each one of us is unique. Put "music for dining" on your tape player, record player or radio. Be good to you!

This is also good advice to the newly widowed, especially widowers. My wife and I only used our dining room for company, and holidays. About 2 or 3 weeks after she died, I decided to use the dining room for my main dinner each evening, complete with candlelight, soft music and gourmet arrangement of the food on the table. I also rearranged the furniture, had all the downstairs rooms papered, got new drapes upstairs and down. Frankly, when I look back, I'm rather surprised that I did those things. We had no widowed support group at that time. About a year and a half later, I helped organize our Widowed Persons Support Group. I still handle the publicity for that group, and am a member of the "I Can Cope" group for cancer patients and their families. We meet monthly. Support groups are so important. I welcome calls from people in either category.

APPETITE- Macrobiotic counselors will never tell you NOT to take chemo, or radiation, but they will suggest what to eat that will strengthen <u>your</u> immune system, help <u>your</u> immune system remain strong. Chemo and radiation destroy cancer cells, and a few others to boot. You can have the best of both systems; one balances the other. Remember what Scripture says, "we are wonderfully made."

APPETITE- I can't write here what you should eat or should not eat. I know what I can and cannot have. I've proven it to myself. I consume no dairy products whatsoever. That includes all milk, be it 1%, 2% or whatever, cheeses or butters, nor any eggs, fats, red meats or fatty fish. After I was declared "in remission" by my oncologist, I tried some of those "no-no's" again. (It was right around the holidays.) To my amazement, and consternation, within 8 weeks, my IgG count (cancer count or immunoglobulin G...malignant melanoma is a cancer of this type of antibody) shot right back up, so I know what my body will tolerate and what it won't. It is MY responsibility. I know that dairy products, sugared sweets, etc. help build up mucous in my body and that mucous in turn feeds cancer cells. So I avoid such foods. I love life, love people and expect to be around here another 30 years or so.

It all adds up. Awareness, plus Attitude, plus Activity, plus Appetite equals peace of mind. And with each part mix in generous portions of humor. Be able to laugh at yourself. See the funny side; the sweet pickle side rather than the sour pickle side of life. When feeling down, play a humorous record, or cassette tape. You can't cry and laugh at the same time. There is nothing as healing, physically, mentally and spiritually as good belly laughs.

The following quote from the magazine "People's Weekly," October 10, 1983 by Dirk Benedict sums it up very neatly:

"The whole point of macrobiotics is to get control of your life and then deal with it yourself. Life belongs to those who are willing to take the responsibility of having it."

-Submitted by Ed (alias "C. Weed Ed")

A NOTE FROM THE AUTHOR

Ed is not my patient and I only saw him briefly once in my life. But he is so adoringly memorable and loving, that I though you would benefit from knowing him, too.

I had gone to the local macrobiotic center for dinner and quite innocently sat next to this older gentleman who had a wonderfully kind, happy and healthy looking face. I asked what a fellow like himself, who was obviously older than the rest of the group, was doing here, eating this strange food. Then he told me that a local oncologist, whom I knew, had diagnosed malignant melanoma with metastases and it had resisted chemotherapy. I knew this was a death sentence and assumed he meant he was just diagnosed. "No. That was when I was 78." It still didn't fit because he looked like a very healthy 70 year old. He was 83.

And the reason he was there that eve is because they were throwing him a surprise birthday. But they got him there under the pretense that it was someone else's birthday. So naturally he had made a huge macrobiotic cake to share with the thirty-odd diners. He's a fabulously loving and giving man with a wonderful twinkle and sparkle.

****

At a macrobiotic luncheon this summer with Michio, I was introduced to a British physician in his 70's who had just cleared himself of any trace of his "untreatable, terminal" cancer of the pancreas. Once you get into this field, there is an overwhelming amount of cases and evidence. But it is persistently stifled by medicine. Many give up talking about it because they meet with such resistance when they try to persuade someone who is in the same death boat. When I mention it to doctors, they look like I had just dropped my drawers.

One doctor wrote up 6 severe cancer cases that had survived because of macro. The response on her rejection slip from the major medical journals to which she had submitted it was that it "would not meet the interest of the readership." I guess we docs are not supposed to be interested in healing!

This next case is a person whom I've never had the pleasure of meeting yet. But when I read of her case, she graciously consented to have it published here, because she is like the others, selflessly eager to help others get well against all odds. (Reprinted with kind permission of the author and editor, Alex Jack of <u>One Peaceful World</u>, Autumn/Winter 1990, #6, pg. 6, Box 10 Becket MA, 01223 where this appeared. <u>One Peaceful World</u> is the newsletter from the Kushi Institute to which you can subscribe.)

<u>HEALING A TERMINAL, INOPERABLE BRAIN TUMOR</u>

In August, 1986, I had just turned 37 and was thoroughly enjoying life. And then the bottom fell out. After a grand mal seizure that sent me sprawling onto an asphalt tennis court, many hospital tests, and two surgeries, I was diagnosed as having a <u>grade 3 anaplastic astrocytoma</u>. This is a fast growing inoperative brain tumor. At that time, it was about the size of a small grapefruit.

The discovery was shattering. One night soon after I experienced a series of physical jolts: nausea, vomiting, and numbness in my right leg.

I had always enjoyed life, living by my own decisions--until now. The doctors' prognoses rang through my mind: "It was bad," "It would never go away," "Chemo might be able to slow it's growth," "It was close to a motor area and I would eventually lose control," "Wheelchair in the future," "Six to eighteen months to live."

When my aunt from New Orleans suggested macrobiotics, I had no idea what she was talking about. But when you have no alternative and a strong desire to live, you do what it takes.

I read several books she recommended, including <u>Recovery</u> by Elaine. Elaine was a housewife like me, but in much worse shape. I reasoned that if she could do it I could, too. It did not matter that I lived in a small town in northeast Mississippi and knew no one who had even heard of macrobiotics at that time.

Before jumping in, I decided to check with the American Cancer Society hotline to see if there was anything else I could do. At this point, I had had 6,000 RADs and two treatments of chemo (PCNU). At least five more treatments were scheduled.

The volunteer's answer was, "Nothing. Good luck." The line went dead. Through clenched teeth my reply was, "We'll see about that!"

Three days later, January 17, 1987, I was on my way to a macrobiotic center in Brookline, Massachusetts (it has since moved to the previously given Becket, MA address). I had trouble understanding the various teachers, as some were from foreign countries, while others were the fast-talking Yankees. And, of course, they couldn't understand my Southern accent. But ingredients for the meals could have come from another planet.

I was on many anti-seizure pills, and my thinking was clouded, to say the least. Luckily, I took my camcorder and videotaped the seminar, because trying to absorb everything sent me to bed with a headache each night.

Looking back, I am able to realize how much I absorbed and credit much of my success to that program. I learned not only the proper way to cook, but also exercises, massage, home remedies, and the power of positive thinking.

Back in Columbus, Mississippi, I quickly learned that cooking for oneself was very different. I started my first solo macro meal at 3 p.m. I finished a little after 8, at which time I was too exhausted to eat!

Another turning point came when I returned to Boston in February to see Michio Kushi. It was then that I fully decided to take charge of my recovery.

I discontinued the chemotherapy and gradually decreased the anti-seizure medication. Dawn, a Kushi Institute cook, came to cook for me for a week, and the food actually started tasting good!

Another angel, whom I'm sure was sent to me by God was Mamie. I had hired her a few days earlier sight unseen, and she was there for Dawn's teaching and absorbed it all. She also was like a mother to me. I truly do not know what I would have done without her guidance and persistence.

A verse from Ephesians became my motto: "Now unto Him that is able to do exceedingly abundantly above all that we ask or think, according to the power that worketh in us."

I also used imaging and constantly imagined that the tumor was decreasing. In my bedroom, I kept a drawing of the tumor that showed it decreasing in size– from the size of a grapefruit to a golf ball to a pinhead and nothing! Amazingly, each test showed the size of the malignancy had diminished just as I had drawn.

The CAT scan in April, 1987, four months after starting macrobiotics, showed no evidence of cancer! And none have since then, either.

One night, two years ago, Parker, my nine year old son, asked, "Mom, do you think you'll ever get cancer again?"

My immediate reply was, "No." After a bit I came back into his bedroom and asked, "But, Parker, don't worry, honey, because if I do, I know what to do."

He smiled and said, "We'll fight like before."

Today with God's help and the love and support of my husband, children, family and friends, I am alive with the chance to work, play, and love. I want to share my experiences with others to spare them the anguish I went through and to offer a practical alternative to degenerative disease.

-Submitted by Mona

****

There are so many more cases, of mine and others, but I hope our limited random selection of various conditions as well as various ages has given you someone with whom to identify, so that you, too, can accomplish the impossible.

****

RECOVERY FROM METASTATIC OVARIAN CANCER

In April 1980, I was diagnosed with uterine cancer. It was a mixed tumor, a carcinosarcoma, and it was embedded in the muscle of the lining of the connective tissue of my uterus. I was treated with external and internal radiation, oral and intravenous chemotherapy, and hormone therapy. In August 1980, I had a radical hysterectomy. I continued to take chemotherapy.

In May 1982, I started having pain in my lower back, which was diagnosed as a compression fracture. Despite strong medication, the pain got progressively worse. I could neither sit nor lie down. In August, after a few days of standing up all day and night, sleeping only on my husband's shoulder in a standing position, I consulted an orthopedist. The orthopedist confirmed the compression fracture and noted that I also had a partially collapsed vertebrae. In order to prevent a total collapse of my backbone, I was put into a brace which extended from below my chest to below my pelvis and wrapped around my back. I wore the brace all day and night.

The pain got worse and spread to my legs. When I could no longer stand, I was placed in a recliner chair, where I stayed in a semi-reclining position taking strong painkillers around the clock. Nothing stopped the pain.

In September, I was carried back to the hospital for more diagnostic procedures. These tests showed that, in addition to the collapsed backbone, I had cancer on my lumber spine, cancer on my thoracic spine, and multiple metastatic deposits in both lungs.

I was given radiation again, then chemotherapy, then more radiation, then more chemotherapy, given at three to four week intervals. Each treatment required an overnight stay in the hospital. I was tired, sick, nauseous, and in pain.

Towards the end of January 1983, after four cycles of chemotherapy, I cut my finger on an envelope. Because my blood levels were so depressed from the heavy chemotherapy, I was unable to fight the infection that set in. The paper cut resulted in a ten-day hospital stay, which included massive doses of intravenous antibiotics, four blood transfusions, and three days in isolation. The doctors then decided that the chemotherapy I was getting was too strong for me. I would be put on something less toxic.

Diagnostic procedures performed during the hospital stay showed unchanged metastatic cancer in both my lungs, and increased activity and progression of the cancer in my spine.

It was then that I realized that conventional medicine was not helping me, and I began to consider an alternative. I chose macrobiotics--based mostly on my reading of other people who had healed themselves with this approach.

In February 1983, I began to practice macrobiotics. I completely eliminated from my diet all meat, poultry, eggs, dairy foods and sugar. I reduced to zero the thirty-eight pills I was taking every day. I decided to stop all chemotherapy, hormone therapy, antibiotics, and vitamin supplements. I started to eat brown rice and cooked vegetables.

I began macrobiotics in a hospital bed, a wheelchair, a brace and in pain. The pain gradually subsided, and I never took another pain killer. After a short time, I was able to take a few steps with the help of a walker. I practiced walking with the walker, then with two canes, then with one can. In April, a urinary problem that had plagued me for three years (a result of the original radiation) disappeared. In mid-May, I took off the brace. On May 22, I walked for the first time in a year all by myself.

In June I put away my wig. My hair, which had all fallen out from the chemotherapy, had grown back enough to be presentable. I returned the hospital bed. I started driving again. I resumed my studies towards my masters degree in nutrition. Within six months, I had changed from a sick depressed, pill-popping invalid, to a happy, optimistic, and very, very grateful pain-free person.

In November 1983, my macrobiotic advisors told me that the symptoms of cancer were gone.

It is now eight years that I have been living the macrobiotic way, and I continue to enjoy good health. I completed the Master's of

Science degree in nutrition. My thesis was entitled, "MACROBIOTICS- An Alternative Treatment for Cancer." I continue to study, practice and teach macrobiotics. I have an active consulting practice, and I also offer macrobiotic cooking classes. My book, RECOVERY (Japan Publications 1986) has inspired thousands of people to improve their health with macrobiotics.

Some important factors in my recovery have included accurate practice of macrobiotic recommendations (no cheating), regular visits with a macrobiotic counselor, shiatsu massage, love and support from family and friends, a lot of prayer and a positive optimistic attitude. My experiences, both personal and professional, have shown me some of the wonderful changes that can occur when living the macrobiotic way.

-Submitted by Elaine

Author's Note

When I read Elaine's book, Recovery, the pain and repeated defeats that she endured made me cry. For 2 years, she had done all that medicine could offer. But when the surgery, chemotherapy and irradiation left her bald and bedridden with the pain of ovarian cancer still viciously spreading throughout her body, medicine gave up. They didn't even dare treat her pneumonia, because she was so destroyed, so fragile, so near death that they feared even the antibiotic might deal the final blow to her life.

She had an expected survival of less than one month, since the cancer and pneumonia were vying for top positions. Yet in spite of this incredibly bleak prognosis, she didn't give up. She bit the macro bullet and healed herself, to the athletic, perky, lovable, dynamic little bundle that I will never forget meeting as she was just coming in from jogging.

****

Although all were invited, some of these people's doctors did not care to add their comments. Also the words 'she' and 'he' have been used arbitrarily here for he, she or it.

CHAPTER 10

THE SALT SOLUTION

by Carlos and Jean Richardson
of The Gold Mine Natural Food Co.
San Diego, CA

Over the last several years, salt has become a very controversial issue. The National Institutes of Health estimates that sixty million Americans have some degree of high blood pressure which, left untreated, may result in heart attacks, stroke and kidney disease. Science and health experts believe that sodium intake is a contributing factor. Excess sodium intake is blamed for many other health imbalances, too, such as fluid retention in premenstrual syndrome. The commonly recommended solution is to cut back on salt. So consumers spend a lot of time reading labels in an attempt to learn where they can cut out excess sodium disguised in "tasty" foods by the food industry.

"Sodium chloride- better known as 'table salt'- is the second most common food additive that is second only to sugar."(1) But sodium chloride or table salt is not the same as natural, unrefined sea salt. And therein lies the critical difference. In his book (Natural Immunity: Insights on Diet and AIDS), Noboru Muramoto says, "Contrary to what we have been led to believe, salt is not just sodium chloride. Good quality salt must include all the various minerals that are found in sea water. Within the last hundred years or so the quality of salt has changed completely. The salt now available in stores is all refined salt. Some labels read "99.999% sodium chloride." It stings the tongue and throat when eaten. For millions of years our ancestors never ate such purified salt; only modern man has broken the millions-of-years-old biological tradition of having true unrefined sea salt in the blood."(2)

By way of further support, Anne Marie Colbin points out in her book, (Food and Healing) we should "not overlook the fact that the commercial land salt generally available today is higher in sodium than traditional sea salt, both because it is land mined and because of the various sodium compounds that are added to it. The presence of these additives must have an effect on the body, perhaps deleterious. The salt that is obtained by evaporation of seawater contains about 78% sodium chloride (NaCl) plus 11% magnesium chloride and smaller amounts of magnesium and calcium sulfates, potassium chloride, magnesium bromide, and calcium carbonate. Land mined salt from Utah (a place that received radioactive fall-out from U.S. nuclear testing, S.R. ed. comment), on the other hand, contains 98% NaCl (plus 0.2% iron, 0.31% calcium and smaller amounts of sulfur, aluminum and strontium).

"USDA standards for "table salt" or "food grade salt" are set at no less than 97.5% NaCl, no more than 2% calcium and magnesium, and up to 2% of "approved additives." The latter include (#1) potassium iodide to supplement the iodine deficient diets of people who have no access to fish, seafood, or sea vegetables; dextrose, a type of sugar, added to keep the iodide from oxidizing; (#2) sodium bicarbonate, to keep the salt from turning purple after the addition of the first two ingredients; and (#3) either sodium silico aluminate, calcium carbonate, sodium ferrocyanide, green ferric ammonium citrate, yellow prussiate of soda, or magnesium carbonate as anti-caking or crystal modifying agents."(3) It is quite a shock when you read the label on your salt box to find it actually contains as aluminum (which is implicated in causing Alzheimer's disease) just so the salt will pour more easily. And that table salt contains sugar!

In 1971, the Japanese government decreed that all salt sold for public consumption be made by the (dubious) ion exchange process, which uses 3,000 volts and 120 amperes of electricity to draw sodium chloride ions out of the sea brine. An atomic physicist who had turned to macrobiotics, Mr. Katsuhiko Tani, became concerned about the health effects of using such salt, and so started the Salt Research Association. The outcome was the creation of a natural salt collection facility, which produces high quality sea salt. (4)

Mr. Tani demonstrated the qualitative difference of natural sea salt with a "clam test." He took five different kinds of salt, added each one to a separate tray of drinking water, duplicating the concentration of salt in sea water. In addition to three samples of natural sea salt, he tested the government ion exchange salt, and a popular salt substitute consisting mostly of potassium chloride. Into each of the five trays, Mr. Tani placed a dozen or so edible long necked clams. Within minutes, the clams in the three natural sea salt solutions had opened, sticking their necks out and nudging around for food. An hour later, the clams in the government ion exchange salt and the popular salt substitute remained closed.(4) They reacted as though they sensed a hostile environment.

The impression visitors receive, in chatting with Mr. Tani, is that natural salt is a "living " food. Its compounds and minerals seem to be transmuting back and forth in a metabolic fashion, in time with environmental influences. The only time the flux might cease would be when the salt is dried completely, when it is highly refined to 99.9% sodium chloride, as is most of the salt available in Japan and the United States.(4)

Interestingly enough, common "table salt," which has per-vaded the U. S. market in the last 50 or so years, appears to be an in-dustrial by-product of weapons manufacture (Morton Thiokol makes rocket fuel. Remember the space shuttle rocket motor that blew up?). The large salt companies refine salt to extract the naturally occurring trace minerals, such as magnesium which sells for much more money than table salt. Magnesium is used in the manufacture of rocket fuel and ammunition. Even if you buy "sea salt" from the bulk bin at the natural food store, you may be purchasing the Leslie Company's in-dustrial byproduct with the magnesium removed.

Be sure to ask if the "sea salt" is unrefined and naturally solar dried. Because during the refining process, common "table salt" is heated to over 1200 degrees F. It recrystallizes into a very hard needle shape instead of its natural cubic shape and becomes insoluble and unavailable to the body. What's worse, according to Miami mac-robiotic counselor and author Lino Stanchich, these crystalline needles stick in the fats, blood vessels, and organs, especially the kid-neys. I suspect that's why, when I eat out at a place that uses com-mon table salt, I subsequently find myself craving excess liquids and desserts, and I get big bags under my eyes the next morning!

So the question of "how much salt" becomes compounded by the issue of quality. Many people who experience difficulty consum-ing "common table salt" find that they not only have no problem with natural sea salt, but in fact that their condition **improves** when they incorporate an appropriate amount of it into their diet. This is possi-bly due to the fact that so many trace minerals are present and available in natural, unrefined sea salt. I received a letter from a man who had suffered for years from excess hydrochloric acid in his stomach. After much experimentation, he finally discovered that using a natural sea salt which contained a high proportion of magnesium solved his problem completely.

The "right amount" of salt is an individual matter. People who eat animal foods already are getting a lot of sodium from the meat, eggs, etc. and may not need any additional salt. In fact, they may be getting more salt (yang) than they need, and thus are attracted to yin foods which also leach excess salt and minerals from the body, such as fruit, alcohol, and desserts. Vegetarians, on the other hand, need some salt (unless they are still carrying excess stored salts from past meat eating days).

"Gustav V. Bunge (1844-1920) carefully studied salt consumption and summarized his findings as follows:

1. Sodium chloride is necessary in mineral form.

2. The requirement for sodium chloride is higher when the diet consists primarily of plant foods.

3. The requirement for sodium chloride is lower when the diet consists primarily of meat and animal foods; in fact, too much salt can be taken in.

4. Sodium chloride and potassium interact within the organism. Plant foods contain three to four times more potassium than meat. The wealth of potassium in plants causes an increased salt requirement for those who eat a primarily vegetarian diet."(2)

Muramoto says, "There is salt and water in all our body fluids--- blood, lymph, mucous, urine, sweat, tears, saliva, and so on. We always lose salt when we urinate and sweat, so it is necessary to replace it by taking a little salt every day.

In Food and Healing, Ms. Colbin states: "Our nutritional need for salt has been established at half a gram daily for the average adult. Three grams (3/5 of a teaspoon) is still considered a reasonable intake. But the average American consumes twelve grams daily, maybe even eighteen---three or more teaspoons!"(3)

In traditional, whole foods cuisine, salt is an integral part of food preparation. Most whole grains tend to be acid forming unless balanced with salt during the cooking process. For thousands of years, food preservation has been methodically controlled through the careful use of salt. Intuitively, traditional cultures have used salty condiments such as miso, soy sauce, and pickles, and sea vegetables to aid in the digestion of their whole grain and vegetable based diet. In contrast, diets heavy in animal foods emphasize sugary condiments (ketchup, Worcestershire sauce, steak sauces, barbecue sauces, syrupy salad dressings, glazes) and, of course, the indispensable "dessert."

In the art of macrobiotic cooking, the experienced cook intuitively takes into consideration who will be eating the food and what their salt requirements are. For example, children and elderly people require far less salt than normal, active adults. Salty condiments on the table allow for individual adjustment to taste.

Over the years that I have been practicing the macrobiotic way, while traveling I have eaten meals prepared by various macrobiotic cooks. I have observed that when the salt content is not right for me, certain predictable symptoms will result. With too little salt, the meal is difficult to digest, even with thorough chewing. With too much salt, I find myself eating too quickly, overconsuming great quantities, craving liquids during and after the meal, and scrambling for the largest dessert.

Lino Stanchich, a longtime friend and macrobiotic counselor, emphatically told me, "I have found out that, without good salt, the macrobiotic diet doesn't work." He went on to explain that, by using good, natural sea salt and eliminating animal foods which contain hormones (e.g. dairy products, eggs, red meat, poultry, honey, etc.), within three months my endocrine system would return to operating as it was designed to, and that I would feel the difference. I did feel the difference, and I felt great! It seemed as if the trace minerals in the salt were making everything function better- the enzymes, glands, organs, nerves- in a more human way. Apparently, even the natural hormones from these animal foods are powerful enough to make one's endocrine system function more like the animal's.

Salt has played an important role throughout history, for both animals and humans. Herbivorous animals search out and visit salt deposits over great distances with the same determination with which they seek out water. Many wars were fought and empires built over the need for salt, and for the lack of it these same empires collapsed. Salt cakes were used as money in early Rome, where soldiers earned a "salary" (from "salarium," money given to Roman soldiers to but salt"). We use our "saliva" to digest our food. Jesus said, "Have salt in yourselves; and be at peace with one another" (Mark 9:50) and "You are the salt of the Earth" (Matthew 5:13). Once a precious and rare commodity, salt has now swung to the opposite extreme of being cheap and plentiful. To quote Ms. Colbin: "As we know that quantity changes the quality of things, it comes as no surprise that the erstwhile magic medicines have of late turned to poison."(3)

BIBLIOGRAPHY

(1) Weiss, Linda, "Salt Is Second On The List of Food Additives," The Nutrition & Dietary Consultant, Volume 11- No. 9, p. 3, September, 1990.

(2) Muramoto, Noboru, Natural Immunity: Insights on Diet and AIDS, Oroville, CA, George Ohsawa Macrobiotic Foundation, 1988, pp. 120-126.

(3) Colbin, Annemarie, Food and Healing, New York, Ballantine Books, 1986, p. 186.

(4) Anonymous, "Natural Salt Processing In Japan: A Remarkable Visit to a Small Island," Chico-San Cracker Barrel, Volume 2, No. 2, a supplement to East West Journal, July 1984.

****

When I was lecturing in San Diego, I heard Carlos Richardson respond to an audience question on salt, and knew he had much to teach me. He graciously agreed with his wife, Jean, to write an article about it.

My goal in this book has been to bring a basic understanding of the strict phase healing diet to the reader who might otherwise have let it pass him by. In attempting to make the healing phase more user-friendly for the average twentieth century person who needs it, there are many intricacies that time and space did not permit. I hope that as a person feels better on the diet, he will continue to study and discover these other facets for himself. For there is a limit to how big a book someone is willing to read.

In fact, for a subsequent book, I plan on having many macrobiotic counselors contribute in their own words what they feel is important to healing. Any wishing to do so may send in their articles (or chapters) now. The address and phone number of where perspective clients can reach them should also be included. It will be a way for all of us to learn and for us to be aware of what counselors are available and their modus operandi.

Meanwhile, this treatise on salt reminds us that if all is not going according to plan, perhaps we had best concern ourselves with some of the "minutia," such as the quality of one's salt. It is easy for us to take salt for granted as a "natural product," because most of us have never seen it any other way than in the grocery store box. But read that label carefully and you'll be in for a surprise. It contains sugar (I couldn't believe it, either) as well as aluminum (as an anticaking agent so that it pours easily). So you have an Alzheimer's potentiating agent (tiny amounts daily over a lifetime do accumulate in the brain) as well as the silent addicting substance, sugar. And as usual, what has been removed (the trace minerals) is never mentioned.

So if your program is solid and the relative proportions are good, but you are not doing well, one of the avenues worth checking is the actual quality of foods. And the quality of salt is a good starting point.

CHAPTER 11
POLITICS OF MEDICINE OR _ _ _ _ WHY
MACROBIOTICS IS POOH-POOHED

There are so many mechanisms that explain why macrobiotics can heal the impossible when all else has failed, that we put over 32 in Tired Or Toxic? In that book, for lay and physician alike, the biochemical explanations are backed by references from the scientific literature. Since that book (1990), I've discovered over a dozen more. But for the person who doesn't want the biochemical detail nor the references, but merely a rough idea, let's start with what strict macrobiotics does not have large amounts of:

Macro does NOT have:	that cause many cases of:
sugar and meat	fatigue
fruit and sugar	hypoglycemia
table salt	puffiness and edema
potato, pepper and tomato	arthritis
milk and ice cream	phlegm and sinusitis
wheat	asthma
citrus, tomato and coffee	acne and eczema
ferments (bread and cheese)	fatigue, brain fog, bloating and irritable bowel
spices	gastritis and irritable colon
soda pop	osteoporosis, mood swings

In other words, it is for many, a great rare food diet which is the basis for diagnosing hidden food allergies (The E.I. Syndrome). For you cut out milk, wheat, eggs, corn, citrus, chocolate, coffee, processed foods, and any foods you normally eat. See what symptoms improve, then put back the foods one at a time to see what triggered the symptoms.

That is how it was found that 73% of people with arthritis, for example, don't hurt nearly as much if they do not ingest members of the nightshade family (potato, tomato, peppers, paprika, eggplant, tobacco). The biggest problem for those who do have this sensitivity is that it takes weeks of being off the foods to simmer down the pain, and one tiny indiscretion can cause a painful flare for weeks and even months.

Some of the most important biochemical mechanisms, without getting into the actual chemistry (all of which are described and referenced in detail in <u>Tired Or Toxic</u>?) stem from the inclusion of:

whole grains and vegetables	* over 3 times the minerals available for regeneration and detoxication compared with ground, processed, bleached and fortified grains and vegetables.
beans	* lecithin for improved membrane function (mitochondrial for energy, endoplasmic reticulum for detoxication, cell membrane for normal cell function and reduced allergic response and brain membranes for prevention of Alzheimer's. * source for molydenum for detox enzymes (aldhyde oxidase) * we actively lose lecithin with the detoxication of chemicals
alkaline diet	* decreases exhaustion of buffer system which improves daily detoxication function and other enzymes
avoids meat	* this decreases the glucuronidase in the gut so intestinal detoxication is more efficient. * unloads xanthine oxidase for detox (for aldehyde path)
cruciferous vegetables (broccoli, cabbage, brussel sprouts, etc.)	* increases sulfur for detox (phase II conjugators) * increases NK and T-helper cells

low in sugar	* decreases fructose-induced (fruit and corn sugar) damage to detox membranes and decreases fructose-induced inhibition of copper absorption for use in super oxide dismutase (anti-inflammatory anti-free radical enzyme)
	* decreases non-enzymatic glycosylation (which can cause gene mutation, arteriosclerosis, and all the damage that chemicals can cause to regulatory proteins)
	* unloads the aldehyde bottleneck, which is one of the steps that causes chemically sensitive people to get progressively worse and react to more chemicals (spreading or snowball phenonomenon)
low in oils	* mobilizes chemicals stored in fat as weight is lost
	* removes excess lipids stored in and retarding function of endoplasmic reticulum
	* unplugs lympatics so cells are not bathed in stagnant wastes

It is basically a high density high nutrient diet that attempts to minimize the metabolic work the body has to do. And as has been observed, the guidelines from every medical association over the last decade have ever so slowly begun to drift further and further into macrobiotic guidelines, as medicine advances. Oddly enough, medicine continues to totally ignore the fact that the biochemical evidence for the beneficial health effects of macrobiotics has been here right under our noses for decades.

Meanwhile, I would love to know how macro was figured

out years before the scientific experiments that decades later came along to substantiate it. And why it is taking so painstakingly long for the guidelines to be "rediscovered" as now everyone knows they should cut back on red meat, fat, sugar, salt and processed foods and opt for more veggies and whole grains?

Renowned microbiologist and author of <u>Man Adapting</u>, Rene Dubos, is quoted " Most microbial diseases today are caused by microbes which... are present all the time in the body of normal individuals... they become the cause of disease when some disturbance occurs which upsets the equilibrium."

The "modern" notion of the germ theory that some microbe (germ) enters the body and disease results is just too simplistically archaic. Why doesn't everyone get the disease? Because, as Pasteur said on his deathbed, "The microbe is nothing, the environment is all important." Germs simply cannot grow if the "terrain" or environment in the body is not conducive to their growth, ie. low nutrient density, high fat and sugar diets, a body overwhelmed with detoxifying too many home, office, traffic air, food and water chemicals. (Lynes, Barry <u>The Healing of Cancer</u>, Marcus Books, P.O. Box 327, Queensville, Ontario, Canada, LOG 1RO. (416 478-2201), 1989).

You see, it matters little what we label or call a disease. What matters is what made the host vulnerable to it, and what can he do to alter his vulnerability. How can he improve his adaptability?

It is all so utterly logical when one understands the chemistry of the body and how we fight disease, but it would appear that those with a vested interest in maintaining a monopoly in the health field would prefer to view our diets and lifestyles as inconsequential to health. It appears they would prefer to have us naively believe that we are victims of "bugs" that work in mysterious ways, attacking us willy - nilly, and that only those with powerful prescription drugs can save the day. Arthritis is a Motrin deficiency and a headache is a Darvon deficiency.

This mindset tenaciously clings to these archaic theories, even to the point of recommending foods like margarines, synthetic eggs and processed foods to help control cholesterol in spite of published evidence (<u>New England Journal of Medicine</u>, August 16, 1990) proving that these chemicalized foods stripped of natural nutrients are more dangerous in terms of causing arteriosclerosis than are the saturated fats of beef, eggs and butter.

Indeed, medicare is riddled with bureaucratic inertia and that scares me as I witness health freedom, freedom of choice concerning how one chooses to treat their disease, erode away with the help of big business. A silent loss of health freedom occurred January 1991, when medicare rules changed. Other groups, such as the cancer treatment monopoly, servicing the 10,000 Americans who die each week of cancer, has seen to it that alternative treatments are steadily legislated against under the guise of protecting the innocent patient against quackery.

Fortunately, one of the single most important factors determining healing and regeneration, is how we eat. And no one can yet legislate against that.

SCIENCE FINDS FAT IS A CAUSE OF CANCER

I never really wanted to go into any of the evidence for macrobiotics in this book because it was assumed that anyone doing the strict healing phase had already read You Are What You Ate, Tired Or Toxic?, as well as Mr. Kushi's The Book of Macrobiotics: The Universal Way of Health, Happiness and Peace (Japan Publications, revised edition 1986) and Dr. Dean Ornish's Program to Reverse Heart Disease (Dean Ornish, MD., Random House Publ., 1990). The majority of evidence for why someone should go on the diet is contained in these four books.

However, I can't help but be overwhelmed as I constantly peruse the scientific literature, that there is progressively more and more evidence for the things that are recommended in macrobiotics. What still baffles me is how were these recommended decades before having been discovered and written about now? And even though they have been written about now, it will be decades more before awareness of these things comes to the medical and public eye in the United States.

For example, take the recommendation in macrobiotics for cancer patients and very sick patients not to watch more than half an hour of T.V. from 15 feet away a day, and not to use computers, water beds, electric heating pads and blankets. One has only to read the books Electromagnetism and Man, or Cross Currents by Robert O. Becker, M.D. or Electromagnetic Man: Health and Hazard in the Electrical Environment by Cyril W. Smith and Simon Best, 1989, J. M. Dent and Sons, to appreciate the myriad of diseases fostered by electromagnetic energies. But macro has recommended EMF avoidance before these books were written.

Likewise, macrobiotics stresses the importance of having plants in the environment. Indeed, out of the NASA's National Space Technology Laboratories in Mississippi, comes the research showing that house plants remove a significant amount of pollutants such as formaldehyde and benzene and other hydrocarbons from the ambient air. The larger the leaf, the larger amount of chemicals removed. For example, a heart leafed philodendron removes 4.99 micrograms per square centimeter of leaf surface. An elephant ear philodendron removes 4.31, a spider plant 4.15, aloe vera 3.27, Chinese evergreen 2.31, mini schefflera 1.96, and so forth (The Human Ecologist #44, Winter 1989, Human Ecology League Inc. P. O. Box 49126, Atlanta, GA 30359-1126).

Probably the most grief you'll receive from people when you're on the healing phase, is the anxiety, worry and resentment that they express when you have lost weight. Medical doctors will try to make you think that it's dangerously unhealthy. But when you study the scientific literature, it shows that cancers often have double the amount of cholesterol in the tissues than do normal tissues. For example, one study of the cholesterol content of all prostatic cancers was double that of the normal prostate (Sporer, A., Brill, D.R., Schaffner, C.P.-Epoxycholesterols in Secretions in Tissues of Normal, Benign and Cancerous Human Prostate Glands, Urology 20, 3, 244-250, September 1982). So it's obvious that these excessive fats need to be dieted off, and the only way you can do that is to first get rid of all of your fat cells. That is why people with cancer get so alarmingly thin as they heal their cancers through macrobiotics. Later on they put back their fat with good, organic wholesome fats.

Many studies correlate high fat diets, such as more butter and dairy product use in women with breast tumors, for example, while other papers show histological progression from normal cells to those with atypical hyperplasia (this can be the precursor to cancerous cells) with progressively increasing concentrations of cholesterol. And cholesterol has even been reported to be mutagenic, carcinogenic and cytotoxic (all changes which can lead toward cancer) (Wrensch, M.R., Petrakis, N.L., Gruenke, L.D., Miike, R., Ernster, V.L., King, E.B., Houck, W.W., Craig, J.C., Goodson, W.H.- Breast Fluid Cholesterol and Cholesterol Beta-epoxide Concentrations in Women With Benign Breast Disease, Cancer Research, 49, 8, 2168-2174, April 15, 1989).

Likewise, other papers show that cholesterol oxide induces chromosome damage similar to that which ultraviolet (UV) light can do (Parsons, P.G., Goss, P. Chromosome damage and DNA Repair Induced in Human Fibroblasts by UV and Cholesterol Oxide, Australian Journal of Experimental Biology in Medical Science, 56, 3, 287-296, June 1978). So the evidence is there: fat predisposes to cancer.

Clearly, fat is where it's at in terms of being one of the factors leading to the changes that occur in cancerous cells. It's one of the reasons why macrobiotics has been so successful for people with cancer, because it diets the person down far enough to get rid of these cholesterol oxides which are deleterious to the cell. Plus the diet is high enough in nutrients to allow the body to heal itself and neutralize free-radicals before they induce oxides.

Isn't it all so beautiful when we begin to understand how it works? Likewise, in Chinese diagnosis, the pulse is very important, in fact, they can feel six pulses. Yet, in the December 1989 Internal Medicine for the Specialist, Vol, 10, #12, an article by Ivan A. D'Cruz entitled "Pulsus Alternans, A Neglected Sign of Left Ventricular Failure" (pg. 57-65) tells us how important just feeling for a pulse that alternates between strong and weak beats is. They even go so far as to use machines to document this. Physical diagnosis if you haven't noticed, is quickly becoming replaced by machines and blood tests.

Now that we have sufficient evidence and sufficient track records, we need to concentrate more on some of the intricacies of macrobiotics. For example, what about the people who cannot tolerate the diet, or who have such violent and swift discharges that we have to back off? There is still a necessity for much individualization. As with anything else in life, there is no blanket prescription for everyone. What do we do with the person who just plain does not like the diet? The multiply food sensitive patient is much easier to deal with than the person who is just plain unhappy with the food. These are all interesting aspects that we must learn to deal with.

The biggest problem that I see with macrobiotics is that you cannot test it double blind to make it scientifically acceptable for some members of the medical community. There is no way to know how carefully anyone has done the diet. And it will certainly be a long time before someone puts money into experimental animals to see if diet will clear their cancers, since there is no money to be made for anyone backing the research.

THE INSURANCE GAME

MEDICARE--IS IT SHORT FOR MEDICAL CARE OR MORE PROPERLY, MEDIOCRE CARE?

Blue Cross just sent a notice to New York State physicians that they are going to instigate a Comparative Performance Report (ironically initialed a CPR--but as you will read it would be more appropriately called a D & C).

At the onset CPR sounds good. They will see what the average standard of care for each medical procedure is and use this for the standard. Then if the doctor tries to do too many tests, he will fall outside of this range and his treatments will not be paid for. It will be a good way for them to save paying you if your doctor does not conform to the average or norm.

But let's look at how it will affect your care. Say you have high blood pressure. The norm says you are recommended certain blood tests, x-rays, and then a low salt diet. If that fails to control your pressure, then you are prescribed a fluid pill or diuretic. If that fails to control it, then stronger (and more expensive) medications are prescribed.

Here is where the clincher lies. One of the commonly missed causes of high blood pressure, or cardiac arrhythmia and many other conditions is hidden magnesium, calcium or potassium deficiency. In fact the U. S. government did a study (SCIENCE NEWS, 1988) that shows the average American diet only provides 40% of the recommended daily allowance for magnesium. This is in part because our foods are so processed. For example, when you eat white flour bread instead of brown rice or cooked whole wheat berries, you lose 80% of the magnesium and other minerals.

The scientific literature is full of reports proving that there is no reliable blood test for magnesium deficiency, but there is a provocation loading test that can diagnose the deficiency (Rogers, SA, Magnesium deficiency masquerades as diverse symptoms, International Clinical Nutrition Review, 11:3, 117-125, 1991). Since most physicians do not read this literature and know this fact, a magnesium deficiency is not looked for and it is said to fall outside the range of norm. So what?, you say.

When you take the diuretic, it causes the loss of potassium and magnesium. So now you get even further in the hole for magnesium. So what is the most common thing to happen next? The magnesium deficiency can now cause other symptoms like muscle cramps, a persistent and uncorrectable potassium deficiency, or a bad back or harmless eye muscle twitches. Or it can cause spasms of the smooth muscles of the coronary arteries and you go into an arrhythmia (irregular or too fast heart beat) and die of sudden death. And nobody knows why you died.

If you want to lose magnesium even faster, have a few I.V.s as you would if you were hospitalized, or do a lot of jogging, for sweating is a great way to lose more magnesium. In fact, this deficiency may be why Jim Fixx and Hank Gathers died. But remember the 1990 Journal of the American Medical Association showed that 90% of the doctors miss or never even think of ordering a magnesium test. Inferior medicine is the norm.

Meanwhile, back at the medicare or mediocre-care ranch, since looking for a biochemical defect is not the norm, it may affect whether or not you can afford to have it done. *You are locked into a system that assures you will only have average or mediocre care, not optimal* _or best_. And it assures that drugs will be the norm. And it assures that the sick get sicker, because the underlying defect is not commonly sought. And to take this one step further, if all else has failed, and you need instruction in a macrobiotic diet to save your life, insurance will not pay for it, and in many states it is even illegal for a doctor to prescribe a diet for cancer!

You see we are in the beginning of a new era of medicine. We are slowly slipping out of the era where a headache is a Darvon deficiency and into the era of molecular and environmental medicine where the cause for many conditions previously thought to be untreatable except for a lifetime of drugs can now have their biochemical defects found and corrected.

John had 57 years of psoriasis. By finding a deficiency in fatty acid, $4.50 worth of a non-prescription oil cleared him and it only recurs if he runs out. But mediocre-care does not pay for that. However, they will pay for years of steroid creams and UV light therapies which also have side effects and do not completely clear the condition like finding the biochemical defect does. They do so because that is the norm or current standard of care. It also pays for coal- tar creams which are commonly used to treat psoriasis and known to cause cancer in years to come. In fact, a common way to get a rat with cancer to test a new cancer drug on is to shave his back and rub on coal tar creams. He will soon develop a cancer (sooner than man because his 76 year life span is compressed into 4 years).

Dr. Alan Levin, a California immunologist through Research On Demand, Inc., Berkeley, CA, found that in 1988, the pharmaceutical manufacturing industry sold $453 million in antihistamines, and $1,000 million in cromolyn (a drug that is used for allergic asthma, nasal congestion and burning eyes). For every dollar that is spent on immunotherapy (allergy injections) this represents $23 that would not have to be spent on antihistamines, cromolyn and other allergy drugs. So for every dollar spent on allergy injections, the drug industry loses $23. And the quickest way I know of to get one step closer to health, that is to not even need allergy injections, is to go on a strict phase macrobiotic diet for a couple of years. It worked for me and hundreds of my patients. Prior to the diet, allergy injections were my life-time. I never even considered being without them.

Likewise, one of the biggest money making prescription drugs is for turning off the acid in the stomach. Yet the savings would be astronomical if the causes of the stomach symptoms of esophagitis were found, like hidden Candida infection from antibiotics and sweets, or hidden food allergy or just getting off coffee, processed foods, etc. Not to mention that shutting off the acid secretion of the stomach with drugs jeopardizes your absorption of vitamins and minerals. This in turn eventually starts an avalanche of seemingly unrelated medical problems. And again, I have witnessed the macrobiotic diet helping people become so healthy that they not only cleared their Candida esophogitis, but they couldn't get Candida if they tried. For remember, bacteria, viruses, and fungi are only able to set up housekeeping in a body that is not optimally healthy. It's the individual's terrain that matters most, not the resiliency of the organism. No wonder those profiting from the current scheme of medicine do not embrace what we do with allergy, nutrition and macrobiotics.

The drug/pharmaceutical industry, agri-business for meat, chemical manufacturers, pesticide manufacturers, construction material manufacturers, and more are locked into profit schemes which have blinders for the big picture.

PEOPLE POWER

On November 11, 1990, the TV show "60 Minutes" did a long overdue exposure on the medical insurance industry scam. They showed normal people who had religiously paid their insurance premiums for years. Then when they got sick, the insurance companies simply disowned them.

They had some of the top doctors from prestigious medical centers testify for them and explain their needs, all to no avail. When they engaged attorneys to help them, it was found that a Supreme Court decision had been silently slipped through that, if found guilty, would only make the insurance companies liable for the monies they should have paid for the medical care. They would not be liable for the attorney fees, the interest accrued from withholding payment, the pain and suffering, or the spread of untreated malignant disease and death resulting from delaying their care. So it is to the insurance industry's benefit to procrastinate in paying as long as possible, which is how many operate today. The trumped up excuses are often even illogical, but earn them millions in interest while they hang on to their money as long as they please with no risk of punishment. We have medical insurance company "procrastination" letters on file showing how blantantly ignorant of basic medical concepts even some "senior" claims adjustors are. So in essence, none of us has insurance that's worth a nickel.

Other legislators are fast at work (and for all but one day nearly got it slipped through) trying to get all vitamin and mineral supplements off the over-the-counter market and onto prescription only. While others want to see supplements off the market entirely until their benefits have gone through prohibitively expensive million-dollar research protocols to prove their worth. The biochemistry of nutrients is already known, but because their use makes many medications unnecessary, it would be to the drug industry's great benefit to make them prescription, since prescription drugs need well over 1/2 million dollars of testing to get on the market and no one would do this for non-patentable supplements. Also supplements work in harmony with one another, not alone as a drug that merely masks symptoms. And as you have seen, many researchers try to use nutrients alone as a drug. This does not work. Also the experiments fail to take people's biochemical individuality into account, i.e. everyone with arthritis does not have the same deficiencies, sensitivities and causes.

Another problem is that no one will sponsor the research because there is no patentable drug or product to make money from that would pay for the millions of dollars of research money needed to substantiate the need for each of the over 40 individual nutrients. Furthermore, by subjecting nutrients to trials individually as though each were a drug, or treating only one type of symptom in everyone, they would never prove to be of much worth. For their usefulness and necessity depend on a complex synergy of action and balance with other nutrients. As well the symptoms produced by a deficiency are as varied as people's biochemical individuality.

What we could end up with is prescription drugs available only: the old "a headache is a Darvon deficiency" type of medical care where the sick get sicker because the causes are not looked for. Symptoms are merely covered up with drugs until something worse emerges. The drug industry (and chemical) will reign superior over the medical domain.

With all that power, how much research do you think will be devoted to chemical sensitivity? And how often will insurance companies deny payments for that diagnosis as many do now? They bank on people being too ignorant to comprehend the overall scheme and too chronically tired or sick to do anything about it. But make no mistake: Your health freedom is quietly being snatched from under your nose. In fact in some states it is illegal for a parent to treat his child with cancer with macrobiotics. The doctors get court orders to have the child removed from the parents to force them to have chemotherapy. If our attorney who cleared her leukemia with macro had been forced to do a third course of chemo, do you think I would have had the pleasure of playing tennis with her last week, 2 3/4 years after her death sentence?

There is only one way out. There is only one thing that can change all of this. There is only one power mightier than all the insurance, chemical and pharmaceutical companies. There is only one power so strong that it can make the Berlin Wall evaporate into thin air. And that is People Power. Informed and united, they have and will continue to succeed in getting what is right and just.

It is alarming to me how many people (including physicians) are not even remotely aware of the continual political battles being fought for health freedom in the U.S. But in order to know one is missing out on something, they first have to know it exists and many people, physicians included, honestly believe that drugs are the best path to health. They are not aware that alternatives exist that are cheaper, safer, freer of side effects and yield more fundamentally healthful and long lasting results.

Some days I have to pinch myself to see if I'm not really dreaming that we're living a scene right out of Ayn Rand's Atlas Shrugged (my all-time favorite book, Random House, NY, 1957). It's scary how far from reality much of the world has strayed.

But people can't correct environmental, social or political injustices until they first get well enough to have the energy to get informed and organized. They can't save the environment or save the earth until they themselves are healthy and have enough energy left to perform. Michio Kushi is right. The most grandiose schemes of man, right up to world peace down to everyday matters like having enough time to cook, all come down to the health of the individual. And each individual, not any doctor or fancy medical specialist, not any insurance company or government, but the individual himself is the only one who possesses the ultimate control over the quality of his health.

WORLD AND PERSONAL ECOLOGY

And in terms of the environment, if you wanted to do one thing that would make the largest impact on the environment, that might be to reduce meat consumption. Let's look at some of the statistics:

(1) Producing enough food to feed a meat-eater requires 4200 gallons of water a day versus 300 gallons to feed a vegetarian.

(2) Nearly 4 billion tons of topsoil are lost each year in the U.S., chiefly because of overgrazing of livestock. This is roughly the size of Connecticut.

(3) It takes 39 times more energy to produce beef than soybeans having the same caloric value.

(4) A pound of hamburger represents 55 square feet of burned-off tropical rain forest.

(5) One acre of U.S. trees disappears every 5 seconds, but one acre of trees is spared for every individual who switches to a vegetarian diet.

(6) Progressive loss of the rain forest damages the ozone layer and causes the loss forever of priceless extinct animals, plants and herbs, many of which have important medicinal properties.

(7) 55% of the total antibiotics used in the U.S. is routinely fed to livestock. This causes the emergence of resistant strains, and the chemical residues are eaten by the consumer.

(8) 20,000 pounds of potatoes can be grown on 1 acre of prime land versus 165 pounds of beef.

(9) A child dies of malnutrition every 2.3 seconds, totalling 38,000 every day.

(10) The world's petroleum reserves would last 13 years if the whole world ate a meat-based diet, versus 250 years if the world ate a vegetarian diet.

(11) 33% of all raw materials consumed by the U.S. are devoted to the production of livestock, compared with 2% needed for the vegetarian diet.

(12) The human U.S. population produces 12,000 pounds of sewage per second, versus the livestock U.S. population that produces 250,000 pounds per second. Yet there are no sewage systems and much of the waste is not recycled but lost in streams and ground water, becoming a source of pollution versus a useful commodity.

(13) The average training in nutrition for a physician in a 4 year medical school program is 2 1/2 hours.

(14) A heart attack strikes every 25 seconds in the U.S. and kills a U.S. person every 45 seconds. Lack of knowledge of nutrient biochemistry for doctors and eating high fat meat based diets have a major bearing on this death rate.

(15) The risk of death from heart attack by the average American meat eating man is 50% versus 15% for the vegetarian, and 4% for the macrobiotic man.

(16) The rate of cancer is 2-4 times higher in meat eaters versus vegetarians.

(17) The chemical pollution of breast milk is 35 times higher in meat eaters versus vegetarians.

(18) David Satt, 6 time winner of the Ironman Triathalon, Sixto Linares, who holds the world record for the 24 hour triathalon, and

many other athletes who hold world records in swimming, cycling, bench press, and more are vegetarians.

In essence, 11 vegetarians can be fed on the amount of land needed to feed one meat eater. Referenced facts from Realities 1990, by John Robbins (author of A Diet For A New America), EarthSave, 706 Frederick St., Santa Cruz CA 95062-2205).

You might be hoodwinked by advertising to think now, "Well, I'll eat more fish. That will be good for me." But one of the problems with meat is not the meat itself, but with the feeding and growing practices that are used for raising commercial beef; the fat is of a different biochemical nature (with more trans fatty acids), due to the artificial substances fed feedlot beef.

And now that Americans have correctly switched to more fish to increase their omega-3 essential fatty acids (remember from Tired or Toxic?, these are the ones that are needed to stave off changes that lead to degenerative diseased like arteriosclerosis, Alzheimers and cancer), big business wants its piece of the pie. So instead of letting commercial fisherman reap the profits, and instead of fish eating other fish high in omega-3's, fish farms have been started where fish are fed chemicalized pellets resembling dog food. This business of man monkeying with food has reduced the amounts of the beneficial cis-form polyunsaturated fats. So the benefit of eating fish has been diminished by the changes resulting in the fish chemistry from commercial fish farming practices (Denton M, Lacey RW, Intensive farming and food processing: Implications for polyunsaturated fats, Journal of   Nutritional Medicine, 2, 179-189, 1991).

Likewise, irradiation of foods (as is commonly practiced now with shrimp, as an example, coming to this country) causes cis-trans isomerization (ibid). This translates again into negating the beneficial effect that the food imparts by abnormally altering the biochemical or molecular structure so that it hastens degenerative disease.

THE TREATMENT OF LAST RESORT

The macrobiotic diet is not a perfect "cure-all" for all people. Gerson and Kelly have certainly cleared many cancers with diets of raw foods, vegetables and fruit juices and even raw liver juice. I'm merely reporting here a diet that I as a physician and person have observed to clear multiple incurable and baffling ailments of my own. Prior to and since doing this, I have personally witnessed many other people do the same. I have deep gratitude for Mr. Michio Kushi and his tireless teaching of a rigidly trained doctor. He showed me that good food can heal where expensive and toxic medicines can fail.

So the bottom line is this:

(1) when your physician and his consultants have exhausted all they know and have nothing more to offer,
(2) when you have arrived at the end of the diagnostic rope,
(3) when you are told you have to take prescription drugs for the rest of your life,
(4) when you are told you'll just have to learn to live with it, or
(5) when you are told your days are numbered,

GO MACRO. What do you have to lose?

Of course, on the basis of what I have observed over 21 years of practicing medicine, I would suggest you try it sooner, not later, but especially when all else fails.

So here you have every reason I can think of to help you make a decision that just may turn out to be the most important decision of your life. For it seems that it doesn't really matter whether one is concerned about world pollution, loss of the ozone layer and tropical rain forests, world peace, the oil crisis, cancer, learning disabilities, heart attacks, arthritis, getting rid of disease and feeling better, reducing high cholesterol or just plain chronic fatigue. What it boils down to is simple: THE CURE IS IN THE KITCHEN.

BIBLIOGRAPHY

Tired Or Toxic? by Sherry A. Rogers, M. D.-This is the first book in history to explain in lay terms the biochemical basis of chemical sensitivity and many diseases such as arteriosclerosis, hypertension and high cholesterol. It provides the evidence plus the directions for your physician so that he will know which tests to draw to check your vitamin and mineral levels. It even provides a test you can give your physician so you know if he understands nutritional biochemistry or not. It also gives over 30 biochemical mechanisms of why macrobiotics is so healing. It provides the scientific backup for all of this so that no physician can put you down again by telling you that there is no evidence for Candida problems, chemical sensitivity, food allergy induced arthritis, brain fog, macrobiotics and much more. It bridges the gap between archaic medicine where a headache is a Darvon deficiency to the new era of environmental medicine and molecular medicine where we can now find the cause of many diseases and get rid of them. (1990)

Macro Mellow (or what I title, "What the hell to feed the rest of the family who hates macro") was designed for people who must go on the healing phase, but whose family members don't want anything to do with macrobiotics. It helps you utilize your macrobiotic foods and kitchen to feed your family more healthfully, but with such delicious foods that they will not even know that they are eating macrobiotically. These foods are not for the healing phase, but they certainly are for the transition phase before or after healing and for family members who must be fed but don't want macro. For example, there are meatless meatballs that you would swear had meat, but they're made from nutritious tofu and sunflower seeds. It is also chock full of garden, storage and kitchen management pearls. Written by Shirley Gallinger and Sherry Rogers, M. D. (1992)

You Are What You Ate is an introductory book to macrobiotics to explain to people why and how to get started in macrobiotics. It's full of cartoons and pearls.   By Sherry Rogers, M. D. (1987)

The E. I. Syndrome is over 650 pages regarding chemical, food, mold and Candida hypersensitivities, the diagnosis and treatment of them, by Sherry A. Rogers, M. D. (1986)

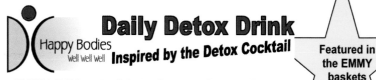

Daily Detox Drink

Happy Bodies well well well **Inspired by the Detox Cocktail**

"YOU REALLY CANNOT AFFORD TO BE WITHOUT YOUR DAILY DETOX COCKTAIL"
-Dr. Sherry Rogers, MD-

The Daily Detox Drink is inspired by the Detox Cocktail recommended by **Dr. Sherry Rogers M.D** in Detoxify or Die & The High Blood Pressure Hoax. It is a blend of Vitamin C (Ascorbic Acid), R-Lipoic Acid & Reduced Glutathione. The Daily Detox Drink by Happy Bodies is the only premixed Detox Cocktail on the market. Dr. Sherry Rogers has featured the Daily Detox Drink in her newsletters & her latest book, *Is Your Cardiologist Killing You?* Dr. Rogers emphasizes taking the Detox Cocktail every day in her books. The ingredients are GMP certified from ISO certified facilities, non-GMO (genetically modified organisms), Kosher/Halal approved, and have no adverse reports on drug compatibility. Until now a consumer would have to buy all the ingredients separately and the cost would be $133 for 30 servings. At Happy Bodies, you can buy these incredible premixed ingredients for only $59! And if you buy the 3 month bulk container you will save another $27, & the shipping is free! That is almost a 300% savings! Additionally, if you have ever mixed this yourself, you know how intolerable the taste is. At Happy Bodies we have solved that problem by adding the natural sweetener stevia & organic lemon flavoring, making The Daily Detox taste good. Stop wasting time & money & enjoy the great tasting high quality Daily Detox Drink.

Reasons for taking the Detox Cocktail are:
- ✓ **Symptoms related to sick building syndrome**
- ✓ **Discarding infections**
- ✓ **Traveler's diarrhea & Flues**
- ✓ **Migraines**
- ✓ **Protecting you from the genetic changes of cancer**
- ✓ **Lowering Cholesterol**
- ✓ **Revving up your detoxification**
- ✓ **Lowering blood pressure**
- ✓ **Protecting blood vessels from aging & becoming hypertensive**
- ✓ **And protecting every organ from premature degeneration**

Ingredients:	
	2,000 mg Vitamin C (Pure Ascorbic Acid)
	800 mg reduced Glutathione
	100 mg R-Lipoic Acid (Stabilized) (**Updated to 100 mg R-Lipoic in High Blood Pressure Hoax, instead of 300-600 mg Lipoic in Detoxify or Die**)

. Ingredients are NOT derived from nightshades.

Daily Detox Drinks saves time and money!
WWW.HAPPYBODIES.COM

How much does it cost to mix your own Detox Cocktail vs taking the Daily Detox Drink from Happy Bodies®?

If you purchased all the ingredients separately and mixed it yourself, it would cost you approximately $133 for 30 servings. That's $4.43 per serving.

At Happy Bodies, you can buy this incredible premixed formula for only $59 for 30 servings! That's only $1.97 per serving.
And if you buy the 3 month bulk container you will save another $27 over 3 months, and the shipping is free!

That's almost a 300% savings!

The organic lemon flavor and the stevia gives the Daily Detox Drink a great taste, far superior to mixing your

---

You can buy this formula with 3 different options:

- 30 packet box
- 30 serving jar with a scoop
- 90 serving jar with a scoop

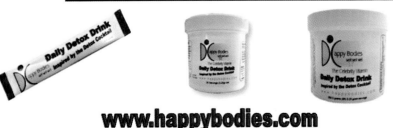

www.happybodies.com

The above are available through:

> Prestige Publishing
> 3502 Brewerton Rd.
> P. O. Box 3161
> Syracuse, NY 13220

Also, all four books can be ordered from the following 14 sources:

N.E.E.D.S.
527 Charles Av.
Syracuse, NY 13209
Ph.   1-800-634-1380 or (315) 488-6300

American Environmental Health Foundation
8345 Walnut Hill Ln. Suite 205
Dallas, TX 75231-4262
Ph.   214 368-4132

Buckingham Healthcare
PO Box 785
Buckingham, England MK18 7JZ
Ph.   0280 813798

Dickey Enterprises
109 W. Olive St.
Fort Collins, CO 80521
Ph.   303 482-6001

East West Books
807 Bloor St. W.
Toronto, Ontario M6G 1L8 Canada
Ph.   416 531-7546

Michael Glasby
221 Wonga Rd.
Warranwood 3134 Australia
Ph.   3-879-7028

Goldmine Natural Food Co.
1947 30th St.
San Diego, CA   92102
Ph.   619 234-9711

Klaire Laboratories
1573 W. Seminole
San Marcos, CA 92069
Ph.   619 744-9600

Mary Jane's Alternative Taste
1313 Hollis St.
Halifax, Nova Scotia B3J 1T8 Canada
Ph.   902 421-1313

Paperback Booksmith
Sarasota Square Mall
Sarasota, FL 34238
Ph.   813 922-5000

Pen. Ent. Plastic Surgery Allergy
1332 Todds Ln.
Hampton, VA 23666
Ph.   804 826-0216

Peter's Cornucopia
60 Genesee St.
New Hartford, NY 13413
Ph.   315 724-4998

Schizophrenia Foundation of NJ
862 Route 518
Skillman, NJ 08558
Ph.   609 924-8607

Smith Pharmacy
3463 Young St.
Toronto, Ontario NYN 2N3 Canada
Ph.   416 488-2600

Whole Health Book Co.
4735 Wunder Av.
Trevose, PA 19047
Ph.   215 322-2880

Also contact your local book-
store or healthfood store and
ask them to order the books
for you, or order direct.

Other books of interest:

The Book of Macrobiotics - The universal way of health, happiness
and peace, by Michio Kushi with Alex Jack. Japan Publications, New
York, 1986.

Aveline Kushi's Complete Guide to Macrobiotic Cooking for Health,
Harmony and Peace- Aveline Kushi with Alex Jack, Warner Books,
New York, 1985.

The Cancer Prevention Diet- Michio Kushi with Alex Jack, Saint Martin's Press, New York, 1983.

Diet For a Strong Heart- Michio Kushi with Alex Jack, Saint Martin's
Press, New York, 1985.

Macrobiotic Home Remedies- Michio Kushi, Edited by Mark Van
Cauwenberghe, M. D., Japan Publications, New York, 1985.

Macrobiotic Pregnancy and Care For the Newborn- Michio and Aveline Kushi, Edited by Edward and Wendy Esco, Japan Publications,
New York, 1984.

How To See Your Health, A Book of Diagnosis- Michio Kushi, Japan
Publications, New York, 1980.

Allergies- Michio Kushi, Japan Publications, New York.

Also get the companion cookbook, Allergies by Aveline Kushi.

    This companion book series is very good. Mr. Kushi writes
about theory, Mrs. Kushi writes about the food. Her part of the series is called The Macrobiotic Food and Cooking Series. There is a
companion book to complement each of Mr. Kushi's books on the
theory of cause. His series is called the Macrobiotic Health Education

Series. The titles of the books are the same as the companion. One theory and diet series is entitled Allergies, another Arthritis, Stress and Hypertension, (1988) another is Diabetes and Hypoglycemia (1985), another is Obesity, Weight Loss and Eating Disorders, and Infertility and Reproductive Disorders (1987). These are highly recommended. Whichever ailment you have and whichever books you decide to get, make sure you get both parts of the series (one part from the Macrobiotic Health Education Series and the other from the Macrobiotic Food and Cooking Series. For example, if you have allergies, I would get both Allergy books. They are in paperback and are relatively inexpensive. As with most other Macrobiotic needs, including books, all of the above are available through N.E.E.D.S. (1-800-634-1380) or (315) 488-6300.

If you're only going to buy one macrobiotic cookbook for the healing phase, you might wish to select The Quick and Natural Macrobiotic Cookbook by Aveline Kushi and Wendy Esco, 1989, Contemporary Books, Inc., 180 N. Michigan Av., Chicago, IL 60601. As you will see, you do not have to have nearly as many dishes at each meal as I have outlined here. It may, however, suffice for many of you, and certainly will be infinitely easier. It also contains the amount of time it takes to make each dish and has recipes and menus for an entire week.

Power Eating Program- You Are How You Eat-Lino Stanchich, Healthy Products, Inc., Miami, FL 1989. This is, believe it or not, a long-needed book on the importance of chewing well.

If you should decide you are not ready for the strict phase, or want to expand the transitional repertoire for the rest of the family beyond the transition phase, there are several other good books on transitional eating, such as:

Food and Healing- Anne Marie Colbin, Ballantine Books, Random House, Inc., NY, 1986. Contains more on balancing out foods by using your cravings to guide you.

The Natural Gourmet- ibid 1989.

The Natural Foods Cookbook- Mary Estrella, Japan Publications, NY, 1985.

The Self-Healing Cookbook by Christina Turner, 1987, Earth Tones Press, P. O. Box 2341-B, Grass Valley, CA 95945.

Working Chef's Cookbook for Natural Whole Foods, J.F. Blackman, Central Vermont Publ., Box 700, Morrisville, VT 05667.

And if you think the government watches out for you to keep your food healthful and clean, read these:

The Mirage of Safety. Food additives and Federal Policy-Hunter, B.T., The Stephen Greene Press, Brattleboro, VT, 1982.

A Diet For a New America- Robbins, J., Stillpoint Publishing, Walpole, NH, 1987.

For cancer cases treated by a physician using macro, Complete Remission of Advanced Medically Incurable Cancer in Six Patients Following a Macrobiotic Approach to Healing, Newbold, Vivien, MD, Townsend Letter for Doctors, 638-692, October 1990. (A. Gaby, M.D., publisher, Maryland)

Other books of importance include, Vibrational Medicine by Richard Gerber, M. D., Bear & Co., Santa Fe, NM 87504-2860.

Faith, Love and Healing- Bernard Segal, M.D.

Cross Currents, The Perils of Electropollution, The Promise of Electromedicine- Robert O. Becker, Jeremy P. Tarcher, Inc., 5858 Wilshire Blvd., Los Angeles, CA 90036

Clear Body, Clear Mind, L. Ron Hubbard, 1990, Bridge Pulications, 4751 Fountain Av., Los Angeles, CA 90029. This is the sauna detoxification program.

RESOURCES

If you go to a weekend Way of Life Seminar in Boston (which I heartily recommend), you'll need a place to stay and eat. I recommend:

Mr. & Mrs. Herbert Walley
29 Buswell Pk.
Newtown, MA 02158
(617) 527-5681

The Way of Life Seminars are a weekend crash course for people with cancer and other serious diseases who must learn macrobiotic theory and cooking quickly. They are held at:

The Kushi Institute
A Division of The Kushi Foundation
P. O. Box 1100, 17 Station St.
Brookline, MA 02147
(617) 738-0045

Week-long residential seminars are also available at the Kushi Foundation in the Berkshires. In the near future, the Brookline facility will totally move to Becket. For information, write:

Kushi Foundation Berkshire Center
Box 7
Becket, MA 01223
(413) 623-5741

They also have week-long seminars for physicians which I highly recommend.

For courses for physicians in nutritional biochemistry and for names of physicians (in various stages of learning) near you who may practice this form of medicine, write to:

The American Academy of Environmental Medicine
P. O. Box 16106
Denver, CO 80216

Support and informational group for people with E.I., regardless of whether or not they use macrobiotics:

Human Ecology Action League
377 Dorthy Dr.
Syracuse, NY 13215

The address of our office is:

Northeast Center for Environmental Medicine
Sherry A. Rogers, M.D., Medical Director
2800 W. Genesee St.
Syracuse, NY 13219
(315) 488-2856

We also have a quarterly health newsletter in which we publish up-to-date findings regarding macrobiotics, nutritional biochemistry (vitamins, minerals, amino acids, essential fatty acids and accessory nutrients) and environmental medicine. There are original and new articles and all is referenced so it is of use for physicians as well. All diseases and aspects of health and medicine as well as politics and insurance items of interest are covered. There is nothing else like it!

The best of health to you.

PRESTIGE PUBLISHING
P. O. Box 3161
Syracuse, NY 13220
(315) 455-7012

Please send the following books:	Quantity	Sub-total
The E.I. Syndrome..........................$14.95	_____	_____
You Are What You Ate.....................9.95	_____	_____
Tired Or Toxic?.. ....17.95	_____	_____
Macro Mellow............................. ..13.95	_____	_____
The Cure Is In The Kitchen..............14.95	_____	_____
Health Letter (quarterly newsletter)14/yr	_____	_____
Mold Plates 20.00	_____	_____
Formaldehyde Spot Test 40.00	_____	_____

Sub-total		_____
*Discount		_____
NY State residents add 7% sales tax		_____
**Shipping/handling each		_____
Total Enclosed		_____

*Discounts available on ten or more books.

**Ship/hand $3.00 each in the continental U.S., $6.00 each elsewhere.

Northeast Center For Environmental Medicine

Statement of Purpose

The goal of the Northeast Center for Environmental Medicine is to help people realize their full health potential, through diagnosis, treatment and extensive education. It especially specializes in difficult to diagnose or apparently incurable medical problems. It does this by taking up where 20th century medicine leaves off by using 21st century molecular and environmental medicine to identify the hidden or unsuspected environmental triggers and biochemical deficiencies that cause most diseases. If there is enough interest in this type of information, we plan to publish it for a nominal sum to cover costs on a quarterly basis initially and then bimonthly.

The health letter is but one facet of our educational thrust, and we welcome your questions, requests, and comments to help us fashion this into the most meaningful health newsletter for you and your family.

- -

NORTHEAST CENTER FOR ENVIRONMENTAL MEDICINE
HEALTH LETTER
P.O. Box 3161, Syracuse, NY 13220
(315) 455 - 7862

_____ Please enter new subscription for_____ years.

Subscription rates: One year, $14.00 Two years, $25.00

_____ Payment enclosed (U.S. Dollars)

_____ Charge to: _____ VISA _____ MasterCard

#_____ Exp._____

Signature: _____

Name _____

Address _____

City _____State _____ Zip _____

Telephone _____

Northeast Center For Environmental Medicine Health Letter is published quarterly by Prestige Publishing, P.O. Box 3161, Syracuse, NY 13220 (315) 455 - 7862

RECENT SCIENTIFIC PUBLICATIONS
THAT DO NOT APPEAR IN PREVIOUS BOOKS:

The first paper on zinc is reproduced with kind permission and was published in International Clinical Nutrition Review, Jan 1990. Subscriptions are available from Integrated Therapies Pty. Ltd., PO Box 370, Manly, N.S.W. 2095, Australia.

The next paper is reproduced with kind permission and was published in Indoor Air '90, The 5th International Conference on Indoor Air Quality and Climate, volume 5, p. 345-349, published by Indoor Air '90 Proceedings Distribution, 2344 Haddington Crescent, Ottawa, Ontario K1H 8J4. This major international indoor air symposium held in Toronto, had multiple sponsors, among which were the World Health Organization, ASHRAE, Canadian Hospital Assoc., U.S.DOE, U.S.EPA, Canadian General Standards Board, Health and Welfare Canada, etc. Key researchers from around the world were invited to present.

The third paper is from Environmental International which goes to 152 countries (P.O. Box 7166, Alexandria, VA 22307). This paper was presented in The Netherlands at the 8th World Clean Air Congress '89 and the proceedings were published as Man and His Ecosystem, vol. 1 (P.O. Box 186, 2600 AD Delft, The Netherlands).

The last paper on the magnesium loading test comes with kind permission also from International Clinical Nutrition Review, July 1991 (ibid paragraph one).

SPECIAL ARTICLE

Zinc Deficiency as Model for Developing Chemical Sensitivity

Sherry A. Rogers, M.D., F.A.B.F.P., F.A.C.A.I., F.A.B.E.M.

Northeast Centre for Environmental Medicine
2800 West Genesee Street,
Syracuse, New York 13219 U.S.A.
Fax: 315 488 7518

ABSTRACT

In 250 randomly selected patients claiming sensitivity to chemicals, red blood cell (RBC) zinc was abnormally low in 54%. Since zinc occurs in over 90 metalloenzymes, a deficiency would be expected to have far reaching effects.

The metabolism of xenobiotics and membrane stability are extremely dependent upon zinc. Since the endoplasmic reticulum is the locus for Phase I detoxication and alcohol dehydrogenase is a zinc-dependent key Phase I detoxication enzyme, increased vulnerability to chemicals because of defective detoxication and faulty membranes could weaken the xenobiotic detoxication system. With a zinc deficiency, several zinc dependent pathways can also explain the nebulous symptoms of the "toxic brain", with its spaciness, or inability to concentrate and mood swings.

Correction of a zinc deficiency is not without problems and must be carefully monitored so as not to create secondary deficiencies of manganese, iron, calcium or copper.

INTRODUCTION

Mental confusion, dizziness, inability to concentrate and unwarranted depression are classic symptoms of central nervous system toxicity (sometimes referred to as "toxic brain") to lipotropic hydrocarbon xenobiotics, and are easily recognized in relation to acute exposures. However, when they occur with greater frequency and severity with seemingly decreasing relation to an obvious cause, they are often attributed to a psychological problem. Such is the plight of the multiply sensitive individual.

Patients who suffer from multiple sensitivities or environmental illnesses (E.I.) display tremendous individual variation in target organ, adaptability, and environmental triggers. For example when a home was insulated with urea foam formaldehyde insulation, almost everyone in the family had dissimilar symptoms and often some members were extremely ill while others were unaffected. Knowledge of the biochemistry of an unsuspected (yet common) deficiency, like zinc, could explain the observations associated with confusing cerebral symptoms as well as the spreading phenomenon.

RESULTS

In a random study of 250 patients presenting consecutively to a private office that only sees allergy and environmental medicine referrals, 54% had an abnormally low zinc level of less than 880 mcg/dl (normal erythrocyte zinc as determined by National Medical Services is 880-1600 mcg/dl) [1].

Many of these patients complained of not only symptoms induced by chemical exposures, but reactions to dusts, moulds, pollens and even foods. Additionally, multiple target organs were involved; usually the sinuses, nose, chest, bowel, brain, skin, metabolic (energy), peripheral and central nervous systems.

DISCUSSION

Literature reports indicate that unsuspected zinc deficiency is relatively common. In one study 13% of randomly selected patients had normal zinc levels, and 68% of the population ingested less than 2/3 the RDA for zinc [2]. Zinc deficiency has been shown to be prevalent througout the world, in all age ranges [3-6], and especially in pregnancy [7], chronic disease [8] and after surgery [9].

Over 90 metalloenzymes are zinc dependent [15]. Because of biochemical individuality, the enzymes affected vary between individuals. There will understandably be no symptoms that are consistently present in all patients exhibiting zinc deficiency. And indeed there were no common symptoms or unifying dietary correlations with any of the subjects with abnormally low levels.

Since zinc deficiency was so prevalent among our chemically sensitive patients and since zinc dependent enzymes are represented in every major metabolic pathway in the body, the following will be an overview that demonstrates how silent deficiency of zinc serves as a model that could account for the chemical sensitivity and cerebral symptoms observed in patients with E.I. (environmental illness, chemical sensitivity or multiply sensitive individual).

Zinc deficiency is prevalent and underrecognized [7-14] for a number of reasons. Zinc is easily washed from the soil by acid rain and is depleted by modern farming practices. Processed foods are notoriously low in zinc. For example, 80% of the zinc in wheat is lost in flour milling. Also, tastes have changed as people become more addicted to the fats, salts and sugars of processed foods.

Xenobiotic overload from air, water and foods, also increases the need for zinc, as do many medications such as diuretics, oral contraceptives and steroids. Alcohol and cigarettes also deplete body zinc (cadmium in cigarettes is preferentially incorporated into zinc metalloenzymes), as do chronic diseases, surgery, sweating, pregnancy and growth [11].

Many factors contribute to poor absorption of zinc e.g. phytates (inositol hexaphosphate) in unleavened bread, self-prescribed vitamins with imbalances of copper (many popular vitamin preparations are disproprotionately higher in copper than zinc), calcium (currently in vogue), iron (frequently self prescribed), and displacement by cadmium from industrial and auto exhausts [12-14]. Zinc is poorly stored in the body and losses need to be replaced daily, so fasting, repeated dieting, many malabsorption disorders, and irregular eating schedules promote development of deficiency.

Zinc is also a requisite for the metabolism of other nutrients that the detoxication system depends upon. For example, pyridoxine kinase, plays a role in the conversion of pyridoxine to pyridoxal-5-phosphate, which is necessary in over 50 enzymes. These include the synthesis of most neurotransmitters such as serotonin, taurine and histamine. A deficiency of serotonin has been noted in some depressions and taurine is an important anti-oxidant, membrane stabilizer and bile component through which many conjugated xenobiotics are excreted [15-17].

Vitamin B6 is also necessary for the conversion of tryptophan to nicotinamide (NAD for detoxication), and for metabolism of cysteine for direct conjugation of xenobiotics in phase II detoxication [18], and the synthesis of anti-inflammatory PGE 1. Clearly defects in the latter biochemistry could account for the defective and easily overloaded detoxication system. And as it continues to be deficient in the wake of continuing xenobiotic exposures, the result could produce progressively exaggerated responses to low level triggers, that previously were tolerated. This spreading phenomenon, as it is called, is frequently observed in chemically sensitive individuals.

Zinc is also crucial in the function of alcohol dehydrogenase, one form of which enables vitamin A to be converted from retinol to retinaldehyde [19]. When zinc is inadequate, vitamin A cannot be utilized. Vitamin A is essential in gene repair, membrane stability, as an anti-oxidant, for synthesis of the Phase II conjugator, PAPS, for mucosal tissue integrity and defense against Candida, T-cell and organ function, as well as the processing of many proteins and in gene expression and adrenal function. Hence, vitamins and neurotransmitters could be affected by zinc deficiency (and it is easily seen how this phenomenon perpetually worsens or spreads).

Thymidine kinase and DNA polymerase are necessary for transcription and repair of genetic material [20]. Moreover, when there is zinc deficiency, the deficiency of alcohol dehydrogenase can lead to further increase in oncogenic epoxides, as metabolism is shifted toward this pathway. In addition, with inadequate zinc, the lowered absorption of vitamin A and E due to deficiency of zinc dependent pancreatic enzymes (like lipase) leaves the genetic material more vulnerable to free radical attack.

The negatively charged DNA molecule is a target for binding a great array of electrophilic free radicals (which are more plentiful when detoxication is not optimally functioning). This interaction of free radicals with DNA modifies the structure and initiates mutagenesis [21].

The shuffling and change in genetic material is an organism's attempt to adapt to its environment, as described by Nobel Prize winners McClintock (1983) and Tonegawa (1987), leads to conjecture as to what may happen as people seemingly become irreversibly sensitized after a particular exposure. Environmental chemicals may trigger the "jumping genes" which then translate into an altered state of reactivity.

Alcohol dehydrogenase is essential in the Phase I detoxication or biotransformation of many xenobiotics [22]. Alcohol intolerance occurs with deficient alcohol dehydrogenase, and this is a common observation among chemically sensitive people. As well they complain of many psychiatric symptoms [5]. But, overloading of the alcohol dehydrogenase pathway shifts metabolism toward chloral hydrate [23] which can account for the symptoms of a "toxic brain" which are reminiscent of the old "Mickey Finn" (chloral hydrate's popular name years ago). [24,25] These symptoms may include confusion, dizziness, paresthesias and mental fatigue. To compound matters, chloral hydrate can be reduced to trichloroethylene [26], a compound with its own similar devastating neuropsychiatric effects [27,28]. These reactions are reversible and could account for the seemingly unexplainable wide mood swings, confusion and disturbed thoughts as the chemistry bounces back and forth between these two compounds. Zinc is also important in Phase II conjugation via glucuronic acid which conjugates with phenols and hydroxyl radicals to facilitate their bowel and urinary excretion.

Formate dehydrogenase actions requires zinc and a deficiency can account for poor tolerance to formaldehydes and other airborne aldehydes of urban pollution.

Glutamate dehydrogenase, another zinc dependent enzyme, is necessary for glutathione peroxidase synthesis; glutathione being a major part of xenobiotic detoxication [29,30]. Furthermore zinc appears to have a direct effect of protecting against carbon tetrachloride-induced liver injury [31].

Many xenobiotics increase acetaldehyde production in the hepatic endoplasmic reticulum as the body attempts to detoxify them after inhalation. For example, disulphiram, a by-product of the manufacture of rubber impairs alcohol dehydrogenase and aldehyde dehydrogenase functions. Vinylidene chloride, used in the manufacture of saran-type plastics is metabolized to monochloroacetate and then to dichloroacetaldehyde. [32] If the xenobiotic detoxication system is malfunctioning and overloaded because of a zinc deficiency, the aldehyde pathways can be stressed and aldehydes accumulate. As a powerful adduct, acetaldehyde can bind to brain membranes [32], cause release of vasoactive substances like catecholamines, condense with catecholamines to form tetrahydro-isoquinolones which in turn become false neurotransmitters, activate the complement sequence, bind to liver membranes, increase peroxidation by binding glutathione and cysteine, further impairing detoxication as well as promoting permanent damage [34]. Aldehydes can also account for the mysteriously prevalent E.I. symptoms of flushing, tachycardia and "toxic brain". Carbonic anhydrase, a zinc dependent enzyme, also plays an important role in the metabolism of aldehydes.

Clearly zinc's importance in detoxication could explain the symptoms of chemical intolerance. The cerebral symptoms can be explained by the formation of chloral hydrate and aldehydes as well as xenobiotic backlog and shift to other metabolites. As areas of the detoxication system weaken, it is easy to see how this would rapidly potentiate faults in other pathways as a side effect of xenobiotic overload. What would clinically be observed is a person who reacts more quickly and more intensely to an ever-increasing number of triggers; this is accompanied by bizarre, fluctuating, unexplainable cerebral symptoms, body perceptions and a heightened sensitivity that makes a victim appear psychotic, since all others about him are seemingly unaffected. This is precisely what is seen in the spreading phenomenon of chemical sensitivity.

Furthermore, gamma amino butyric acid (GABA) is an inhibitory cerebral neurotransmitter, necessary for calming or modulating anxiety, and known to be disturbed by ethanol intoxication [35]. Zinc is necessary for the binding of GABA to synaptic membranes for normal inhibitory CNS tone [36]. Perhaps this mechanism relates to the cerebral symptoms observed in people reacting to chemical exposures, since they complain of unwarranted anxiety and even panic attacks.

One important caveat is that with correction of zinc deficiency, every two or three months the RBC zinc level as well as the serum copper and iron levels should be monitored, since there is a reciprocal relationship between zinc, manganese, copper, calcium, molybdenum and iron [37]. With the presence of a zinc deficiency, there is already an imbalance within the system, so reciprocally, a highly unbalanced prescribed regimen is necessary for correction (often we had to use levels in excess of 100mg of zinc to correct the deficiencies over three months). However, the mark can be overshot, and the creation of secondary deficiencies could go undetected without proper monitoring.

Case Example of Corrected Zinc Deficiency Improving Xenobiotic Metabolism

A.R. was a 53 year old women who had complained of headaches at home and at work for eleven years. She had worked for the last 15 years in a factory where she shaped wax forms with a hot tool before they were used near her station to cast plastic parts. She had

had a complete workup by her internist including a computerized axial tomography (CAT) scan. Four years prior to this she had had another such workup before she then consulted an allergist. Injections for four years were of no help. Recently she consulted another allergist who told her there was nothing wrong and returned her to her family doctor who advised her to see a psychiatrist.

Single-blind testing to chemicals provoked her headache and the neutralizing dose terminated it when trichloroethylene was tested. Formaldehyde, toluene and normal saline control were negative [54]. A blood level of trichloroethylene after a day at work was 26.1 ng/dl (population average 1.1 ng/dl) [38]. After two weeks at home, it was 18.3. The headaches were not as severe at home, but persisted for the next eight months while she remained out of work. They were noticeably worse if she went into certain stores or offices or returned to visit her friends at her place of employment. At this time, an RBC zinc level was found to be 870 mcg/dl (normal; 880-1600 mcg/dl). She was placed on 105 mg of zinc gluconate a day in divided doses as well as multiple minerals and vitamins. Within two months she had corrected the zinc deficiency to 1060 mcg/dl and reported that she was markedly improved. The headaches had totally cleared at home and she was able to do her housework. Stores and offices that were intolerable before this, now caused no headaches. Also she no longer had leg aches, insomnia, periorbital oedema nor a shakey, jittery feeling.

Her serum tetrachloroethylene level had dropped to 1.3 ng/dl (ppb). One month after this she was again tested with trichloroethylene, only this time it was done double-blind. Again she had no reaction to normal saline given twice. With the provoking intradermal dose she reported a headache, then the normal saline control was given twice and there was no change. Next, the neutralizing dose was given and she reported termination of the symptom.

The important point of all this is that a person who had elevated xenobiotic levels and who had reacted to this chemical in blinded intradermal testing, could not clear her blood levels after two weeks at home. During the next 8 months at home, while she had relief from the previous horrible headaches if she stayed out of work and stores, she still was too ill in her own home to do housework. However, within two months of correcting the zinc deficiency, all this was corrected (the blood level as well as reactivity in stores and at home). So a person who had been labelled as incapacitated by previous chemical exposures was able to resume normal life. However, the suggestion of a possible genetic change is supported by the fact that double-blind testing can still produce the symptoms, as can re-entering the work environment.

CONCLUSION

We did not attempt to do a clinical efficacy study because all patients wanted as quick relief from symptoms as possible. Therefore, the total load was addressed. Sensitivities to inhaled dusts, moulds, mites and pollens were sought and environmental controls for dusts and moulds were implemented.

Immunotherapy to positive reacting inhalant allergies was begun [39]. The diagnostic rare food diet [40] was initiated in order to determine if hidden food sensitivities existed. Other nutrient deficiencies, as well as chemical hypersensitivities were also sought and corrected [41]. Environmental controls, including avoidance where possible, were instituted. In other words, no patients elected to merely treat the zinc deficiency, since like our example, they had exhausted all that medicine had to offer. Instead they all chose to explore and treat the total body burden of problems for as quick and complete relief of symptoms as possible. Using this protocol, they all reported at least positive, if not total improvement in their symptoms. How much of the improvement is due to correction of the zinc deficiency is unknown.

It has been shown that a solitary, "subclinical", unsuspected deficiency of zinc is capable of initiating a cascade of malfunctions. Furthermore, a zinc deficiency will not be found unless it is looked for, since the deficiency is a protean disease and any symptoms are possible and are usually non-specific. As the more readily available plasma zinc is not adequate for diagnosis [42], a special erythrocyte zinc must be requested.

The biochemistry of zinc is not alone in being able to serve as a model for the spreading phenomenon and other symptoms of E.I. Likewise, if one were to follow the enzymes that are magnesium dependent, or the pathways that are B6 dependent, for example, one could probably explain the spreading phenomenon with either of these deficiencies. And yet both of these can become deficient eventually as zinc deficiency worsens. (Vitamin B6 conversion is compromised with poor levels of pyridoxine kinase and magnesium ingestion suffers if carbonic anhydrase is insufficient). It goes without saying that singular deficiencies are unlikely. Furthermore, in the case of multiple deficiencies, an even more devastating and puzzling scenario could evolve, especially when one also considers individual biochemical needs and target organ relativity.

Unfortunately, as zinc deficiency occurs, the symptoms can progressively worsen when multiple systems become defective and then further deficiencies arise as a consequence, causing a vicious downward spiral that many of us have personally experienced in ourselves and our patients as the spreading phenomenon. These victims become increasingly sensitized to a wide range of substances as major detoxication mechanisms are jeopardized.

When the faulty, overloaded detoxication system is further stressed, the ability to handle daily neurotropic xenobiotics dwindles, leaving one's sanity in doubt. Yet, it is merely the combination of twentieth century lifestyles (depleted soils, processed foods, xenobiotic overloads in the air, water, and food as well as medicine's emphasis on prescribed drugs to mask the symptoms of chronic illness) that create this deficiency. Obviously, even the staunchest person with this disease risks eventual mental decompensation, due to the exorbitant stresses of the symptoms. For after all, in an era of exceptional medical technology, it is inconceivable to him that he could have an undiagnosable condition. Then when medications make him worse (as they also can serve to increase xenobiotic overload), family, friends and physicians become frustrated and begin to doubt him.

But if one does look at the worldwide socioeconomic factors leading to poor soil and poor food quality, in terms of zinc, and look at the xenobiotic overload in our air, water and food, as well as look at all of the symptoms simultaneously and then relate them to human biochemistry and the xenobiotic detoxication pathways, the cerebral symptoms are more easily understood.

REFERENCES

1. National Medical Services, Inc., 2300 Stratford Ave. P.O. Box 433A, Willow Grove, PA 19090, a reference lab through Smith Kline Bio-Science Laboratories, King of Prussia,PA.
2. Elsborg L, The Intake of vitamins and minerals by the elderly at home. Int J Vit Nutr Res 53, 321-329 (1983).
3. Hambridge KM, Walravens PA, Brown RM, Webster J, White S, Anthony M, Roth ML. Zinc nutrition of preschool children in the Denver Head Start Program. Am J Clin Nutr 29, 734-738 (1976).

259

4. Sanstead HH, Henriksen LK, Gregor JG, Prasad A, Good RA. Zinc nutriture in the elderly in relation to taste accuity, immune response and wound healing. Am J Clin Nutr 36, 1046-1059 (1982).

5. Klevay LM, Reck SJ, Barcome DF, et al. Evidence of dietary copper and zinc deficiencies. JAMA 241, (18), 1916-1918 (1979).

6. Gregor JL, Prevalence and signficance of zinc deficiency in the elderly. Geriatr Med Today 3 (1), 24-30 (1984), J Am Diet Assoc 82, 148-153 (1983).

7. Hambridge KM. Zinc nutritional status during pregnancy: A longitudinal study. Am J Clin Nutr 37, 429-442 (1983).

8. Prasad AS. Zinc in Human Nutrition, CRC Press, Boca Raton, FL 33431, 16-30 (1979).

9. Van Rij AM. Zinc supplements in surgery. Current Topics in Nutrition and Disease: Chemical, Biochemical and Nutritional Aspects of Trace Elements, Prasad AS, ed., Alan R. Liss, Inc., 150 Fifth Ave, New York, NY 10011, 6: 14, 259-276 (1982).

10. Rennert OM, Chan WY, Metabolism of Trace Elements in Man: Developmental Aspects, Vol1, CRC Press, Boca Raton, FL 33431 2-3 (1984).

11. Sanstead HH, Availability of zinc and its requirements in human subjects. in ibid (9), 83-101.

12. Mills CF. Dietary interactions involving the trace elements. Am Rev Nutr, Annual Reviews, Inc., 4139 El Camino Way, Palo Alto, CA 94306, 5: 173-193 (1985).

13. ibid (10), 102-103.

14. Spivey Fox MR, Biochemical basis of cadmium toxicity in human subjects. in ibid (9), 537-547.

15. Gelder NM. A central mechanism of action for taurine: osmoregulation, bivalent cations and excitation threshold. Neurochem Res 8(5), 687-699 (1983).

16. Brewer GJ. Calmodulin, zinc, calcium in cellular and membrane regulation: An interpretive review. Am J Hematol 8, 231-248 (1980).

17. ibid (9), 205-206.

18. Orten JM, Neuhaus OW. Human Biochemistry, 10th ed.,, C.V. Mosby, St. Louis, 775-776(1982).

19. Smith JC. Interrelationship of zinc and vitamin A metabolism in animal and human nutrition: A review. in ibid (9), 239-258.

20. Martin DW. DNA organization and replication. Harper's Review of Biochemistry, Martin DW, Mayes PA, Rodwell VW, Altos CA 94023, 386-404 (1985).

21. Castro E. Nutritional influences on chromatin; Toxicologic implications. Nutritional Toxicology, Hathcock JN, Academic Press, NY, 2: 129-156 (1987).

22. Barron WF, Li TK. Alcohol dehydrogenase. Enzymatic Basis of Detoxication, Vol I, Jakoby WB, ed., Academic Press, NY 231-250 (1980).

23. Leibman KC, Ortiz E. Metabolism of halogenated ethylenes. Envir Health Persp 21, 91-97 (1977).

24. Reynolds, et al. Hepatotoxicity of vinyl chloride and I,I-dichloroethylene. Am J Pathol 81(1) 219-231 (1975).

25. Parke DV. Mechanisms of chemical toxicity: A unifying hypothesis. Regulatory Toxicology and Pharmacology 2, 267-286 (1982).

26. Homburger F, Hayes JA. Pelikan, A Guide to General Toxicology, Karger NY, 177-181 (1983).

27. Feldman RG, Meyer RM, Taub A. Evidence for peripheral neurotropic effects of trichloroethylene. Neurology 20, 599-606 (1970).

28. Feldman RG, Ricks NC, Baker EL. Neuropsychological effects of industrial toxins: A rev v. Am J Industr Med 1, 211-277 (1980).

29. Reeves AL. The metabolism of foreign compounds. Toxicology: Principles and Practices, Vol.I, Reeves AL, ed., John Wiley and Sons, NY 1-28 (1985).

30. Levine, SA, Kidd PM. Antioxidant Adaptation, Biocurrents Division, Allergy Research Group, 400 Preda St, San Leandro, CA 94577, 48-521 (1985).

31. Chvapil M, Ryan JN, Elias SL, Peng YH. Protective effect of zinc on CCl4-Induced liver injury in rats. Exp Mol Pathol 19, 186-196 (1973).

32. Costa AK, Ivanetich KM. Vinylidene chloride: Its metabolism by hepatomicrosomal cytochrome P-450 in vitro. Biochem Pharmacol 31(11), 2083-2092 (1982).

33. Tottmar O. Biogenic Aldehyde: Metabolism, binding to brain memoranes, and electrophysiological effects. Aldehyde Adducts in Alcoholism, Collins MA, Ed., Alan R. Liss, NY, 57-66 (1985).

34. ibid (25), P. 65-88.

35. Hakkinen HM, Kuloner E. Ethanol intoxication and acivities of glutamine decarboxylase and gamma-amino-butyric amino transferase in rat brain. J Neurochem 33, 943-946 (1979).

36. Baraldi M, Casilgrandi E, Santi MS. Effect of zinc on specific binding of GABA to rat brain membranes. The Neurobiology of Zinc, Part A, Frederickson GA, ed., Howell GA, Kasarskis EJ, NY, Alan R. Liss, 59-71 (1984).

37. Cunnane SC. Zinc: Clinical and Biochemical Significance, CRC Press Inc., Boca Raton, FL 68, 118, 115-119, 127-128 (1988).

38. Accu-Chem Laboratories, a division of E.H.S. Inc., 990 Bowser, Ste 800, Richardson, TX 75081.

39. Rogers SA. Resistant Cases: Response to mold immunotherapy and environmental and dietary controls. Clinical Ecology V(3) 115-118 (1987-88).

40. Rogers SA. The E.I. Syndrome, Prestige Publishing, P.O. Box 3161, Syracuse, NY 13220, 481-487 (1986).

41. Rogers SA. Diagnosing the tight building syndrome. Env Health Persp 76, 195-198 (1987).

42. Spencer H, Kroner L, Osis D. Zinc balances in humans. ibid (14), 4, 103-116.

A PRACTICAL APPROACH TO THE PERSON WITH
SUSPECTED INDOOR AIR QUALITY PROBLEMS

Sherry A. Rogers, M.D.
Northeast Center For
  Environmental Medicine
2800 West Genesee St.
Syracuse, New York 13219

From   Indoor Air '90

vol. 5, 345-349, 1990

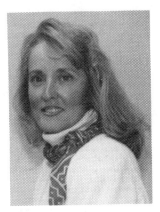

Because we are the first generation of man ever exposed to so many chemicals, and to tighten our buildings to conserve energy, we have accelerated the problems associated with poor indoor air quality (IAQ), which can present as nearly any symptom. This paper will show how we approached over one hundred patients, 90% of whom were markedly improved, with a step-wise approach to sort out whether environmental factors were due to mold, dust or chemical sensitivities. Once the culprit was established, the methods to bring about improvement in 90% of the people will all be described in detail. This should provide a basis for ruling out whether undiagnosable symptoms can be secondary to poor IAQ, and if so, how to help people get well again.

INTRODUCTION

Yearly seminars, throughout the world, in the last decade have demonstrated the emergence of symptoms in people that can be traced back to problems of indoor air quality (IAQ) (1,2,3,4,5). Because these victims exhibit a broad range of symptoms, and no two people are exactly alike, generic terms such as sick building syndrome, tight building syndrome, chemical sensitivity, and universal reactor have evolved in attempt to explain this twentieth century malady.

Because we have had the privilege of successfully diagnosing and treating well over a thousand of these people, and the author herself was severely afflicted, the emergence of specific patterns has enabled us to formulate an approach that might be useful for others.

METHODS AND MATERIALS

A retrospective analysis of the last one hundred patients was performed. They represented people from fourteen states, ages three through seventy eight years. The reasons for presenting to the center were many, and divided into six major categories. In Category I, they had upper airway symptoms including chronic nasal congestion, recurrent sinus infections, headaches, dizziness, recurrent pharyngitis, recurrent ear infections, hoarseness, or burning of the eyes or nasal membranes.

In Category II, they had lower airway symptoms of chronic asthma, bronchitis, throat spasms, chest tightness, or cough. Category III was what we called the toxic brain syndrome. In this category we lumped symptoms of inability to concentrate, spaciness, dizziness, headache, mood swings, unprovoked irritability and unwarranted depression.

Chronic fatigue was a fourth category, and a fifth included musculoskeletal symptoms of arthritis, arthralgia, muscle spasms, and flu-like body aches. A sixth category was for the remaining symptoms such as eczema, irritable bowel, recurrent vaginitis, recurrent cystitis, adult enuresis, hyperactivity, panic attacks, infertility, and much more. Over 90% of the subjects had symptoms referable to more than one category.

Most people were referred by "word of mouth", and had had a minimum of six evaluations by different specialists. Many lacked a definitive diagnosis and treatment, and came not because they suspected that they had problems initiated by poor indoor air quality, but because it was their last resort and they wanted to rule out potential causes that had not been considered in the conventional medical workup.

An eight page questionnaire was filled out which included their six worst symptoms, the duration of time for which they had had them, and the time of day, week, month, or year that they were more prevalent, as well as whether they were worse at home, work, in schools, shopping malls, churches or other places. Another two pages allowed them to list all of their symptoms, not just the six worst ones, and the average person listed over one dozen symptoms.

We then proceeded to work through a four stage program to determine which aspects of IAQ were the culprits that could be contributing to their symptoms:

Stage 1: To rule out dust mold and pollen hypersensitivity, patients were screened to a seven grass mix, house dust, both forms of house dust mite, and seven common fungi (molds). If these were positive, a fuller testing was done which included 10 tree mix, ragweed mix, 3 weed mix, goldenrod, mattress dust, twelve more fungi, and lake algae. The technique for testing and treating has been described in detail (6).

To assess which environment was the source of excess mold, petri dishes were exposed in the bedroom, family room, and office. The methodology has been fully described (7,8). Methods to lesson the molds were explained to the patient (9).

Stage 2: To determine whether unsuspected chemical sensitivity was a culprit, a detailed history of exposures was taken. The suspected xenobiotics were measured in the blood. They were often measured after a day at work, toward the end of the work week, and then again after a weekend at home to determine which area was the source of contamination (10).

Single, and/or double-blind testing in the office was also done to determine which symptoms might be triggered by specific chemicals. The technique is described in detail (11,12).

Then the patient was instructed in how to reduce his exposure to these chemicals (9,13). Even if the offending exposure was at work, he was instructed in how to reduce his exposures even at home, also, to give his detoxication system a maximum rest, and allow it to function better in time of demand (13).

Stage 3: If the person was demonstrated to have problems with chemical sensitivity (stage 2), it was rationalized that it was because his xenobiotic (foreign chemical) detoxication pathways to metabolize chemicals were somehow defective, since many other people in the same environment tolerated the same exposures without symptoms. Blood and urine tests were done to assess the adequacy of nutrients that were crucial in the enzymes that detoxify the chemicals identified in the blood, and identified to cause symptoms with skin chemical testing. Those nutrients that were found to be abnormally low were corrected. The commonest ones evaluated were intracellular (rbc or red blood cell) zinc, thiamine (vitamin B1), rbc copper, rbc selenium, B6, B12, folic acid, iron, vitamin A, and the magnesium loading test (13, also submitted for publication).

Stage 4: If the person was still chemically and/or dust/mold sensitive in spite of environmental controls, immunotherapy, and biochemical corrections, a special diet was prescribed which has helped over 450 patients increase their tolerance and maximize their xenobiotic detoxication (13,14).

RESULTS

After six months on this program, over 90% rated themselves as at least 50% improved overall, many for the first time in years. Fifty percent rated themselves as at least 75% improved, stating that when they were more adherent to the diet, they were even better than 75%. For less than 5% there was no improvement, whatsoever.

Although a step wise approach was attempted, it was found that marked improvement did not occur in many people unless multiple stages were used simultaneously. Less than 30% had marked improvement with just one stage. As a rule there was step wise improvement as each stage was evaluated, but for others there was no improvement until the last stage was completed. If the preceding, seemingly non-effective, former stages were then omitted from the program, there was an increase in symptoms. This lead us to appreciate that there was, indeed, a total overload that needed to be addressed.

Sometimes one stage made a very dramatic difference. For example, one woman had severe headaches, fatigue and nasal congestion for eleven years. She had been evaluated by otolaryngologists, neurologists, internists, psychiatrists, and family doctors. We had tested molds, dust and pollens, and started administering those that were positive by injection. We then found her level of trichloroethylene after a day at work to be 26 times normal, after two weeks at home it was 18 times normal; after eight months at home she was still plagued by symptoms, but not as bad as she had been, had she been attending work. The intradermal (skin) tests for the chemical trichloroethylene could also provoke the very headaches she was complaining of.

Since trichloroethylene is metabolized first by the hepatic enzyme, alcohol dehydrogenase, and requires zinc for its action, an rbc zinc was measured. It was found to be low, and it was supplemented. In one month she was well (15) and no longer reacting.

DISCUSSION

Clearly, there are three problems here that combine to create this 20th century malady which we are forced to diagnose and treat when we see victims of poor IAQ (1).

347

We are the first generation of man ever exposed to so many chemicals (2). This has created a strain on the detoxication system.

We are the first generation of man to ever tighten his buildings to conserve energy. This has effectively prolonged the abnormal concentrations of these hundreds of new chemicals in construction materials, furnishings, and more.

And if that were not enough, we are the first generation of man to ever eat so many processed foods. This has lead to a plethora of hidden nutrient deficiencies. For example, the United States government has shown that the standard American diet provides only 40% of the recommended daily allowance for magnesium (16). In one study (17) we found over ten patients out of one hundred were markedly less chemically sensitive after their magnesium deficiencies had been identified and corrected.

In essence, we have a detoxication system that is under-nourished and over burdened. This initiates poor metabolism of chemicals and ushers in symptoms that we, as physicians, are untrained in diagnosing and treating. In this study we merely whittled through the total load of potential environmental and biochemical causes, pealing away the layers of symptoms as one would peal away an onion. This need to whittle away at the total load may in part be explained by the fact that in many studies it is rarely just one chemical that is causing the problems. But it is small doses of many chemicals that contributes to the measurable blood overload of chemicals and symptoms (18).

Many patients described themselves as 30-50% improved once we had started immunotherapy for their dust, mold, and pollen sensitivities. Then when we identified chemical sensitivity through blood tests and/or provocational intradermal (skin testing) for chemicals, and instructed them in environmental controls to reduce their exposure to them, they improved even further. As we went to other stages, such as looking for any biochemical defects or nutrient deficiencies in the detoxication pathway, they gained even further tolerance to their environments. The prescribed diet provided even further benefits, and even enabled many to discontinue other parts of the program.

SUMMARY

We have provided here a model with which the physician can successfully diagnose and treat the majority of people with potential symptoms from poor indoor air quality.

BIBLIOGRAPHY

1. Brasser LJ, Mulder WC, eds., Man And His Ecosystem, Proceedings Of The 8th World Clean Air Congress 1989, vol. 1-4, Elsevier, NY, The Hague, Sept. 11-15, 1989.
2. Indoor Air '87, Proceedings of the 4th International Conference on Indoor Air Quality and Climate, Institute for Water, Soil and Air Hygiene, Vol. 1-4, Coirensplatz 1, D-1000 Berlin 33, 1987.
3. Healthy Buildings '88, Abstract guide, Swedish Council for Building Research, Stockholm, 1988.
4. The Annual International Symposium, Man and His Environment in Health and Disease, by American Center for Environmental Medicine, Dallas, 1982-1990.
5. American Academy of Environmental Medicine Annual Scientific Sessions, Denver, 1969-1989.

6. Rogers SA, Resistant cases: Response to mold immunotherapy and environmental and dietary controls, Clinical Ecology, V, 3:115-120, 1987/1988.
7. Terracina F, Rogers SA, In-home fungal studies: Methods to increase the yield, Ann Allerg, 49:35-37, 1982.
8. Rogers SA, A thirteen-month work-leisure-sleep environment fungal survey, Ann Allerg, 52:338-341, 1984.
9. Rogers SA, The E.I. Syndrome, Prestige Publishing, Box 3161, 3502 Brewerton Rd., Syracuse, NY 13220, 1986.
10. Rogers SA, Diagnosing the tight building syndrome or diagnosing chemical hypersensitivity, Environment International, 15:75-79, 1989.
11. Rogers SA, Provocation-neutralization of cough and wheezing in a horse, Clinical Ecology, V, 4:185-187, 1987/1988.
12. Rogers SA, Diagnosing the tight building syndrome, Environmental Health Perspectives, 76:195-198, 1987.
13. Rogers SA, Tired or Toxic?, Prestige Publishing, Box 3161, 3502 Brewerton Rd., Syracuse, NY 13220, 1990.
14. Rogers SA, You Are What You Ate, Prestige Publishing, Box 3161, 3502 Brewerton Rd., Syracuse, NY 13220, 1988.
15. International Journal of Clinical Nutrition Reviews, in press, #16.
16. Anonymous, New misgiving about low magnesium, Science News, 133, 23:356, June 4, 1988.
17. Rogers SA, Is is chemical sensitivity or magnesium deficiency? Presented at the 8th Annual International Symposium on Man and His Environment in Health and Disease, Feb. 22-23, 1990, Dallas, also available on audio tape (1-800-Now Tape).
18. Sheldon LS, Handy RW, Hartwell TD, Whitmore H, Pellizzari ED, EPA Project Summary: Indoor Air Quality In Public Buildings, vol. 1:1-6, United States Environmental Protection Agency, Office of Acid Deposition, Environmental Monitoring and Quality Assurance, Washington, D.C., 20460, EPA/600/S6-88/009a, Sept. 1988.

Environment International, Vol. 17, pp. 271-275, 1991
Printed in the U.S.A. All rights reserved.

INDOOR FUNGI AS PART OF THE CAUSE OF RECALCITRANT SYMPTOMS OF THE TIGHT BUILDING SYNDROME

Sherry A. Rogers

Northeast Center For Environmental Medicine, Syracuse, NY 13219, USA

EI 9003-035M (Received 19 March 1990; accepted 10 October 1990)

As buildings are tightened to conserve energy, moisture and fungi as well as outgasing xenobiotics are trapped. It becomes necessary to have a method that will differentiate whether complaints blamed on poor indoor air quality are due to chemicals or molds, especially since many of the symptoms are identical. Patients whose symptoms were unrelieved by regular medical treatments were tested to the fungi chosen on the basis of previous research. Of 100 random cases out of 2000 that are annually asked to review their progress, 61% rated themselves as having markedly reduced symptoms while at the same time being able to reduce or completely discontinue all symptomatic medications. Case examples will demonstrate the diverse symptoms that improved, many of which had previously exhausted all that medicine had to offer. For some, double-blind placebo substitution was used and symptoms recurred. Upon reinstitution of injections, symptoms again were relieved. This therapy provides a method with potential to help differentiate whether complaints regarding indoor air quality are due to chemical hypersensitivty or an individual's mold sensitivity.

INTRODUCTION

Molds can produce some of the most potent toxins, hallucingens, and antibiotics known to man, while, at the same time, they are indispensible to the food industry (Beuchat 1978). They can thrive in conditions inimicable to many other living organisms (such as jet fuel lines) and, under certain climatic conditions, can produce billions of spores. During the height of the pollen season it is not unusual for the ratio of *Cladosporium (Hormodendrum)* spores to pollen to be 1000:1 (Lehrer et al. 1983). Fungi have been shown to produce many symptoms in the allergic individual (Holst et al. 1983; Mazar et al. 1981; Salvaggio and Aukrust 1981; Holst et al. 1990). Al-

lergists usually test a patient's degree of sensitivity to the major molds, *Hormodendrum, Aspergillus, Alternaria,* and *Penicillium,* and test a dozen or fewer other fungi on an individual basis.

In a previous study (Terracina and Rogers 1982), substituting a medium of malt agar extract for Sabouraud's medium, increasing petri dish exposure time from 10 min to 1 h, and saving plates for up to three weeks to allow the slow growers to appear, resulted in a 32%-higher yield of fungi isolated and identified. It was then observed that the fungal flora was in a state of constant change, and that for best results, gravity plates should be placed during periods of human activity, between knee and shoulder height (Rogers 1983). A third paper updated fungal flora, revealing many fungi that were previously not monitored (Rogers 1984).

The purpose of this study was to determine the practical and clinical significance of incorporating these newly identified fungi into the regular pollen, dust, mite, and mold testing to determine if additional benefit in symptom improvement would occur. Since these people suspected their symptoms were worse indoors, and these fungi were isolated from indoor cultures, it was a logical next step to see if incorporating these into their testing (and treatment if the skin tests were positive) would provide symptom relief.

MATERIALS AND METHODS

Twenty-one fungi were selected for this trial and divided into mixes as shown in Table 1. The patients to be tested had a large range of symptoms, and most had undergone a variety of specialty and general workups, including conventional allergy workups. They were still not well. Since they spent the majority of their time indoors and suspected indoor air as a source of problem, they were skin-tested to these fungal antigens along with local pollens, house dust, and house dust mite, *Dermatophagoides pteronyssinus*, according to our previously published protocol (Rogers 1988). All antigens that were positive were included in the patient's prescribed medication to be administered by intradermal (skin) injection twice weekly for one month and then weekly thereafter.

Trichophyton, Candida, Epidermophyton, Rhizopus, and *Sporobolomyces* were tested individually.

At the beginning of the test period, patients were also placed on a major elimination diet which prohibited such commonly consumed foods as milk,

Table 1. Components of mold mixes.

Mix A	*Aspergillus, Alternaria, Hormodendrum (CladosPorium), Penicillium*
Mix B	*Epicoccum, Fusarium, Pullularia (Aureobasidium)*
Mix D	*Fomes, Mucor, Poma, Rhodotorula*
Mix E	*Cephalosporium, Botrytis, Geotrichum, Helminthosporium, Stemphyllium*

wheat, corn, processed sugars, and ferments (bread, cheese, alcohol, vinegar, salad dressing, mayonnaise, ketchup, mustard, chocolate, and processed foods). They were allowed to eat foods they knew to be safe and that they did not normally eat more than once a week. This was done with the rational that elimination of ingested potentially cross-reacting fungal antigens and possible hidden food antigens might strengthen the therapeutic result. Questionnaires were mailed to patients yearly to evaluate their progress. They were asked to rate their symptoms according to whether they (1) were worse, (2) were the same, (3) experienced some improvement and rated themselves as less than 50% improved, still experiencing frequent symptoms and requiring chronic medications, (4) rated themselves as 50-75% improved with a definite reduction in symptoms and a marked reduction in medications, or (5) rated themselves as 75-100% better with no medications and with a marked reduction in symptoms.

RESULTS

Of 100 randomly selected subjects, 21% were male, 79% female. The age range was 12-66 y, and the duration of treatment by injection ranged from 1-10 y with an average of 5 y. Thirteen questionnaires were not fully answered, and so were not included in the statistics, even though all subjects were improved. None of the subjects felt worse, one person felt no change, and 15 thought they had some improvement, but not enough to decrease any medications, and definitely less than 50% improvement. Forty-five rated themselves as 50-75% improved with a marked reduction in symptoms and, consequently, a reduction in medication. Sixteen rated themselves as 75-100% better with no medications and indicated a marked reduction in symptoms. Thus 61% of 100 patients rated themselves as at least 50% improved with a marked reduction in symptoms. Consequently, they reduced medications or no longer needed medications.

CASE STUDIES

Since this program has been ongoing for over 10 y, and over 2000 patients have been successfully treated in this manner, a number of case examples will illustrate the improvement of a wide range of symptoms. Of the following cases, many were selected because of their uniqueness. They were not all part of the mailed questionnaire survey reported in this paper. They are by no means the entire program which covers over 2000 patients.

Certain patients (as designated) received double-blind substitution of their injections with placebo (normal saline). All of those worsened within two weeks and after re-institution of the injections, they again gained control of their symptoms. This also happened occasionally when they veered from the diet.

To obtain double-blind two-week substitution of active injections with the placebo, the syringes were prepared by the author without the knowlege of the patient or the nurse administering injections. This practice was a good way also for determining the time for discontinuation of the injections.

Chronic fatigue and nasal congestion

Twenty patients had complained of chronic fatigue and nasal congestion. Before the program, many related their symptoms to being inside a particular environment, usually home or office. All subjects rated themselves as at least 50% improved within four months of starting the program. However, many had a recurrence of symptoms if they were late for an injection. The time of symptom recurrence varied from one day to three weeks. Some were incapacitated by fatigue. For example, J.M. (30-y-old) had 5 y of symptoms. He had consulted several physicians for treatment of recurrent skin infections and chronic fatigue that left him unable to work. After 4 months of injections, he was so well that he was able to return to exercising, lifting weights, and teaching gymnastics.

Migraines

Four people with incapacitating migraines were also treated. One 48-y-old barber had a 6-y history of being bedridden 50% of the time with facial swelling, photophobia, tearing, glassy eyes, and a headache that left him threatening suicide. Narcotic analgesics, beta blockers, vasoconstrictors and antihistamines provided no relief. With the injections all symptoms ceased, and recurred only once in 3 y when he vacationed two weeks and missed one injection.

Eczema

Four people had intractable atopic dermatitis or eczema, and two had concomitant hyper-IgE. One of these, S.B., a 51-y-old teacher's aide, had received 15 y of conventional allergy injections which helped her nasal congestion partially, but did not improve her scaley, lichenified, cracked, bleeding, and brilliant red eczema. It involved the skin of her neck, upper chest and back, face, antecubital and wrist areas, and popliteal areas. It caused such constant pain that she rarely moved her neck if she could avoid it. Her skin burned more when in indoor environments which were perceived by her to have a musty odor. Her IgE was 75 082 I.U. (normal 14-100). After two months of injections her skin was clear of disease for the first time since it had begun, and in 8 months, her IgE was 30 006 I.U.

A 33-y-old snow ski laminator had facial, arm, torso and leg eczema since childhood. For the previous 11 y so severe that thick scales covered his body. He also suffered from chronic diarrhea and had been thoroughly examined and treated by four allergists and three dermatologists. He had used many dangerous medications to no avail, including high doses of steroids. He lived in the woods in a tight trailer and suspected that molds were part of his problem.

Laboratory findings revealed an IgE of 33 088 I.U., increased T-4 cells of 60.2% (normal 38-53%) and B cells of 18.9% (normal 7-11%), decreased T-8 cells of 10.3% (18-30%), and NK cells of 2.1% (6-13%). Unlike the typical patient with hyper-IgE syndrome, he had not had even one cold in the last 5 y. He also knew that milk caused severe exfoliation within a day, and his milk RAST (radio allergosorgent test) was moderately positive for milk. Within 13 d of participation in the program, his skin was totally clear for the first time in 11 y. His IgE dropped to 8809 I.U. after four months, and to 6456 after six months. After 1 y it was 2305 and after 2 y 1231. He has remained clear for over 6 y except for one time when a double-blind substitution of his injections was administered using normal saline placebo. It took two weeks to clear his symptoms again. His dermatitis flared up if he ingested certain foods he avoided.

C.V., a 37-y-old housewife had 6 y of severe pustular erythematous eczema. Her IgE was unremarkable at 17. She knew her face would burn and tingle and erupt more when in indoor moldy environnments and in the fall. She has remained clear, except with dietary indiscretion or single-blind placebo substitution.

Asthma

Six cases of asthma included R.S., a 36-y-old woman who worked in the family-owned bakery. Wheat RAST was strongly positive and her IgE was 70 I.U. Cultures from her bedroom yielded 16 colonies of *Sporobolomyces*, 1 *Fusarium*, 48 bacteria, 2 yeasts and one sterile fungus. The bakery yielded 1 *Penicillium*, 1 *Rhodotorula*, 3 bacteria, and 4 *Sporobolomyces*.

After two months of the program, her asthma was clear and she has had no recurrence, needed no further asthma medications, and has continued to work in the bakery for the last 4 y.

S.K., a 57-y-old carpenter, was disabled by asthma who became visibly cyanotic just walking across the room. He was maximally medicated for asthma (maximum therapeutic blood levels of theophylline, inhaled beta-agonists, inhaled steroids, and inhaled chromolyn) including oral steroids. Pulmonologists had hospitalized him for bronchoscopies and bronchograms and his prognosis was guarded. His IgE was 5666 I.U. After 1 y with the program, his IgE dropped to 2146, and he no longer needed steroids and some of his other medications. After 2 y, his IgE was 1370 and his only medication was a few puffs of albuterol a week compared to daily.

M.G., a 26-y-old man, had 4 y of asthma, exhaustion, headaches, nasal congestion, and recurrent sinus infections. He could no longer run his 10 mi/d. His PEF (peak expiratory flow) was 37% of predicted normal level with 47% improvement post bronchodilator. He was able to resume cross country racing after three months of the program.

Urticaria

Five patients with urticaria (hives) included M.D., a 30-y-old patient with 5 y of chronic total body pruritis, headaches, and rhinitis. All symptoms were gone in two months of participation in the program. Likewise, K.L. had seven months of giant urticaria, 20 y of headaches, and perennial rhinitis. All were clear in two months.

Lupus

Three people were diagnosed with systemic lupus erythematosis. G.H., a 36-y-old restaurant manager, received this diagnosis from a major medical center and returned yearly, for 5 y, for an update. She required monthly 40 mg of injected steroids to function. In spite of this, she had a chronic erythematous (red), pustular malar rash, daily joint pain, asthma, irritable bowel, and chronic fatigue. In two months she was off all steroids, and well, and has remained medication- and symptom-free for 4 y.

Miscellaneous

C.H., an 8-y-old boy was receiving 10 mg of a commonly used amphetamine derivative, prescribed three times a day by the pediatric neurologist to subdue his hyperactivity. In spite of this, he would throw the iron at his father, pour hot water on his baby sister and was unteachable, with failing grades

in school. Testing for molds by the provocation technique, previously described (Rogers 1987), enabled his behavior to be provoked and neutralized. He was placed on immunotherapy for the positive molds, and within one month he was able to discontinue the amphetamine, his attention span had improved to the point to where he was teachable, his behavior was markedly improved, he grew in height and his teeth erupted after a 2-y arrest. After four months of the program, the boy was earning high grades in school.

One year later, a placebo was substituted for two weeks, double-blind. Within two weeks, his mother came in wearing a black eye that he had given her in an unprovoked attack, and stated that his entire behavior had changed and it was as though he was no longer receiving his injections. Also during that period, the teachers had gone to the principal of the school requesting that he not return to the school for the following year, and the police had been to the house twice to warn his parents about not allowing him to use the phone to call them for fabricated emergencies. When his injections were reinstated, his former improvement returned.

M.E., a 68-y-old orthopedic surgeon, had experienced cardiac arrhythmia accompanied by diarrhea and weakness over the previous months. The weakness had become incapacitating to the point where he feared walking across a room. After one week of mold injections, he described himself as 80% improved over anything he had experienced over the last 10 y. Also 30 y of anosmia (inablity to smell things normally) had returned to normal.

Post-viral syndrome

Four patients who were diagnosed as having a flu, never recovered, and complained of persistent symptoms that were actually worsening.

W.B., a 41-y-old college professor and chairman of his department had developed what he thought was a flu 18 months prior, but it had never resolved. He complained of constant non-vertiginous dizziness, headache, and incapacitating weakness that would fluctuate in intensity without ever completely abating. His prior treatments included hospitalization with CAT scans of the brain and a lumbar puncture. He reported a distinct improvement after being tested with the mold extracts and receiving his first therapeutic injection. The second injection, a few days later, cleared all the remaining symptoms for the first time since the onset 2 y previously. His symptoms recur every fourth day and disappear within 30 min after an injection. He remains clear as long as he obtains his injection twice a week. Double-blind placebo substitution for his injections caused the symptoms to recur.

DISCUSSION

Sixty-one of 100 randomly selected ongoing patients rated themselves as at least 50% better with a marked reduction in symptoms and a partial or total reduction in medications. An obvious defect of the current study is that it does not allow for the number of dropouts. The case histories reported here represent another 55 patients who were successfully treated by this method. An obvious major flaw of this part is that it is in no way a statistically rigid study, nor is it randomly selected. Many of these people were blaming home or work environments for their recalcitrant symptoms, but were actually more suspicious of indoor chemicals as the cause and were surprised when the culprit turned out to be a much more easily remedied cause, mold allergy.

We have already reported the variety of symptoms that can be precipitated by indoor chemicals (Rogers 1989), including approaches for diagnosis of suspected chemically-induced symptoms (Rogers 1986; Rogers 1990). But when the symptoms go beyond what the individual can handle or when the problem creeps into the legal arena, a method is needed to separate chemically-induced from mold-induced symptoms.

This paper suggests a treatment method for a variety of disorders which have failed to respond to other forms of treatment, and/or which have been blamed on indoor chemicals. The indications for the specificity and appropriateness of the immunotherapy with fungal antigens were reinforced by the use of double-blind placebos and the serendipitous failures of patients who were unable to maintain what proved to be criti-cal restrictive diets. It also demonstrates that mold sensitivity is responsible for a wider range of symptoms than is commonly perceived. Although more rigid studies are needed, this provides another tool to define, and in many cases treat, the cause of problems presumed to be secondary to poor indoor air quality.

REFERENCES

Beuchat, L.R. Food and beverage mycoloqy. Westport, CT: AVI Publ.; 1978.

Holst, P.E.; Coleman, E.D.; Sheridan, J.E.; O'Donnell, T.V.; Sutthoff, P.T. Asthma and fungi in the home. New Zealand Med. J. 96:718-720; 1983.

Horst, M.; Hejjaoue, A.; Horst, V.; Michel, B.; Bousquet, J. Double-blind, placebo-controlled rush immunotherapy with a standardized Alternaria Extract. J. Allergy Clin. Immunol. 85:460-472; 1990.

Lehrer, S.B.; Aukrust, L.; Salvaggio, J.E. Respiratory allergy induced by fungi. In: Symp. on immune factors in pulmonary disease. Clin. Chest Med. 4:23-41; 1983.

Mazar, A.; Baum, B.C.; Segal, E.; Glazer, I.; Schur, S.; Markus, J. Antibodies to inhalant fungal antigens in patients with asthma in Israel. Ann. Allergy 47:361-364; 1981.

Rogers, S.A. A comparison of commercially available mold survey services. Ann. Allergy 50:37-43; 1983.

Rogers, S.A. A thirteen-month assessment of local work-leisure-sleep fungal environments. Ann. Allergy 52:338-341; 1984.

Rogers, S.A. The E.I. syndrome. Syracuse, NY: Prestige Publ.; 1986.

Rogers, S.A. Diagnosing the tight building syndrome. Env. Health Persp. 76:195-198; 1987.

Rogers, S.A. Resistant cases: Response to mold immunotherapy and environmental and dietary controls. Clin. Ecol. 5:115-120; 1988.

Rogers, S.A. Diagnosing the tight building syndrome or diagnosing chemical sensitivity. Environ. Int. 15:75-79; 1989.

Rogers, S.A. Tired or toxic? Syracuse, NY: Prestige Publ.; 1990.

Salvaggio, J.E.; Aukrust, L. Mold-induced asthma. Allergy Clin. Immunol. 68:327-364; 1981.

Terracina, F.; Rogers, S.A. In-home fungal studies. Ann. Allergy 49:135-137; 1982.

ORIGINAL RESEARCH

Unrecognised Magnesium Deficiency Masquerades as Diverse Symptoms: Evaluation of an Oral Magnesium Challenge Test

Sherry A. Rogers, M.D.

Northeast Centre for Environmental Medicine,

2800 West Genesee St,

Syracuse NY 13219 USA

ABSTRACT

It is becoming increasingly apparent that magnesium deficiency (MD) is under appreciated and under diagnosed. At the same time, it can be responsible for a vast array of seemingly unrelated symptoms, including arteriosclerosis, the leading cause of morbidity and mortality. To compound the problem, medications that are usually prescribed for these symptoms have the side affect of further lowering the magnesium. Since there is no reliable blood test for MD, we devised a magnesium loading test (MLT) with a before and after 24 hour urine magnesium. Additionally, a two week trial of magnesium at a reduced dosage was evaluated. Fifty one percent of patients had marked relief in over 40 different symptoms. Ten percent of the patients reported marked reduction in chemical sensitivity. Clearly, this test was useful in relieving 51% of the patients of long-standing symptoms (in some cases potentially lethal) for which no effective treatment was available, and should be evaluated in all patients with chronic medication or symptoms.

INTRODUCTION

The U.S. government collected data showing that the average American consumes only 40% of the recommended daily allowance for magnesium.[1]

It is the fourth most abundant cation in the body, and the second most plentiful intracellularly. Bone contains about half of the total magnesium, while liver and muscle have the highest concentrations. A third of the ingested magnesium is absorbed mainly in the proximal small intestine.

Magnesium is essential in over 300 reactions. It is in enzymes that hydrolyse and transfer phosphate groups (ATP for glucose utilization, fat, protein, nucleic acid and co-enzyme synthesis, muscle contraction, methyl group transfer, sulphate, acetate and formate activation), hence, it is critical for energy storage and utilization. Also, it contributes importantly to macromolecular structure, especially the synthesis, transcription and translation of DNA and RNA in ribosomes, as well as protein synthesis and genetic repair.

It is essential for the release of acetyl choline across the motor endplate and, thus, neuronal excitability and enhanced neuromuscular transmission and excitability. [2,3] It is essential for the sodium potassium pump and is a physiological calcium channel blocker. Since it is crucial to over 300 reactions in the body, it is surprising that a deficiency could manifest as one or more of a staggering array of diverse symptoms.

Many researchers label it as the most recognized electrolyte abnormality in clinical practice today. [4,5,6,7] To compound the problem, there are no current blood (serum, plasma, or intracellular) levels or urine tests that can assess absolutely the adequacy of the magnesium pools. In fact there is universal agreement that the best way to define a deficiency is with a challenge. [6,7,8,9,10,11,12]

Even with looking at serum magnesium only, which is known to be extremely insensitive and unreliable, a minimum of 10% of patients in tertiary care hospitals have serious symptom producing deficiencies that are often overlooked. This can have a staggering effect on hospital stay and additional studies of the patient, not to mention morbidity and mortality. Whenever hypokalaemia or hypocalcaemia are present, it is even more likely that hypomagnesaemia is present. [13]

When one remembers that blood levels miss many cases of magnesium deficiency, current statistical studies which are based on blood levels take on even greater significance, such as those demonstrating that 11-49% of hospitalized patients have magnesium deficiencies. As would be expected, there is wide variation in symptomatology from patient to patient. [14,15]

It is obvious that magnesium should be determined on a routine basis because of the frequency of the occurrence of hypomagnesaemia in hospitalized patients. [16] The question is how to determine adequacy conveniently when blood tests are not sufficient.

As with most deficiencies, the causes can be grouped as due to either decreased intake, decreased absorption, or excessive urinary loss. Under the decreased intake, most reviewers mention prolonged intravenous therapy, starvation with metabolic acidosis, protein and calorie malnutrition, kwashiorkor, and alcoholism. [17] Most surveys, however, overlook a major culprit which appears to be decreased intake secondary to poor selection of nutrient dense foods, with a preference for high fat, sugar and salts of processed foods over whole grains and vegetables.

The processing of whole grains has made a major five-fold decrease in magnesium availablity. Furthermore, as a factor that constitutes often 50% of a normal diet, this has a vast influence. For example, changing from brown rice to polished rice, the magnesium dropped from 1477 to 251mcg/dm. Likewise, changing from whole wheat to refined flour, it dropped from 1502 to 299mcg/dm. Other unprocessed whole grains are even more magnesium-rich, such as millet with a content of 1670mcg/dm of magnesium and buckwheat with 2526. [18]

Surveys show now that many people eat as much as four meals or more in restaurants each week, and restaurants do not serve whole grains. Use of medications can decrease intestinal absorption, as well as increase renal loss, as can many chronic disease states. [19] Thiazides, the aminoglycosides, cis-platin and cyclosporines are among the medications that can significantly reduce magnesium. Since these are used on more seriously ill patients it behooves us to be sure that they have sufficient stores with which to fight their illnesses.[20,21]

As well, exercise, through sweating, can deplete magnesium for months at a time.[22,23] This may explain why several joggers of national acclaim died of sudden cardiac arrhythmia, yet showed no cardiovascular changes on autopsy.

METHODS AND MATERIALS

Since there is no blood test to adequately assess the prevalence of magnesium deficiency, we wanted to devise a before and after 24 hour urinary magnesium assay to determine the adequacy of the magnesium pool. As a confirmatory test, we added a two week trial of magnesium, after which symptom relief was assessed.

Patients were instructed in the collection of a 24 hour urine. This was done before any oral magnesium and they were to eat regularly and take no other supplements or medications. Then they were instructed to take two 64 mg magnesium chloride enteric coated tablets three times daily before meals, for two days; this provided a total of 384 mg, or an average RDA. (In preliminary trials we found a dose larger than that was not tolerated by many, as it caused diarrhoea.) On day two of the magnesium loading, subjects were to collect a second 24 hour urine beginning at 8 a.m. and to continue taking the magnesium throughout the day as they were collecting the urine.

To determine if a trial made any change in symptoms, after that they were to drop the dose to two tablets, twice daily, for two weeks and report any symptom change at the end of the two week trial.

Before and after 24 hour urine magnesium levels were used to assess the percentage retention; before divided by after equals the percent retention. An arbitrary cut-off of 50% retention was considered acceptable. Any retention exceeding 50% was considered as reflective of either retention due to deficiency or defective absorption:

$$\frac{\text{Before 24 hr urine magnesium}}{\text{After 24 hr urine magnesium}} \times 100 = \% \text{ retention}$$

It was assumed that if the magnesium pool status was normal, this extra 384 mg per day, times two days, would be seen as excessive by the body and excreted. If the body was deficient, however, the vast majority of magnesium should be retained.

Phase II of the test, not yet reported here, involved a 2 month trial of magnesium in those patients who exhibited over 50% retention or marked improvement in a symtom during the initial two week trial. The MLT was again repeated to assess the change in percent retention.

RESULTS

From 100 randomly selected patients, exactly 51 patients (51%) reported improvement in symptoms. 16% had no change in symptoms, and 33% did not report either way. It was later found after the cut-off date of the trial, that of the 33% that did not report their symptoms, several failed to do so either because of diarrhoea induced by the magnesium chloride tablets, so that they did not finish the trial, or they reported improvement but it was too late, after the termination of the data collection. Many of the 33% who reported too late stated that even though they did have marked improvement in a number of symptoms they had delayed in reporting their improvement because they assumed that we would know they were going to be better, since we prescribed this for them, and hence, there was no urgent need to report to us.

Of the 16% who had no change in symptoms, many of these had a 50% or greater retention of magnesium. Many of these people also reported marked symptom improvement. However, the statistics were not carried through for these two categories of delayed responses to the study. Clearly, however, in reality many more than 51% of the subjects had improvement in symptoms.

In many cases, the symptoms that improved were not the chief complaints of these patients for which they had presented to the office. They had already had many negative previous investigations through the years (often with multiple specialists) in attempts to define the causes of these symptoms, and had given up mentioning these symptoms to subsequent physicians.

Of the responders with improvement in symptoms, 91.9% was the average percent of magnesium retention, with a range of 10-428%. Of those that responded, but had no improvement in symptoms in the two week trial, 77% retention was the average, with a range of 21-140. 25% of these people had retentions over 100%, as did 29% of those with improved symptoms (Table1).

It appears that the symptom improvement was a much more reliable guide than the percent retention. This may be for a number of reasons that were observed later:

TABLE 1:   *The results of the magnesium loading test.*

Symptoms	Number of Patients	Average % Retention of Magnesium	Range of % Retention of Magnesium	% of Patients with over 100% Retention
Improved Symptoms	51	91.9	10-428	29
No Symptom Change	16	77	35-140	25
Did Not Report	33	80.6	22-224	42

1. There may have been poor absorption rather than increased retention, neither of which can be differentiated by this test as it stands alone.
2. It may have required a longer trial of magnesium to improve the symptoms and saturate the magnesium pool.
3. There may have been other nutrient deficiencies that needed correction along with the magnesium before symptom improvement could occur.
4. The patient may have not followed the written directions for the test adequately.

We saw case examples of all of these.

Table 2 shows the distribution of the top ten symptom categories that were relieved in the 51 patients after the two week trial of two 64 mg magnesium chloride tablets, twice daily (a total of 256 mg per day). The questionnaire was open ended, it did not give the patients a list of symptoms from which to choose, but allowed the patients to use, in their own words, the symptoms that improved.

Of the 51% who reported spontaneous improvement in symptoms with the two week trial, 70% reported improvement in the category labeled central nervous system or peripheral nervous system (CNS/PMS) symptoms, which included the following patient reports:

depression	confusion	insomnia
disorientation	headache	chemical sensitivity
dizziness	panic attacks	paresthesia
irritability	learning disorder	anxiety
violence	mood swings	autism
PMS	poor memory	hyperacusis

TABLE 2: Breakdown of systems in which improvement was reported among the 51% of patients who had improved symptoms. Most patients had improvement in more than one category.

Symptoms Relieved	% of Positive Responders
CNS/PMS	70%
Increased Energy	50%
Musculoskeletal	38%
ROAD	18%
IBS	14%
Arrhythmia	8%
Dental	6%
Urinary/Bladder	4%
Miscellaneous	6%

Many of these symptoms were known to be induced by exposures to chemicals in shopping malls, traffic, homes and businesses.

A feeling of increased energy, well-being and strength were reported in 50% of the positive responders. Many stated that they had not felt this much energy in decades. Thirty eight percent were grouped in the musculoskeletal category because they reported reduction in leg cramps, back pain, hip pain, shoulder pain, arthralgia, or were able to discontinue pain medication and/ or chiropractic manipulations. Many of these symptoms had also been present for years.

Eighteen percent of the positive responders reported reduction in asthma, chest pain related to asthma, and/or throat spasms that were known to be induced by chemical exposures. These were grouped under reversible obstructive airway disease (ROAD). Fourteen percent reported reduction in abdominal pain, intestinal spasm, diarrhoea, and/or irritable bowel syndrome (IBS) symptoms. Eight percent had cessation of cardiac arrhythmia, six percent had reduction in tooth pain, burning tongue, or reported the healing of long-standing denture sores. This represented the dental category.

Four percent reported relief from interstitial cystitis symptoms, and/or bladder spasms. Six percent wrote miscellaneous changes which included decreased pruritus, normalization of previously chronically elevated formic acid and SGPT, and one patient who had had three unsuccessful fertility workups in the past, became pregnant.

Many patients had positive results in more than one category, and were surprised by the abrupt and dramatic cessation of symptoms that had been present for years. Within a few days, these symptoms had cleared. After several exhaustive consultations, these people had learned to accept that there was no known cause for these symptoms. They were not expecting relief of these long-standing problems. Many also called the office immediately when the two week trial was finished, because upon discontinuing the magnesium, some of their symptoms had returned. When the magnesium was recommenced the symptoms were again terminated.

The MLT numerical results were not an absolute guide to response, since some with a high percentage of retention had no improvement. But it did lead us to attempt to slowly saturate their magnesium stores over two months and this did lead to significant improvement, although we did not keep statistics on this. Also, some people with retention in the 50 percentile felt such dramatic relief in symptoms with recurrence after the cessation of the oral trial, that we had to resume treatment. The MLT was useful, however, in following the correction of an individual's magnesium deficit. In many cases, other nutrient deficiencies complicated the picture we were attempting to simplify.

Four patients obtained total relief from years of panic attacks which had required psychiatric investigation and tranquilizers. Abruptly after the magnesium correction they no longer had the panic attacks, nor did they require any further medications.

Ten patients were no longer chemically sensitive. Previously they had experienced a variety of symptoms from inability to concentrate, extreme fatigue, spaciness, dizziness, to a sensation that the throat was closing when they were in areas where they could identify chemicals, such as in new buildings, traffic exhaust, or in rooms with new carpeting. These patients had marked reduction in these symptoms.

Many other people had had years of muscle twitching about the eyes, or years of low back pain, neck pain, other joint pains, and flu-like body aches that were relieved immediately. Many reported a good sleep for the first time in years, plus marked relief from depression, confusion, tiredness, irritability and a hopeless feeling, dizziness and weakness. Many felt that their thinking was clearer, they felt stronger and had much more energy.

Some were magnesium renal wasters, and after correction of the magnesium, they were no longer wasters. One physician's wife, when she was called to tell her that she was a waster, was actually hospitalized at that moment for a myocardial infarction with recalcitrant cardiac arrhythmia. As soon as the attending physician gave magnesium, upon our recommendation, the arrhythmia ceased, along with six other symptoms. One lady had been bedridden for six months, and one man for two weeks, because of back pain attributed to bulging discs and they were about to have surgery; for both, the pain ceased on the magnesium within one week. All of the above symptoms recurred when the two week trial was finished, alerting us to the probability that the magnesium stores had not been satiated.

DISCUSSION

Clearly, as other researchers have confirmed, magnesium is a prevalent, yet relatively undiagnosed or unthought of deficiency. When the U.S. government finds the average diet only provides 40% of the RDA, it makes identification of the problem even more imperative. Not only is the range of symptoms in the literature staggering,[24] but also the amount of money spent in drug therapy to disguise the symptoms, not to mention the progression of the morbidity due to the undiagnosed basic cause of disease and the eventual premature mortality. As well, many of the medications prescribed further depleted the magnesium, thus assuring a downward spiral or more symptoms and the need for more medications.

For example, arteriosclerotic vascular disease is the number one cause of chronic illness and death in the United States; yet it is clear than in an undertermined percentage it is due to undiagnosed magnesium deficiency leading to hypertension, cardiac arrhythmia, increased cholesterol, vascular calcifications and even sudden death.[25,26,27,28,29, 31,32,33,34,35,36,37,38,39,40,41,44,45,59] Furthermore, the first line of treatment of a disease, like hypertension, or fluid retention (that can be caused by an unsuspected magnesium deficiency), is often diuretics which have repeatedly been shown to not only further deplete magnesium, but cause secondary resistant (magnesium dependent) hypokalaemia, and raise serum cholesterol and triglyceride levels.[42,43,44]

Since magnesium is nature's calcium channel blocker,[28] and a deficiency can mimic the senile organic brain syndrome and toxic brain, [17,45] accentuate histamine release,[46] compromise xenobiotic (foreign chemical) detoxication, osteoporosis,[48] retard the correction of other nutrient deficiencies,[49,50] and increase the release of catecholamines,[3] it is easy to appreciate why the drug industry thrives on selling calcium channel blockers, antihistamines and tranquilizers, not to mention the afore-mentioned diuretics, antihypertensives and arrhythmia control medications.

Fortunately, chemically sensitive patients are made worse or are intolerant of further chemical prescription drugs, so we were forced to identify an underlying biochemical defect.

Clearly, a look at the magnesium status, as well as other nutrients, may change the way medicine is practiced and open up an era of molecluar medicine where the biochemical defect as the cause of symptoms is sought before merely diagnosing and medicating, as is often currently practiced.

It is interesting how a vast array of prescription medication has evolved to mask the symptoms that an unsuspected magnesium deficiency can cause. Indeed, many researchers are now realizing that nutrition is the single most important component of preventive health.[51]

REFERENCES

1 Anonymous, **Science News 133(23)**, 356 (1988)

2 Wacker WEC, Parisi AF. Magnesium metabolism. **N Engl J Med 278**, 658-663 (1968)

3 Graber TW. The role of magnesium in health and disease. **Comprehensive Therapy 13(1)**, 29-35 (1987)

4 Wang R. Prevalence of magnesium deficiency, in Giles TD, Seelig MS. Monograph: The Role of Magneisum Chloride in Clinical Practice, 5-6, Oxford Health Care Inc., Clifton, NJ (1988)

5 Seeling CB. Magnesium deficiency in hypertension uncovered by magnesium load retention. **J Am Coll Nutr 8(5)**, 455. Abstract 113 (1989)

6 Rea WJ, Johnson AR, Smiley RE, Maynard B, Dawkins-Brown O. Magnesium deficiency in patients with chemical sensitivity. **Clinical Ecology 4(1)**, 17-20 (1986)

7 American College of Nutrition 26th Annual Meeting,a nd the Fourth International Symposium on Magnesium. **J Am Coll Nutr 4**, 303-405 (1985)

8 Ryzen E, Elbaum N, Singer FR, Rude RK. Parenteral magnesium tolerance testing in the evaluation of magnesium deficiency. **Magnesium 4**, 137-147 (1985)

9 Elin RJ. The status of mononuclear blood cell magnesium assay. **J Am Coll Nutr 6(2)**, 105-107 (1987)

10 Rhinehart RA. Magnesium metabolism: A review with special reference to the relationship between intercellular content and serum levels. **Archives of Internal Medicine 148**, 2415-2420 (1988)

11 Wacker WEC, Parisi AF. Magnesium metabolism. **N Engl J Med**, 712-717 (1968)

12 Reyes AJ, Leary WP. Pathogenesis of arrhythmogenic changes due to magnesium depletion. **SA Med J 64**, 311-312 (1983)

13 Flink EB. Magnesium deficiency causes and effects. **Hospital Practice** 116A-116P (1987)

14 Nicar MJ, Pak CYC. Oral magnesium load test for the assessment of intestinal magnesium absorption. **Mineral Electrolyte Metabolism 8**, 44-51 (1982)

15 Wang R. Routine serum magnesium determination, a continuing unrecognized need. **Magnesium 6**, 1-4 (1987)

16 Wang R, Oei TO, Aikawa JK, Watanabe A, Vannatta J, Fryer A, Markanich M. Predictors of clinical hypomagnesaemia: hypokalaemia, hypophosphotaemia, hyponatraemia, hypocalcaemia. **Archives of Internal Medicine 144**, 1794-1796 (1984)

17 Juan D. Clinical review: The clinical importance of hypomagnesemia. **Surgery 91(5)**, 510-517 (1982)

18 Schroeder JA, Nason AP, Tipton IH. Essential metals in man, magnesium. **J Chron Dis 21**, 815-841 (1969)

19 Giles TD, ed. The Role of Magnesium Chloride Therapy in Clinical Practice. Oxford Health Care Inc., 1425 Broad St, Clifton NJ 07013 (1988)

20 Zemba-Palko V, Lacher D. Serum magnesium as affected by drugs. **Clinical Chemistry 34(9)**, 1913 (abst) (1988)

21 Rodrigeuz M, Salanki DL, Whang R. Refractory potassium depletion due to cisplatin-induced magnesium depletion. **Arch Intern Med 149**, 2592-2594 (1989)

22 Stendig-Lindberg G, Scipirro Y, Epstein Y, Galun E,Schonberger E, Graff E, Wacker WE. Changes in serum magnesium concentration after strenuous.exercise. **J Am Coll Nutr 6(1)**, 35-40 (1987)

23 Liu L, Browski G, Rose LI. Hypomagnesaemia in a tennis player. **The Physician and Sportsmedicine 11(5)**, 79-80 (1983)

24 Chernow D, Smith J, Rainey TG, Finton C. Hypomagnesaemia: Implications for the critical care specialist. **Critical Care Medicine 10**(3), 193-196 (1982)

25 Rayssiguier Y. The role of magnesium and potassium in the pathogenesis of arteriosclerosis. **Magnesium 3**, 226-238 (1984)

26 Wacker WEC, Vallee BL. Magnesium metabolism. **N Engl J Med 259**(9), 431-438 (1958)

27 Meema HE, Oreopoulos DG, Rapport A. Serum magnesium level and arterio calcification in end-stage renal disease. **Kidney International 32** (3), 388-394 (1987)

28 Iseri LT, French JH. Magnesium: Nature's physiologic calcium blocker. **Am Heart J 108**(1), 188-192 (1984)

29 Drisco AM, Reagan C. The effect of magnesium on calcium metabolism in man. **Am J Clin Nutr 19**, 296-306 (1966)

30 Leonard F, Boke JW, Ruderman RJ, Hegyeli AF. Initiation and inhibition of subcutaneous calcification. **Cal Tiss Res 10**, 269-279 (1972)

31 Lowenhaupt E, Schulman M, Greenberg DM. Basic histologic lesions of magnesium deficiency in the rat. **Arch Pathol 49**, 427-433 (1950)

32 Cachs JR. Interaction of magnesium with the sodium pump of the human red cell. **J Physiol 400**, 575-591 (1988)

33 Altur BM, Altur BT, Gerrewold A, Ising H, Gunther T. Magnesium deficiency in hypertension: Correlation between magnesium deficient diets and microcirculatory changes in situ. **Science 223**, 1315-1317 (1984)

34 Motoyama T, et al. **Hypertension 13**, 227-232 (1989)

35 Rayssiguier Y, Gueux E, Weiser D. The effect of magnesium deficiency on lipid metabolism in rats fed a high carbohydrate diet. **J Nutr 111**, 1876-1883 (1981)

36 Rasmussen HS, Aurup P, Goldstein K, McNair P, Mortensen PB, Larsen OG, Lawaetz H. Influence of magnesium substitution therapy on blood lipid composition in patients with ischaemic heart disease. **Arch Intern Med 149**, 1050-1053 (1989)

37 Cannon LA, Heiselman DE, Dougherty JM, Jones J. Magnesium levels in cardiac arrest victims: Relationship between magnesium levels and successful rescusitation. **Annals of Emergency Medicine 16**, 1195-1198 (1987)

38 Rasmussen HS, Morregard P, Lindeneg O, McNair P, Backer V, Balselv S. **Lancet**, 234-235 (1986)

39 Rasmussen HS, McNair P, Goransson L, Balslov S, Larsen OG, Aurup P. Magnesium deficiency in patients with ischaemic heart disease, with and without acute myocardial infarction uncovered by an intravenuos loading test.

40 Anonymous. Hypertensives tend to be glucose intolerant and hyperinsulinaemic. Vol.4 #21, Internal Medicine World Report, p.23, reporting on Dr. Swislocki et al. **American Journal of Hypertension 2**, 419-423 (1989)

41 Steidl L, Tolde I, Svomova V. Metabolism of magnesium and zinc in patients treated with antiepileptic drugs and with magnesium lactate. **Magnesium 6**(6), 248-249 (1987)

42 Calssen HG. Magnesium and potassium deprivation and supplementation in animals and man: Aspects in view of intestinal absorption. **Magnesium 3**, 257-264 (1984)

43 Pollare T et al. A comparison of the effects of hydrochlorothiazide and ketopril on glucose and lipid metabolism in patients with hypertension. **N Engl J Med 321**, 868-873 (1989)

44 Anonymous. Hypertension, heart disease and diuretics, **Science News 136**, 254 (1989)

45 Hall RCW, Joffee JR. Hypomagnesaemia, physical and psychiatric symptoms. **JAMA 224**(13), 1749-1751 (1973)

46 Rolla G, et al. Reduction of histamine induced broncho constriction by magnesium in asthmatic subjects. **Allergy 42**, 186-188 (1987)

47 Hsu JM, Rubenstein B, Paleker AG. Role of magnesium in glutathione metabolism of rat erythrocytes. **J Nutr 112**, 488-496 (1982)

48 Cohen L, Kitzes R. Infrared spectroscopy and magnesium content of bone mineral in osteoporotic women. **Isr J Med Sci 17**, 1123-1125 (1981)

49 Zieve L. Influence of magnesium deficiency on the normalization of thiamine. **Ann NY Acad Sci 162**, 732-743 (1969)

50 Zieve L. Role of cofactors in the treatment of malnutrition as exemplified by magnesium. **The Yale Journal of Biology and Medicine 48**, 229-237 (1975)

51 Sauberlich HE. Implications of nutritional status on human biochemistry, physiology and health. **Clin Biochem 17**, 132-142 (1984)

Reader's Notes